BREAST CANCER

Its Link to Abortion and the Birth Control Pill

Chris Kahlenborn, M.D.

ISBN 0-9669777-3-4

One More Soul
1846 North Main St.
Dayton, Ohio 45405
800-307-7685
www.OMSoul.com
OMSoul@OMSoul.com

Cover art taken from various drawings
of Michelangelo Buonarroti (1475–1564)
and composed by Cindy Turner.

Printed
in New Hope, Kentucky, U.S.A.

To: the Truth

Acknowledgements

I wish to thank the following people for their prayers, their time and their love:

All of the researchers who have had the courage to publish their findings despite the negative repercussions; the wonderful librarians without whom this work would have taken twice as long: Sonya Koros, Nancy Zachocki, Michelle Burda, Susan McKinney and Virginia A. Lingle; editors Dorothy Dugandzic and Carolyn; John McTernan, who gave me the impetus to "put it all together"; the "angels" at Prime Care; all of the wonderful people at PCUC, especially Helen Cindrich; the wonderful researchers and lay people who patiently reviewed this book, especially Joan and Walt; Teresa Donovan, Teresa Menart, Steve Koob and his staff, particularly Vince Sacksteder; Lucille Canty for her research; Doug Ednie, Mildred Tapparo, Paul Hofbauer and our "burger time," Father Silvan Rouse, Nina Partovi, and my family. A special thanks to Kevin E. Slattery† (4/26/61-5/23/00) whose zeal encouraged me often.

Private Dedication: TtLJCatTOHCAC;atisr

— Chris Kahlenborn

BREAST CANCER

Its Link to Abortion and the Birth Control Pill

Appendices:

Introduction

Almost every reader of this book has a mother, a sister, an aunt or a friend who has or had breast cancer. Breast cancer is the most common cause of cancer death in the U.S. in women ages 20 to 59. In the U.S. *nearly 1 out of every 8 women* will develop breast cancer over the course of her lifetime. Each year about 175,000 women develop breast cancer and more than 43,000 women die from it in the U.S. In addition, the mortality rate from breast cancer in the U.S. *increased* by 4% in females from 1960 through 1992, while it *declined* by over 30% in males during the same period [1]. <u>Medical epidemiologists</u> (ie, those researchers who study trends and patterns regarding various medical phenomena) have noted that the rate of breast cancer has steadily been increasing throughout the world over the last 4 decades and that rates have increased even faster in more advanced countries, as noted in Table A on page x. *These phenomena, among others, have prompted researchers to search for factors which could explain the increase in breast cancer rates in women.* Are there specific risk factors that have been "overlooked"?

In 1993, I attended a meeting in which the speaker noted that if a woman had an induced abortion she sustained an increased risk of developing breast cancer. I was skeptical. I reviewed the pertinent studies and came to the conclusion that this statement was indeed supported by the medical literature; however, one thing bothered me. That "one thing" was the issue of hormonal birth control, specifically "the Pill." The fact is that many women who had an early abortion *also* took the birth control pill (also known as the oral contraceptive pill [OCP] or "the Pill") or other forms of hormonal birth control. This made me wonder whether it was indeed induced abortion or use of "the Pill," or both, that increased a woman's risk of developing breast cancer. I decided to review the literature regarding breast cancer and the birth control pill and specifically sought answers to the following two questions:

1) Do women who use oral contraceptive pills prior to their first full-term pregnancy (FFTP) have an increased risk of developing breast cancer?

2) Do women who undergo an elective abortion before their first full-term pregnancy (FFTP) have an increased risk of developing breast cancer?

The answers to these two questions are the subject of this book. After 6 years of analyzing the data contained within the hundreds of medical studies that pertain to these two questions, I have come to a definite conclusion. *I believe that the evidence contained within this book will convince the lay person and the professional that both an induced abortion and use of the birth control pill are independent risk factors for the development of breast cancer, especially if the woman has participated in either of these factors at a young age. The fact that few women have been informed of this, is, in my opinion, a very, very serious "mistake"* — one with worldwide implications.

One of the goals of this book is to make this complicated subject understandable. Too often, "experts" (the researchers behind the studies) not only tell us what a study means — they tell us what "*they think*" the implications of the study are. The readers are often left in the frustrating position of trusting the researchers' opinions and are unable to critique the results for themselves. This subject is too important to leave the facts *and their interpretation* in the hands of a few experts, many of whom are subject to intense political and financial pressures. It is time for the people to decide for themselves whether or not today's women are at significantly increased risk for breast cancer because of having an induced abortion at an early age and/ or by taking oral contraceptives at a young age.

It is my hope that women and men will now have a book that will help *them to understand the link between the Pill, breast cancer, and abortion.* They will learn what to look for in a medical study and how better to understand statistical data and methods. They will then be able to *understand what separates a good medical study from a bad one,* so they will know "how much stock" to place in the results of a particular study. A second hope is that they will share this resource and its information with interested family members and friends, especially those who have a family history of breast cancer or have daughters, nieces, or granddaughters who may be, or have been, on the Pill or had an abortion. Ideally, the laity, nurses, physicians, and pharmacists will use this book as a reference to clear the air of myths and fill it with factual references based on documented studies. Hopefully, the ping-pong match which pitted "this study" against "that study" will be replaced with thinking based on the facts from the most recent and best done studies. This book will take some time to read and carefully study, but it is important, and may be life-saving for the woman who believes that she or a friend/relative may be at increased risk for breast cancer based on her sexual history.

The reader is therefore asked to go through this book with patience. One of the dilemmas that I had when deciding to present the data and arguments of this very technical area is exactly how to do it. If I went into "too much detail," it would be useless as a resource. If I oversimplified the subject, medical researchers could challenge the basis of my arguments. Therefore, I decided to state the major arguments in "layman's terms" while placing the more technical arguments at the end of certain chapters or in appendices. It may also be noted that *certain parts of this book are repeated and that certain chapters have a "chapter bibliography." These aspects are intentional,* not only for emphasis, but because *some readers may wish to copy certain whole chapters for educational purposes* (eg, especially Chapters 2, 3, and 11). I have made an effort to use AMA formatting consistently in the references and in other relevant places. (*Any part of this book may be copied so long as it is used for educational purposes and the source is properly cited.*) In addition, the medically-trained person is asked to be patient when seemingly obvious medical terms are defined for the layperson. *Chapters 2 and 3 will present a simplified overview of the answers to the two main questions of this book. In fact, the first three chapters of this book will give a fairly good understanding of why (and how much) abortion and use of the birth control pill increase the risk of breast cancer.* Presenting this overview in the initial chapters will help the reader "see the picture" of what is admittedly a challenging subject.

Given the extremely controversial nature of this book, I expect that both the criticism and support will be intense. I anticipate that some in the audience will criticize the work on grounds other than its content. There are those who will agree and disagree with my viewpoint, but few will disagree that too many women are developing and dying from breast cancer around the world. It is my hope that all readers will be open-minded enough to judge this work solely on its content.

Chris Kahlenborn, M.D.

Table A:

PERCENTAGE INCREASE IN BREAST CANCER RATES FOR VARIOUS COUNTRIES FROM TIME PERIODS 1968-72 TO 1983-87*

COUNTRY	PERCENT INCREASE
JAPAN	114%
U.S. (FILIPINOS)	110%
RUSSIA	74%
(SINGAPORE) CHINESE	63%
U.S. (HAWAIIANS)	52%
PUERTO RICO	50%
U.S. (BLACKS)	42%
ICELAND	41%
U.S. (WHITES)	31%
NEW ZEALAND	23%

*Kelsey et al. [2, p.10] and Remennick [3, p.500]

References:

1. Landis SH, Murray T, Bolden S, Wingo PA. Cancer statistics, 1999. *CA Cancer J Clin*. 1999; 49: 8-31.

2. Kelsey J, Horn-Ross P. Breast cancer: Magnitude of the problem and descriptive epidemiology. *Epidemiologic Reviews*.1993; 15: 7-16.

3. Remennick L. Reproductive patterns and cancer incidence in women: a population-based correlation study in the USSR. *Int J Epidemiol*. 1989; 18: 498-510.

Chapter 1:
Essential Background

Over the past few decades, researchers have noted that the normal development of a woman's breast depends on a number of factors. Central factors in this process include two classes of female sex hormones called estrogens (estrogens are spelled oestrogens by the British) and progestins and a pheromone (ie, similar to a hormone, but is secreted by one member of a species and affects another member) called hCG (human Chorionic Gonadotropin). In the human body, estradiol (which is a type of estrogen) and progesterone (which is a specific type of progestin) are referred to as the dominant sexual hormones. *The breast requires a proper level and balance of both of these hormones if it is to develop normally.* However, when the breast is exposed to synthetic estrogens and/or progestins, or to a rapid fall in hormone levels, it may be at risk of becoming cancerous as noted in animal studies [1, 2, 3, 4, 5].

Oral contraceptives are composed of a synthetic estrogen/progestin combination and put the breast cells of a young woman at risk, because these hormones increase the rate of cell division, a process called mitosis [6, p.375]. In general the higher the mitotic rate of a cell, the higher the risk that it will turn into a cancer cell.

In regard to abortion, when a woman becomes pregnant she experiences a dramatic increase in her hormone levels of estradiol, progesterone, and hCG. The initial increase in hormone levels induces breast cells to divide and undergo a maturing process called differentiation, which lasts throughout a woman's pregnancy and is completed only after her first term baby is delivered. Hormone levels fall rapidly if she has an induced abortion, leaving her breast cells in a <u>transitional state</u> where they have not completely matured (differentiated) and are vulnerable to <u>carcinogens</u> (ie, factors that cause cancer).

On this note, a number of researchers have studied the effects of having an abortion at a young age and/or taking oral contraceptive pills (OCPs), in relation to an increased risk of developing breast cancer. Dr. Emily White, a researcher from Washington State, observed in 1987: "Recently, two other factors have emerged as possible risk factors for breast cancer: oral contraceptive use before first pregnancy and abortion before first term pregnancy." She adds, "Exposure to induced abortion and oral contraceptives has increased dramatically" [7, p.242]. Let us now explore in more detail the background of these risk factors and the settings in which they influence a woman's risk for developing breast cancer.

Q-1A: What happens to the breast during pregnancy?

The anatomy of the normal breast is depicted in Figure 1A. The mature breast consists of about 15 to 25 alveolar (ie, grape-like) glands, called mammary lobules, which drain into the lactiferous ducts. These in turn empty the mother's milk through small pores in the areola — the pigmented area of skin which surrounds the nipple.

During a woman's pregnancy, her breasts are influenced by many hormones including prolactin, cortisol, insulin, human Chorionic Gonadotropin (hCG) and others, but *the main three hormones are estradiol, progesterone, and hCG.* These particular hormones reach levels that are far higher than those experienced by a woman at any other time of her life and cause a particularly rapid growth and maturation of the breast cells, especially during the first trimester of pregnancy. This is why women note breast tenderness and swelling during pregnancy. The combination of the high levels of estradiol, progesterone, and hCG during pregnancy serve to help complete the maturation process in the latter half of a woman's pregnancy.

Figure 1A: Normal Breast Anatomy

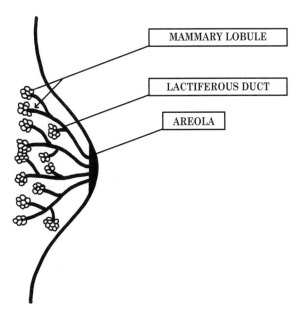

MAMMARY LOBULE

LACTIFEROUS DUCT

AREOLA

Figure 1B compares two stages of a woman's breast. The first, is the virginal stage, which is found in women who are <u>nulliparous</u> (ie, they have not borne children). Here one notes that most of the ends of the ducts, called <u>terminal ducts</u>, are still immature and have not sprouted into fully formed lobules as noted in Figure 1B-2. These terminal ducts contain many more immature or undifferentiated cells than are found in the mature lobule.

After a woman delivers her first child, we can see in Figure 1B-2, that the breast has formed many mature lobules. These mature cells are more protected from <u>carcinogenic</u> (ie, cancer producing) influence because many of them are fully differentiated (matured). Most cancers begin in *immature* terminal ducts in cells that are *not* fully differentiated.

Figure 1B1: Breast Development (Early)

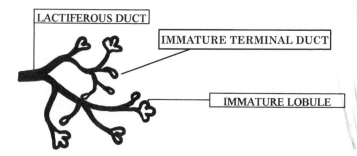

Figure 1B2: Breast Development (Late)

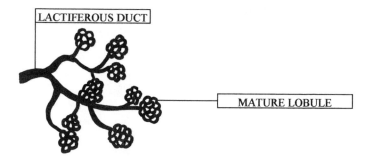

Q-1B: *What is breast cancer?*

What is it about the cells of a woman with breast cancer that make them different from normal breast cells? The main difference is that breast cancer cells tend to grow rapidly and uncontrollably. Normal breast cells will stop growing when the area in which they are growing gets too crowded. Breast cancer cells continue to grow in an uninhibited fashion even when they have little room to continue to grow. Breast cancer then is composed of millions of breast cancer cells that literally do not know when to quit growing.

Q-1C: *Where did the breast cancer cells come from?*

Breast cancer cells actually came from normal breast cells through a process called <u>carcinogenesis</u>. Normally, cells divide and grow by a process called <u>mitosis</u>. During this process the original cell divides, resulting in two cells with the same nuclear material as the original cell. The nucleus contains the chromosomes that in turn contain the genes. The chromosomes are composed of strands of genetic material called <u>DNA</u> (deoxyribonucleic acid). During the mitotic process a "mistake" may occur in which one of the cells gets damaged DNA, often because of the influence of a carcinogen, such as radiation or certain chemicals called "super-oxides." These injuries may result in an abnormal cell — that is, one that tends to grow and divide <u>much more rapidly</u> than normal breast cells.

The initial factor that starts the process of changing a normal breast cell into a cancerous one is called an <u>initiator</u>. The factors which continue the process of converting the now changed cell into a full blown cancer are called <u>promoters</u>. Unfortunately, the original cancer cell divides rapidly, forming a mass or cluster of abnormal cells. After enough time elapses, these cells will form into a mass that is large enough to be felt or detected by mammography (clinically, cancer usually feels like a rock in the breast). The time between the formation of the original abnormal cancer cell and the point at which it has divided and grown large enough to be felt as a lump is usually several years.

The cells of a woman's breast depend on a number of hormones to complete their maturation (differentiation) process. The principal ones are <u>estradiol</u>, <u>progesterone</u>, and especially <u>hCG</u> (human Chorionic Gonadotropin). The breast cells undergo the greatest amount of maturation when a woman's first full-term pregnancy (FFTP) is completed, as was noted in Figure 1B2. Two prominent cancer researchers, Jose and Irma Russo, have demonstrated this phenomenon in their classic work, both in the rat model as well as in humans [1, 2, 8]. In their research, the Russos meticulously documented the microscopic changes that occur in both the rat and human breast during the various stages of life, specifically, before, during and after pregnancy and lactation. They state: "The human breast undergoes a complete series of changes from birth to senility but the *differentiation* process only takes place through pregnancy and lactation." [1, p.56].

Q-1D: What factors are known to cause or influence the risk of breast cancer?

There are several factors that cause breast cancer (either by initiation or promotion) or increase a woman's tendency toward it (eg, having a strong family history of breast cancer). The following list includes most of the known risk factors and/or causes of breast cancer:

> *Note*: Often people get confused with the concept of "increased risk." If a particular risk factor increases the risk of getting breast cancer for a group of women by 50%, *it does not mean that 50% of that group of women will get breast cancer.* It means that the group of women in question will have a 50% higher incidence of getting breast cancer than the general population. If the general population of women in the U.S. has a lifetime breast cancer risk of 12.5%, a 50% increased risk would mean that the affected group would have an 18.75% overall lifetime risk. A 100% increased risk would mean a 25% lifetime risk.

Age:

In the U.S., and in most parts of the world, the incidence of breast cancer increases dramatically as a woman ages. The table below based on data from the National Cancer Institute (1997), shows the percentage of U.S. women who get breast cancer in the various age groups [9, p.9].

Table 1A:
RISK OF BREAST CANCER FOR VARIOUS AGE GROUPS (U.S. WOMEN)

AGE→	1→39 YEARS	1→59 YEARS	1→79 YEARS	LIFETIME RISK
Percent of women who get breast cancer →	0.47% (1 out of 213)	4.38% (1 out of 23)	11.31% (1 out of 9)	12.64% (1 out of 8)

Source: Cancer Statistics, 1996. American Cancer Society.

Family history:

In general, women who have a first degree relative (eg, a mother or a sister) who has or had breast cancer, have a 2- to 2.5-fold greater risk of developing breast cancer [10, p.2127]. This risk increases to a 4-fold risk if the particular relative developed the cancer before menopause or in both breasts (ie, bilateral breast cancer) [11].

Country of birth:

The rates of breast cancer vary tremendously from country to country. For example, the *U.S. has at least a 5-fold higher rate compared to countries such as Iceland or Japan.* Dr. Kelsey wrote: "Low rates are found in most Asian and African countries, intermediate rates in southern European and South American countries, and high rates in North American and northern European countries." [11, p.75] It is interesting to note that when a group of people migrate from a country with a low rate of breast cancer to a country with a high rate such as the U.S., the original group will begin to approach a similar incidence of breast cancer as is in the country to which they migrated after living there for two or three generations. For example: "Native Japanese women who migrate to the U.S. as young adults have a small increase in their breast cancer rates while living in the U.S., whereas Japanese women born in the U.S. have rates approaching those of their white counterparts" [12, p.S11-12]. This indicates that there are certainly factors in addition to genetics that influence a woman's risk of developing breast cancer.

Estrogens in general:

For a long period of time it was thought that estrogens were the only female hormone that increased a woman's risk of breast cancer. As noted below (under progestins), this is no longer the case. Nevertheless, estrogens are still considered to play a major role. It became obvious over the years that women who experienced less "total estrogen exposure," either because of an early hysterectomy with removal of the ovaries, or because of late onset of menarche (ie, the start of menses) or early onset of menopause, all had a decreased risk of getting breast cancer. In general, women whose bodies experience more exposure to estrogens, whether natural or synthetic, have a higher risk of breast cancer than women who experience less exposure.

Progestins in general:

Twenty years ago, most researchers paid little attention to progestins as a major factor in the development of breast cancer [11], yet today, few would disclaim their role as a significant factor. Progestins seem to increase the risk of breast cancer at least as much and possibly more than estrogens. Animal studies have shown that progestins increased the risk of breast cancer in rodents and dogs [13, 14]. Experiments by the World Health Organization (WHO) on women around the world showed that women who had been injected with long-lasting progestin contraceptives such as Depo-Provera (depot-medroxyprogesterone acetate) for at least 2 years before the age of 25 had a 190% or more increased risk of developing breast cancer [15]. Furthermore, Anderson et al have shown that the rate of cell division in the breasts of <u>nulliparous</u> women (ie, women who have not borne children) is highest in the phase of the menstrual cycle in which progesterone levels are highest [1, p.1140].

Induced abortion (in young women):

There have been several prominent studies which show that women who had an induced abortion at a young age have an increased risk of developing breast cancer. A team of researchers (Russo and Russo) have also shown that rats who had a surgical abortion before giving birth or those who were never pregnant (ie, virgin rats), were both at far higher risk of getting breast cancer than rats who gave birth, when all groups were exposed to the same carcinogen (ie, cancer producing agent) [2]. The most prominent and meticulous <u>meta-analysis</u>* in the medical literature on breast cancer risk due to induced abortion was performed by Brind, Chinchilli, Severs and Summy-Long in 1996. These investigators reported a conservative increased risk of 50% to women who had had an induced abortion prior to their <u>first full-term pregnancy</u> (FFTP) and a 30% increased risk for women who had an induced abortion after their FFTP [16].

*A meta-analysis is a particular type of study which pools together the results of most of the major studies in a field of medicine and then gives an overall risk for the risk factor in question based on the collective data and/or results of those studies.

Oral contraceptive use at a young age:

"Several studies have suggested that the use of oral contraceptives in the early teen years may increase the risk of subsequent breast cancer." [Haskell 17, p.327]. Obviously the focus of this book will be to explain why, and how much, early use of oral contraceptives contributes to the development of breast cancer. There have been a number of meta-analyses [18, 19, 20, etc.] that have tried to measure the risk of using oral contraceptive pills (OCPs) on breast cancer, but unfortunately they do not always test for the risk in women *who used them prior to their FFTP.*

For example, the largest meta-analysis done to date, a study that was published both in *The Lancet* and in *Contraception*, had *no data on the risk of contraceptive use in women who used them prior to their FFTP.* (For a detailed analysis of this study see Appendix 4.) The last meta-analysis which specifically examined the risk of OCPs to women who used them for 4 or more years prior to their FFTP was done by Dr. Isabelle Romieu in 1990 [18]. *She noted that women who had taken OCPs for 4 or more years prior to their FFTP had a 72% increased risk of developing breast cancer [RR (relative risk)=1.72 (1.36-2.19)].* (See Chapter 4, question 4D, for a definition of the term "relative risk.")

Miscarriage:

Several studies have noted an increased trend or risk of developing breast cancer when a woman has a miscarriage *before her FFTP* as noted in Table 1B. Further research or a meta-analysis is urgently needed to verify if this is indeed a true risk factor.

Table 1B:
RISKS OF BREAST CANCER TO WOMEN WHO HAD A MISCARRIAGE BEFORE THEIR FFTP

AUTHOR	YEAR OF PUBLICATION	PERCENT CHANGE	CONFIDENCE INTERVAL
Pike et al [21]	1981	151% increase[A]	unknown
Brinton [22]	1983	9% increase*	0.8-1.5
Hadjimichael [23]	1986	250% increase	1.7-7.4
Rosenberg [24]	1988	10% (decrease)*	0.7-1.4**
Ewertz/Duffy [25]	1988	163% increase*	0.83-8.32***
Adami [26]	1990	20% increase*	0.7-2.0
Daling [27]	1994	10% (decrease)*	0.6-1.3
Rookus [28]	1996	40% increase*	1.0-1.9

[A] Calculation of this at end of chapter.

* This result reflects a trend toward an increased or decreased risk but does not attain statistical significance.

** Inappropriate age matching in study: median age of "cases" was 52; median age of "controls" was 40.

*** First trimester miscarriage in nulliparous women.

It should be noted that women who have miscarriages *after* their first full-term pregnancy do not seem to have a significantly increased risk of developing breast cancer.

Menopause:

"It has been estimated that women whose natural menopause occurs before age 45 have only one-half the breast cancer risk of those whose menopause occurs after age 55." [12, p.S13]

Menarche (ie, the start of a woman's menstrual cycles in life):

A number of studies have noted that having a later onset of menses confers a small decrease in breast cancer risk — usually about 20 to 25%, although many of these results are not statistically significant [27, 29, 30, 31, 32, 33]. Of note, young women who are obese and/or sedentary tend to have an earlier age of menarche, whereas women who exercise consistently tend to delay the age of menarche.

Parity (refers to how many children a woman has):

Several studies have noted that the risk of breast cancer decreases as a woman has more children. In general, women who have more children have a lower risk of breast and ovarian cancer. Women who have five or more children have about a 50% decreased risk of breast cancer [34, 35, 36, 37, 38, 39, 40]. In contrast women who are nulliparous have about double the risk of attaining breast cancer compared to the general population [11].

Age at first birth:

Researchers have noted that the risk in mothers who give birth at a young age (ie, under the age of 20) is about one-half to one-third of that of women who deliver their firstborn child after the age of 35 [34, 36, 37, 39, 40, 41]. The main reason for this is that when a younger woman has a child the cells in the small ducts of her breast mature (differentiate) and are less susceptible to cancer producing agents (carcinogens) [see Figure 1B].

Certain types of fibrocystic disease:

Many women have been told that they have "fibrocystic breasts" or "fibrocystic breast disease." There are four types: 1) fibrosis; 2) cyst formation; 3) sclerosing adenosis; and 4) duct epithelial hyperplasia. A woman is said to have duct epithelial hyperplasia if a biopsy of one of her breast nodules reveals "hyperplastic cells" — that is, cells which proliferate more abundantly than normal breast cells. Sometimes these hyperplastic cells display "atypical features" when viewed under a microscope, that is *atypical hyperplasia*. Dr. Colditz, from Harvard, noted that atypical hyperplasia is associated with a 3.7 fold risk of developing breast cancer [42]. Henderson [10] noted that women with atypical hyperplasia had a 4.4-fold risk, which increased to almost a 9-fold risk if a woman also had a family history of breast cancer.

Previous personal history of breast cancer:

The cumulative lifetime incidence rate of a second breast cancer occurring in women who have already had one breast cancer has been reported to be about 25% [10].

Laterality:

Most investigators have noted that breast cancer is found about 10% more often in the left breast than in the right [11]. This may be due to a higher tendency to breastfeed with the right breast.

Long-term breastfeeding:

In a large study, Newcomb et al [43] noted that premenopausal women (ie, women who have not experienced menopause yet) who breast fed for more than 4 months in their lifetime, had at least a 22% *decreased* risk of breast cancer, whereas postmenopausal women showed no obvious benefit from a history of breastfeeding [43]. In a study of 329 women, McTiernan et al [44] noted that premenopausal women who breast fed for more than 13 months had a 55% decreased risk, whereas postmenopausal women who did so [in their reproductive years] had a 62% decreased risk. Byers et al [45] also noted a decreased risk of breast cancer in premenopausal women who breastfed, but failed to find it in postmenopausal women. Wang also noted that women who breastfed more than 6 years had a 60% decreased risk. Mayberry et al [46] noted that parous black women (ie, black women who have had children) who breastfed for more than 16 months had half the risk of breast cancer compared to black women who breastfed less than 4 months. In general, breastfeeding (lactation) appears to reduce the risk of breast cancer in premenopausal women but further studies are needed to assess how much benefit it has in postmenopausal women.

[In addition, for researchers: It should be pointed out that prolonged lactation (ie, greater than 25 weeks) results in a 40% reduction [RR=0.6 (0.3-1.0)] of the risk of p53+ tumors [47] (a decrease in the p53 [over expression] level means an increase in the amount of tumor suppressor gene, which is beneficial)].

Postmenopausal hormone use (ie, hormone replacement therapy [HRT]):

Most major studies show that women who take *artificial* estrogen and/or progestin for a number of years after menopause have a significantly increased risk of breast cancer. Yang, Daling and colleagues [48] noted that women who had taken estrogen for more than 10 years had a 60% increased risk 1.6 [1.1-2.5] of breast cancer. Colditz et al in a study of 1,935 women who developed breast cancer, noted that women who were currently taking hormonal therapy had a 41% increased risk in getting breast cancer [RR=1.41 (1.15-1.74)] and that women who were taking progestins alone had a 124% increased risk [RR=2.24 (1.26-3.98)] [49, p.1590]. Finally, in an extremely large meta-analysis Beral noted that women who had used estrogen replacement within the last 4 years had a 35% increased risk of developing breast cancer if they had taken the estrogen for 5 years or more [50].

Religion:

Jewish women seem to have a 2.8-fold increased risk of getting breast cancer, perhaps because of their higher rate of the defective BRCA1 gene and/or environmental factors [36].

Alcohol:

Longnecker et al [51] in his meta-analysis in 1994 noted that women who drank about two drinks a day had a 25% increased risk of breast cancer ("one drink" would be the equivalent of one beer or one mixed drink or one 4 oz. glass of wine). His large study in 1995 [52] noted that this risk increased even further if the daily consumption of alcohol was greater than two drinks. For example the risk went to a 75% increase when women consumed four or more drinks per day. Alcohol is theorized to cause breast cancer by raising a woman's estrogen levels.

Vitamin A:

Colditz et al [42] noted that the women in the Nurses' Health study who took *more* Vitamin A were noted to have 22% *less* breast cancer than women who took smaller or no doses of Vitamin A. (Note: taking more than 10,000 units of Vitamin A during pregnancy may increase the risk of birth defects [53]).

Obesity in postmenopausal women:

Fat (adipose) tissue converts a hormone produced by the adrenal gland called <u>androstenedione</u> to estrone, a type of estrogen. Theoretically, women with higher estrogen levels should have a higher incidence of breast cancer. In a large study of 570,000 Norwegian women Tretli et al [54] found that postmenopausal women who were in the top 25th percentile of weight had an 18% increased risk of breast cancer over women who were at the lower 25th percentile.

History of having had certain "other cancers" in the past:

Women who have or had cancer of the ovary and/or uterus appear to be at increased risk of developing breast cancer. A history of ovarian cancer puts a woman at about twice the risk of developing breast cancer, whereas a history of endometrial (uterine) cancer raises the risk by 50% compared to the general population [11]. In addition, having a personal history of malignant melanoma, colon cancer, cancer of the salivary glands, or Hodgkin's lymphoma appears to increase the risk of getting breast cancer in the future [55]. (Conversely, having a history of breast cancer is associated with an increased risk of getting ovarian, uterine, colon or thyroid cancer [55]).

Oncogenes:

Certain people carry genes which may either predispose them to or against breast cancer. <u>BRCA1</u> and <u>BRCA2</u> are examples of the former and are thought to make up 80% of the "gene-linked" breast cancer cases. Usually women inherit a normal BRCA1 and BRCA2 gene. These particular genes — <u>tumor suppressor genes</u> — act like "brakes" against breast cancer. If a woman inherits a defective BRCA1 or BRCA2 gene, she will have a markedly increased risk of developing breast cancer. Women with an abnormal BRCA1 gene have an 85% chance of getting breast cancer during their lifetime (ie, 85 out of 100 will get it during an average woman's life span) and a 60% chance of getting ovarian cancer. Jewish women of

Ashkenazic descent (ie, most Jewish women in the U.S.) have a higher incidence of carrying a defective BRCA1 gene. The defective BRCA2 gene also confers an 85% lifetime risk of breast cancer. In fact, women who have a defect of this gene are at much higher risk of developing bilateral premenopausal breast cancer. These women also have an increased risk of ovarian cancer — estimated at 15 to 20% in a lifetime. BRCA2 also confers a 50-fold increased risk of developing breast cancer in the male population so that men carrying the gene have an overall lifetime risk of 6%. In spite of all the news about the discovery of the new genes, it is important to keep in mind that only about 5 to 6% of women with breast cancer are thought to have the type that is caused directly by specific gene defects [56,57].

Radiation:

Women who are exposed to radiation, especially before the delivery of their firstborn child, are at increased risk of developing breast cancer. Sadly, this was proven when researchers found that young women who were exposed to radiation doses of 10 rads or more at the time of the atomic blast in Japan, suffered a far higher incidence of breast cancer as they grew older [58]. The increased incidence of breast cancer was smaller in older women who already had children (because they had more fully matured breast cells). The effects of radiation appear to be permanent and are still apparent for as long as 40 years after exposure [11]. Women who have received routine x-rays are probably at little risk of developing cancer from them because they contain small amounts of radiation (e.g., a chest x-ray contains 0.01 rads) whereas a mammogram contains 0.45 rads (based on data from Paul and Juhl's *Radiological Imaging*, 1993).

Dense mammography:

A woman's mammogram may vary in the "density of its appearance." A researcher named Dr. Wolfe [59] has noted that women with extremely dense looking mammograms have more than five times the incidence of cancer than women with breasts whose mammograms show a minimally dense appearance.

DES (Diethylstilbestrol):

This artificial estrogen was given to about 2 million women, especially diabetics, to prevent premature labor and miscarriages in the 1940s and was used until the late 1960s [60]. Overall it increases a woman's risk of breast cancer by 35% [61].

Being a twin:

In one study, Hsieh et al [62, p.1321] noted that women who are twins, especially if their twin was a male, experienced a higher in-utero (ie, "when in the uterus") estrogen level and have noted a trend toward a slightly increased breast cancer risk in these women.

Smoking:

Smoking *does not* appear to increase the risk of breast cancer. Several well designed studies have failed to find a link [29, 30, 63, 64, 65, 66, 67, 68]. A single study in the *Journal of the National Cancer Institute* (May, 1998) has noted that women who carry the BRCA1 or BRCA2 gene mutation may have a decreased risk of breast cancer if they have a history of smoking.

Addendum:

In 1981, Pike et al [21] noted that women who had either an induced abortion or a miscarriage prior to their FFTP had an increased risk of breast cancer. The information given in Table IV of their paper enables one to calculate the odds ratio (estimated relative risk) of a miscarriage prior to a FFTP. The number of women with breast cancer who had a miscarriage prior to their FFTP was 13, and the number of "controls" who had a miscarriage prior to their FFTP was 9. The total number of "cases" who did not have a miscarriage before their FFTP was 139 in addition to the 11 women who had induced abortions prior to their FFTP (ie, the latter did not have a miscarriage prior to their FFTP) or 139 + 11 = 150. The number of "controls" who had no miscarriage prior to a FFTP was 261 (253+8).

Using the equation for estimating the relative risk (RR) given in Chapter 4 we obtain:

Estimated [RR = 13/150 divided by 9/261 = 2.51] or a 151% increased risk of breast cancer for women who have a miscarriage prior to a first birth.

References:

1. Russo J, Tay TK, et al. Differentiation of the mammary gland and susceptibility to carcinogenesis. *Breast Cancer Research and Treatment*. 1982; 2: 5-73.

2. Russo J, Russo IH. Susceptibility of the mammary gland to carcinogenesis. *Am J Pathol*. 1980; 100: 497-512.

3. Kirschstein RL, et al. Infiltrating duct carcinoma of the mammary gland of a Rhesus monkey after administration of an oral contraceptive: a preliminary report. *J Natl Cancer Inst*. 1972; 48: 551-553.

4. Geil, et al. FDA studies of estrogen, progestogens, and estrogen/progesterone combinations in the dog and monkey. *J Toxicol Environ*. 3: 1979.

5. Shubik P. Oral contraceptives and breast cancer: laboratory evidence. In: Interpretation of Negative Epidemiological Evidence for Carcinogenicity. *IARC Sci Pub*. 1985: 65; 33.

6. Harlap S. Oral contraceptives and breast cancer. Cause and Effect? *J Reprod Med*. 374-395.

7. White E, Daling J, et al. Rising incidence of breast cancer among young women in Washington State. *J Natl Cancer Inst*. 1987; 79: 239-43.

8. Russo J, Russo IH. Toward a physiological approach to breast cancer prevention. *Cancer Epidemiology, Biomarkers and Prevention*. 1994; 3: 353-364.

9. Parker S, Tong T, et al. *Cancer Statistics, 1996. American Cancer Society*. 1996; 46: 1-23.

10. Henderson IC. Risk Factors for breast cancer development. *Cancer* (Supplement). 1993; 71: 2127-2140.

11. Kelsey J. A review of the epidemiology of human breast cancer. *Epidemiologic Reviews*. 1979; 1: 74-109.

12. Henderson B, Bernstein L. The international variation in breast cancer rates: An epidemiological assessment. *Breast Cancer Research and Treatment*. 1991; 18: S11-17.

13. Lanari C, Molinolo AA, et al. Induction of mammary adenocarcinomas by medroxyprogesterone acetate in balb/c female mice. *Cancer Letters*. 1986; 33: 215-223.

14. Laarsson, KS, et al. Predictability of the safety of hormonal contraceptives from canine toxicology studies. In: Michal, F. ed. *Safety Requirements for Contraceptive Steroids*. Cambridge: Cambridge University Press; 1989: 203-269.

15. Skegg DCG, Noonan EA, et al. Depot medroxyprogesterone acetate and breast cancer [A pooled analysis of the World Health Organization and New Zealand studies]. *JAMA.* 1995: 799-804.

16. Brind J, Chinchilli M, et al. Induced abortion as an independent risk factor for breast cancer: a comprehensive review and meta-analysis. *J Epidemiol Community Health.* 10/ 1996; 50: 481-496.

17. Haskell CM. *Cancer Treatment.* 4th ed. Philadelphia: WB Saunders Company; 1995.

18. Romieu I, Berlin J, et al. Oral contraceptives and breast cancer. Review and meta-Analysis. *Cancer.* 1990; 66: 2253-2263.

19. Thomas DB. Oral contraceptives and breast cancer: review of the epidemiologic literature. *Contraception.* 1991; 43: 597-643.

20. Collaborative Group on Hormonal Factors in Breast Cancer. Breast cancer and hormonal contraceptives: further results. *Contraception.* 1996; 34: S1-S106.

21. Pike MC, Henderson BE, et al. Oral contraceptive use and early abortion as risk factors for breast cancer in young women. *Br J Cancer.* 1981; 43: 72-76.

22. Brinton LA, Hoover R, et al. Reproductive factors in the aetiology of breast cancer. *Br J Cancer.* 1983; 47: 757-762.

23. Hadjimichael OC, et al. Abortion before first live birth and risk of breast cancer. *Br J Cancer.* 1986; 53: 281-284.

24. Rosenberg L, Palmer JR, et al. Breast cancer in relation to the occurrence and time of induced and spontaneous abortion. *Am J Epidemiol.* 1988; 127: 981-989.

25. Ewertz M, Duffy SW. Risk of breast cancer in relation to reproductive factors in Denmark. *Br J Cancer.* 1988; 58: 99-104.

26. Adami HO, Bergstrom R, Lund E, Meirik O. Absence of association between reproductive variables and the risk of breast cancer in young women in Sweden and Norway. *Br J Cancer* 1990; 62: 122-126.

27. Daling J, Malone K, et al. Risk of breast cancer among young women: relationship to induced abortion. *J Natl Cancer Inst.* 1994; 86: 1584-1592.

28. Rookus M, Leeuwen F. Induced abortion and risk for breast cancer: reporting (recall) bias in a Dutch case-control study. *J Natl Cancer Inst.* 1996; 88: 1759-1764.

29. Brinton LA, Daling JR, et al. Oral contraceptives and breast cancer risk among younger women. *J Natl Cancer Inst.* 6/7/1995; 87: 827-35.

30. Ewertz M. Oral contraceptives and breast cancer risk in Denmark. *Eur J Cancer.* 1992; 28A: 1176-1181.

31. Chilvers C, McPherson K, et al. Oral contraceptive use and breast cancer risk in young women (UK National Case-Control Study Group). *The Lancet.* May 6, 1989: 973-982.

32. Rookus MA, Leeuwen FE. Oral contraceptives and risk of breast cancer in women ages 20-54 years. *The Lancet.* 1994; 344: 844-851.

33. Thomas DB, Noonan EA. Breast cancer and combined oral contraceptives: results from a multinational study (The WHO collabora-

tive study of Neoplasia and steroid contraceptives). *Br J Cancer.* 1990; 61: 110-119.

34. Lowe CR, MacMahon B. Breast cancer and reproductive history of women in South Wales. *The Lancet.* Jan. 24, 1970: 153-157.

35. Mirra AP, Cole P, et al. Breast cancer in an area of high parity: Sao Paulo, Brazil. *Cancer Research.* 1971; 31: 77-83.

36. Helmrich S, Shapiro S, et al. Risk factors for breast cancer. *Am J Epidemiol.* 1983; 117: 35-45.

37. Lin TM, Chen KP, MacMahon B. Epidemiologic characteristics of cancer of the breast in Taiwan. *Cancer.* 1971; 27: 1497-1504.

38. Rao DN, Ganesh B, et al. Role of reproductive factors in breast cancer in a low-risk area: a case-control study. *Br J Cancer.* 1994; 70: 129-132.

39. Soini I. Risk factors of breast cancer in Finland. *Int J Epidemiol.* 1977; 6: 365-373.

40. La Vecchia C, et al. General epidemiology of breast cancer in northern Italy. *Int J Epidemiol.* 1987; 16: 347-355.

41. Yuasa S, MacMahon B. Lactation and reproductive histories of breast cancer patients in Tokyo, Japan. *Bull World Health Org.* 1970; 42: 195-204.

42. Colditz G. Epidemiology of breast cancer. *Cancer.* 1993; 71: 1480-1489.

43. Newcomb PA, et al. Lactation and a reduced risk of premenopausal breast cancer. *N Engl J Med.* 1994; 330: 81-87.

44. McTiernan A, Thomas DB. Evidence for a protective effect of lactation on risk of breast cancer in young women. *Am J Epidemiol.* 1986; 124: 353-358.

45. Byers T, Graham S, et al. Lactation and breast cancer. *Am J Epidemiol.* 1985; 121: 664-674.

46. Mayberry RM, Stoddard-Wright C. Breast cancer risk factors among black women and white women: similarities and differences. *Am J Epidemiol.* 1992; 136: 1445-1456.

47. Van der Kooy K, Rookus MA, et al. P53 protein overexpression in relation to risk factors for breast cancer. *Am J Epidemiol.* 1996; 144: 924-933.

48. Yang CP, Daling JR, et al. Noncontraceptive hormone use and risk of breast cancer. *Cancer Causes and Control.* 1992; 3: 475-479.

49. Colditz G, Hankinson S, et al. The use of estrogens and progestins and the risk of breast cancer in postmenopausal women. *N Engl J Med.* 1995; 332: 1589-93.

50. Beral V, et al. Breast cancer and hormone replacement therapy: collaborative reanalysis of data from 51 epidemiological studies of 52, 705 women with breast cancer and 108,411 women without breast cancer. *The Lancet.* 1999; 350; 1043-1047.

51. Longnecker MP. Alcoholic beverage consumption in relation to risk of breast cancer: meta-analysis and review. *Cancer Causes and Control.* 1994; 5: 73-82.

52. Longnecker M, Newcomb PA, et al. Risk of breast cancer in relation to lifetime alcohol consumption. *J Natl Cancer Inst.* 1995; 87: 923-929.

53. Rothman K, et al. Teratogenicity of high vitamin A intake. *N Engl J Med.* 1995; 333: 1369-1373.

54. Tretli S, et al. The effects of premorbid height and weight on survival of breast cancer patients. *Br J Cancer.* 1990; 62: 299-303.

55. Horn-Ross PL. Multiple primary cancers involving the breast. *Epidemiological Reviews.* 1993; 15: 169-176.

56. Feldman G. Is genetic testing right for you? *Self.* October,1996; 187-190.

57. Greene MH. Genetics of Breast Cancer. *Mayo Clinic Proceedings.* Jan. 1997; 72: 54-64.

58. McGregor DH, et al. Breast cancer incidence among atomic bomb survivors, Hiroshima and Nagasaki 1950-1969. *J Natl Cancer Inst.* 1977; 59; 799-811.

59. Wolfe JN. Risk for breast cancer development determined by mammographic parenchymal pattern. *Cancer.* 1976; 37: 2486-2492.

60. Malone K. Diethylstilbestrol (DES) and breast cancer. *Epidemiologic Reviews.* 1993; 15: 108-109.

61. Colton T, Greenberg ER, et al. Breast cancer in mothers prescribed diethylstilbestrol in pregnancy. *JAMA,* 1993; 269: 2096-3000.

62. Hsieh C, et al. Twin membership and breast cancer risk. *Am J Epidemiol.* 1992: 136: 1321-1326.

63. Gomes L, Guimaraes M, et al. A case-control study of risk factors for breast cancer in Brazil, 1978-1987. *Int J Epidemiol.* 1995; 24: 292-299.

64. Jick SS, Walker AM, et al. Oral contraceptives and breast cancer. *Br J Cancer.* 1989; 59: 618-621.

65. Maybery RM. Age-specific patterns of association between breast cancer and risk factors in black women, ages 20 to 39 and 40 to 54. *Ann Epidemiol.* 1994; 4: 205-213.

66. Paul C, Skegg DC, et al. Oral contraceptives and breast cancer: a national study. *Br Med J.* 1986; 293: 723-726.

67. White E, Malone K, Weiss N, Daling J. Breast cancer among young U.S. women in relation to oral contraceptive use. *J Natl Cancer Inst.* 1994; 86: 505-514.

68. Daling J, Brinton L, et al. Risk of breast cancer among white women following induced abortion. *Am J Epidemiol.* 1996; 144: 373-380.

Chapter 2:
Overview:
Breast Cancer and Abortion

Q-2A: Why would a woman who has an induced abortion before her _first full-term pregnancy_ (FFTP) suffer an increased risk of developing breast cancer?

A woman's breast is especially sensitive to <u>carcinogenic</u> (ie, cancer producing) influences before she delivers her first child. When a woman becomes pregnant, a number of hormone levels increase dramatically in her body. Three especially notable ones are <u>estradiol</u>, <u>progesterone</u> (ie, the female sexual hormones), and <u>hCG</u> (human Chorionic Gonadotropin). All of these hormones, especially the latter, serve to stimulate immature breast cells to mature into fully differentiated cells [1]. If this process is artificially interrupted by way of an induced abortion, the hormone levels drop suddenly and dramatically, thereby suspending the natural process of maturation of many of the woman's breast cells. This is referred to as a "<u>hormonal blow</u>" by researchers. These cells are now "vulnerable" to carcinogens because they started the maturation process but were never able to complete it. (Cells that have fully matured are less vulnerable to carcinogens than cells that are in the process of maturation).

Q-2B: Do any animal models support the claim that abortions early in life increase breast cancer risk?

Yes. Russo and Russo, in their classic work published in 1980 [2], studied several groups of rats which were given a specific <u>carcinogen</u> (cancer producing agent) called DMBA. They noted that 77% of the rats who underwent an abortion developed breast cancer and 69% of the virgin rats developed breast cancer, but 0% of the rats who were allowed to complete their pregnancy developed breast cancer.

Q-2C: Could you tell me about the history of the abortion/breast cancer debate?

As early as 1957, Segi et al noted that women who had induced abortions had at least a 2-fold increased risk of breast cancer [3]. In 1981, Pike et al [4] published their notable work showing that young women (under the age of 32) who had experienced an abortion before their <u>first fullterm pregnancy</u> (FFTP) had a 140% increased risk of breast cancer. A number of studies followed but in 1994, Daling et al [5] published a large study which noted that women who had an abortion before their FFTP suffered a 40% increased risk. This risk increased to 150% if the adolescent had her abortion before the age of 18. In addition, Daling et al noted that if adolescents under the age of 18 aborted a baby that was more than 8 weeks old, *they suffered an 800% increased risk of developing breast cancer.*

Finally, in 1996, in what is openly regarded as the most meticulous and comprehensive <u>meta-analysis</u> (ie, a synthesis of all the major studies done in a particular field concluding in an overall risk for the pooled studies) of all the abortion/breast cancer research articles ever done, Brind et al [6] found *that women who had an abortion before their FFTP had a 50% increased risk of developing breast cancer whereas women who had an abortion after their FFTP sustained a 30% increased risk.*

Q-2D: If Dr. Brind et al's study was so conclusive, then why is the subject still being debated?

Because of the controversy regarding abortion, Dr. Brind's study came under intense scrutiny; however, the results seemed irrefutable. Janet Daling — a prominent epidemiologist (a researcher who studies trends in the medical field) — was quoted in the *Wall Street Journal* as stating that Brind et al's results were "very objective and statistically beyond reproach." [7] Then in early 1997, the *New England Journal of Medicine* published the results of a large prospective study by Melbye et al [8] which claimed to show that abortion did not increase the risk of breast cancer.

Q-2E: Was there any problem with the study by Melbye?

Yes. It is astonishing that the *New England Journal of Medicine* allowed it to be published in its submitted form. It had several glaring problems that have been pointed out in a follow-up letter to the *New England Journal of Medicine* [9]. The main ones include the following: 1) Melbye's data actually pointed to a 44% increased risk of breast cancer due to abortion, *but they never printed this result*; 2) The follow-up period for the "cases" (ie, women who had an induced abortion) *was less than 10 years,* whereas it was over 20 years for the "controls" (ie, women who did not have an induced abortion). *A follow-up period of less than 10 years is not long enough to show the effect of an abortion (ie, too short of a latent period);* 3) Over 30,000 women in the study who had abortions were "misclassified" as not having them — thus 30,000 women were counted as not having abortions, when in fact they really had abortions; and 4) The study did note that women who had an abortion after the 12th week sustained a 38% increased risk of breast cancer, whereas *women who had late-term abortions (ie, after 18 weeks) had a statistically significant increase of 89%.* Both of these results received little media attention.

Q-2F: Dr. Melbye claimed that his study did not suffer from "recall bias." What did he mean by this?

Some researchers have claimed that retrospective studies suffer from "recall bias." (An example of a retrospective study is one in which women with breast cancer would be interviewed and asked questions about their risk factors such as family history, induced abortion, etc.) The recall bias hypothesis can be defined as the following: "The hypothesis that people who develop a disease (eg, breast cancer) are more likely than people who do not develop that disease to admit that they participated in a 'controversial risk factor' (eg, an induced abortion or oral contraceptive pill [OCP] use) for that disease." In essence they claim that women who have breast cancer are more likely to be truthful about the fact that they had an induced abortion than women who do not have breast cancer.

Q-2G: On what basis do such researchers make such a claim?

This *claim* of recall bias is based on a study by Lindefors-Harris et al [10] from Sweden. She compared the responses of "cases" and "controls" to the national register which reportedly keeps an accurate record of all women who had an abortion. The study *claimed* to show that in the group of women who indeed had an induced abortion (according to the national register), the women who had breast cancer were about 50% more likely to admit that they had the abortion than the women who did not have breast cancer. The study has been criticized by Daling, a prominent epidemiologist, who noted that the study actually showed only a 16% "recall bias" (versus the reported 50% figure), when analyzed properly [5].

Q-2H: Were there any problems with the study?

Yes. The study noted that 7 out of the group of 26 women with breast cancer who stated that they had an abortion at a young age, actually did not have an abortion according to the national register. This implies that 7 women out of the 26 women, or 27% of these "cases," stated that they had an abortion at a young age, when they really did not. Obviously, this undermines the credibility of the study. Who would place any confidence in a study in which more than one quarter of a group of women with breast cancer reportedly lied and said they had an abortion when they actually had not?

Q-2I: Is there any way to get around the "recall bias" problem?

Yes. A direct way to "get around it" is to *measure it*. Researchers did this already in the oral contraceptive and breast cancer debate in which some researchers claimed that women with breast cancer would be more honest about their history of oral contraceptive use. A number of studies refuted this claim by going back to a woman's medical records and comparing the results of her interview response to that of the written record. All three of the studies that did this found less than a 2% difference between "case" and "control" responses [11,12].

Q-2J: Can the same technique be used in regard to the abortion and breast cancer studies?

Absolutely. *Most good obstetricians and gynecologists obtain a thorough medical history of their patients especially on their initial visit.* A standard question would be to ask a woman how many miscarriages and/or induced abortions she had. If one wished to measure the degree of "recall bias" between "cases" and "controls," one could simply compare their oral responses to that of the written medical record. Any degree of bias would be recorded and accounted for.

Q-2K: This seems so basic. Why has it not been done?

That is a good question. Perhaps the question that should be asked is: Has someone done it and not reported it for fear of going against the bureaucratic forces within the political and medical establishments?

Q-2L: Do women who had an abortion or miscarriage, or used oral contraceptive pills (OCPs) early in their reproductive life develop a more aggressive breast cancer?

Yes. Olsson et al has noted [13]: "These results indicate that the rate of tumor cell proliferation [ie, rate of growth of cancer cells] is higher in patients with breast cancer who have used oral contraceptives at an early age or who at a young age have had an early abortion. . ."

Q-2M: Do miscarriages carry the same risk of breast cancer as induced abortion?

Women whose pregnancies end in miscarriage usually do not experience the same increase in estradiol and progesterone (ie, the female sexual hormones) or hCG levels that would result from a healthy pregnancy. Therefore, when a woman experiences a miscarriage, there is a less dramatic shift in hormone levels and less of a "hormonal blow" to the breast. Studies have shown that miscarriages, in general, have less of a risk than induced abortions. However, *several studies show that miscarriages before a first full-term pregnancy (FFTP) may still carry a significant risk of developing breast cancer as noted in Table 2A below. (Further research in this area is critical to determine if an early miscarriage does indeed increase the risk of breast cancer.)*

Table 2A:
RISKS OF BREAST CANCER TO WOMEN WHO HAD A MISCARRIAGE BEFORE THEIR FFTP

AUTHOR	YEAR OF PUBLICATION	PERCENT CHANGE	CONFIDENCE INTERVAL
Pike et al [4]	1981	151% increase	unknown
Brinton [14]	1983	9% increase*	0.8-1.5
Hadjimichael [15]	1986	250% increase	1.7-7.4
Rosenberg [16]	1988	10% decrease*	0.7-1.4**
Ewertz/Duffy [17]	1988	163% increase*	0.83-8.32***
Adami [18]	1990	20% increase*	0.7-2.0
Daling [5]	1994	10% decrease*	0.6-1.3
Rookus [19]	1996	40% increase*	1.0-1.9

* This result reflects a trend toward an increased or decreased risk but does not attain statistical significance.

** Inappropriate age matching in this study: median age of "cases" was 52; median age of "controls" was 40.

***First trimester miscarriage in nulliparous women.

Q-2N: Is the prognosis of a pregnant woman who currently has breast cancer improved if she has an induced abortion?

No. Clarck and Chua noted that: "Those (pregnant women with breast cancer) undergoing a therapeutic abortion had a poorer prognosis compared to a live birth and even a spontaneous abortion." [20] King et al obtained a similar result. ". . .patients who had termination of the pregnancy had a five year survival rate of 43 percent, whereas patients who underwent mastectomy and who went to term had a five year survival of 59 percent." [21].

Q-2O: What should women be told in general about having an abortion at a young age and the risk of breast cancer?

Women who have an elective abortion before their firstborn baby suffer at least a 50% increased risk of developing breast cancer according to the best meta-analysis done to date. The risks are almost certainly higher for women who have had an abortion before the age of 18, or those who have additional risk factors, such as a positive family history or use of oral contraceptives before a FFTP. (The person who is interested in an excellent review article describing the physiologic reasons behind the link between abortion and breast cancer should see Canty's article [22].)

References:

1. Russo J, Russo IH. Toward a physiological approach to breast cancer prevention. *Cancer Epidemiology, Biomarkers and Prevention.* 1994; 3: 353-364.

2. Russo J, Russo IH. Susceptibility of the mammary gland to carcinogenesis. *Am J Pathol.* 1980; 100: 497-512.

3. Segi M, et al. An epidemiological study on cancer in Japan. *GANN.* 1957; 48: 1-63.

4. Pike MC, Henderson BE, et al. Oral contraceptive use and early abortion as risk factors for breast cancer in young women. *Br J Cancer.* 1981; 43: 72-76.

5. Daling J, Malone K, et al. Risk of breast cancer among young women: relationship to induced abortion. *J Natl Cancer Inst.* 1994; 86: 1584-1592.

6. Brind J, Chinchilli M, et al. Induced abortion as an independent risk factor for breast cancer: a comprehensive review and meta-analysis. *J Epidemiol Community Health.* 10/ 1996; 50: 481-496.

7. Lagnado L. Study on abortion and cancer spurs fight. *Wall Street Journal.* Oct. 11, 1996.

8. Melbye M, Wohlfahrt J, et al. Induced abortion and the risk of breast cancer. *N Engl J Med.* 1997; 336: 81-85.

9. Brind J, et al. Induced abortion and the risk of breast cancer. *N Engl J Med.* 1997; 336: 1834.

10. Lindefors-Harris BM, Eklund G, et al. Response bias in a case-control study: analysis utilizing comparative data concerning legal abortions from two independent Swedish studies. *Am J Epidemiol.* 1991; 134: 1003-1008.

11. Chilvers C, McPherson K, et al. Oral contraceptive use and breast cancer risk in young women (UK National Case-Control Study Group). *The Lancet.* May 6, 1989: 973-982.

12. Rookus MA, Leeuwen FE. Oral contraceptives and risk of breast cancer in women ages 20-54 years. *The Lancet.* 1994; 344: 844-851.

13. Olsson H, Ranstam J, et al. Proliferation and DNA ploidy in malignant breast tumors in relation to early contraceptive use and early abortions. *Cancer.* 1991; 67: 1285-1290.

14. Brinton LA, Hoover R, et al. Reproductive factors in the aetiology of breast cancer. *Br J Cancer.* 1983; 47: 757-762.

15. Hadjimichael OC, et al. Abortion before first live birth and risk of breast cancer. *Br J Cancer.* 1986; 53: 281-284.

16. Rosenberg L, Palmer JR, et al. Breast cancer in relation to the occurrence and time of induced and spontaneous abortion. *Am J Epidemiol.* 1988; 127: 981-989.

17. Ewertz M, Duffy SW. Risk of breast cancer in relation to reproductive factors in Denmark. *Br J Cancer.* 1988; 58: 99-104.

18. Adami HO, Bergstrom R, Lund E, Meirik O. Absence of association between reproductive variables and the risk of breast cancer in young women in Sweden and Norway. *Br J Cancer.* 1990; 62: 122-126.

19. Rookus M, Leeuwen F. Induced abortion and risk for breast cancer: reporting (recall) bias in a Dutch case-control study. *J Natl Cancer Inst.* 1996; 88: 1759-1764.

20. Clarck RM, Chua T. Breast cancer and pregnancy: the ultimate challenge. *Clinical Oncology.* 1989; 1: 11-18.

21. King RM, Welch JS, et al. Carcinoma of the breast associated with pregnancy. *Surgery, Gynecology and Obstetrics.* 1985; 160: 228-232.

22. Canty L. Breast cancer risk: Protective effect of an early first full-term pregnancy versus increased risk of induced abortion. *Oncol Nurs Forum.* 1997; 24: 1025-1031

Chapter 3:
Overview:
Breast Cancer and the Pill

Q-3A: What is an oral contraceptive pill?

An oral contraceptive pill is usually a combination of a synthetic estrogen and progestin (ie, the two major types of female hormones) which women take for 21 days out of a 28-day cycle. These hormones work by suppressing, but not eliminating ovulation, thickening cervical mucus, and by changing the lining of the uterus.

Q-3B: Is there any evidence that OCP (oral contraceptive pill) use causes breast cancer in animals?

Yes. Concerns were raised in 1972 when it was noted that an oral contraceptive pill containing the artificial hormones mestranol and norethynodrel appeared to cause a case of metastatic breast cancer in a group of six female rhesus monkeys [1]. This was especially worrisome because rhesus monkeys rarely develop breast cancer. Until that time, only three cases of breast cancer in rhesus monkeys were reported. Although some argued that this was simply a "chance finding," concern grew further when it was noted that both beagles and rodents developed breast cancer when exposed to the hormones contained in today's OCPs [sources: 2, 3, 4, 5, 6].

Q-3C: How might OCP use cause breast cancer in humans?

In 1989, Anderson et al [7] published a classic paper regarding the influence of OCP use on the rate of breast cell division. They found that nulliparous women (ie, women who have not had children) who took OCPs had a significantly higher rate of breast cell division than nulliparous women who did not take them. This was especially important because it is known that in general, cells that divide more rapidly are more vulnerable to carcinogens (ie, cancer producing agents) and thus more likely to become cancerous.

Q-3D: Does OCP use cause an early abortion and if so, could this also be playing a role in the increased risk of breast cancer?

Both pro-life and pro-abortion groups openly admit that OCP use causes early abortions, with the latter doing so publicly in testimony before the Supreme Court in 1989 [8]. Induced abortion before a woman's first full-term pregnancy (FFTP) has been noted to increase a woman's risk of breast cancer by 50% [9]. Could an abortion (defined to be the death of the zygote, embryo or fetus after conception has occurred) within the first week after conception have a deleterious effect as concerns breast cancer? The hormonal physiology of early pregnancy is difficult to measure but Stewart et al [10] and Norman et al [11] have shown that estradiol and progesterone levels (ie, the female hormones) start to rise above baseline levels within 4 days of conception, thus prior to implantation and before hCG levels begin to rise. An early abortion would cause a sudden fall in the levels of these hormones. Could this early "hormonal blow" be playing a role? To this author's knowledge, no one has asked or studied this question.

Q-3E: Can you give a brief history of the studies that showed a link between OCP use prior to a first full-term pregnancy (FFTP) and the increased risk of breast cancer?

In 1981, Pike et al [12] found that women who took OCPs for 4 years before their first full-term pregnancy (FFTP) had at least a 2.25-fold (125%) increased risk of developing breast cancer before the age of 32. This startled the research world and led to additional studies, including a very large American trial called the CASH study (ie, Cancer And Steroid Hormone study). In 1993, the CASH study showed that women who took OCPs prior to their FFTP and were under 44 years of age had a 40% increased risk of breast cancer, which reached statistical significance in the 35 to 44 year-old age group [13].

Later in England, Chilvers et al [14] published the results of another large study called the United Kingdom National Study. She showed that young women under the age of 36 who had used oral contraceptives for at least 4 years before their FFTP had at least a 44% increased risk in breast cancer. The last large study was performed in 1995 by Brinton et al [15]. It showed a 42% increased risk for women who used OCPs for more than 6 months prior to their FFTP.

Q-3F: If the major studies showed the risks that have been mentioned, then why do doctors and pharmacists fail to inform their patients of those risks?

That is a good question. Major journals and major medical associations (eg, the AMA [American Medical Association], the ACOG [American College of Obstetricians and Gynecologists], and the AAP [American Academy of Pediatrics]) have failed to stress or properly note this risk. Part of the problem is that because the OCP/breast cancer debate is complicated, most people have to rely on what "the experts" tell them.

A good example of this occurred recently in the Oxford study reported in a condensed version in *The Lancet* [16] and in complete form in *Contraception* [17]. This study was and remains the largest meta-analysis (ie, a synthesis of all the major studies done in a particular field, concluding in an overall risk for the pooled studies) regarding the studies of OCPs and breast cancer. Researchers from around the world studied and combined the data from 54 studies, involving 25 countries and 53,297 women who had breast cancer. It concluded that: *"Women who are currently using combined oral contraceptives or have used them in the past 10 years are at a slightly increased risk of having breast cancer diagnosed, although the additional cancers tend to be localized to the breast. There is no evidence of an increase in the risk of having breast cancer diagnosed 10 or more years after cessation of use...*" Unfortunately, this study is known more for what it did say, than what it did not say! There were *several major weaknesses* of the study.

Q-3G: What are the weaknesses of the Oxford study and what implications do they have?

The main weakness was *the failure to report any evidence of what the pooled risk of oral contraceptive use before a first term pregnancy was in women less than 45 years old.* Another major weakness is that the Oxford study pooled data from studies which looked at women with breast cancer from the early and mid 1970s [17, p.5S].

A woman's breast is especially sensitive to <u>carcinogenic influence</u> (ie, cancer producing influence) *before* she has her first child because the breast undergoes a maturing process throughout a woman's first pregnancy. By failing to measure the effect of OCP use *before* a premenopausal woman's first full-term pregnancy (FFTP), the Oxford study failed to give data on the one group of women who are most likely to get breast cancer from oral contraceptives, namely, those women who used them before their FFTP (eg, many teenagers and women in their 20s).

The second weakness is that the Oxford study used data from older studies which took some of their data from the mid and early 1970s. This does not leave a long enough latent period. A <u>latent period</u> is the time between exposure to a suspected risk factor (eg, early OCP use) and the cancer which it increases (eg, breast cancer). Often the latent period between a risk factor and a cancer is 15 to 20 years or more (eg, cigarettes and lung cancer). Although women in the U.S. began taking OCPs in the 1960s, they only began taking them for longer periods of time at younger ages in the 1970s. Thus, only studies which include data from the 1980s and 1990s or beyond would allow a long enough latent period to pick up the influence of early OCP use.

Q-3H: Why is it important to study women who are under the age of 45?

Women who are under the age of 45 are more likely to have used OCPs prior to having a child than woman over the age of 45. For example a 55-year old woman who had breast cancer in 1990 would have been very unlikely to have taken the OCP for a significant period of time prior to giving birth because OCPs were just coming to the U.S. in the early 1960s when the cited woman would have been in her late 20s.

Q-3I: What do the four largest studies, which take the bulk of their data after 1980, state regarding women who used OCPs prior to their first full-term pregnancy (FFTP)?

Table 3A: RISK OF BREAST CANCER TO WOMEN WITH OCP USE PRIOR TO THEIR FFTP

AUTHOR	YEARS STUDIED	SIZE OF STUDY	FINDINGS
Wingo [13] CASH Study	12/80-82	2089 less than age 45	40% increase; ages 20-44
Rosenberg [18]	1977-1992	1427 less than age 45	88% increase*
White [19]	1983-1990	747 less than age 45 (Parous women)	50% increase: for use within 5 years of menarche
Brinton [15]	5/90-12/92	1648 less than age 45	42% increased risk*

*Computed from data from study, increase reflects the odds ratio.

The four largest retrospective studies** of parous women under the age of 45 all show *at least a 40%* increased risk for women who took OCPs prior to their FFTP or within 5 years of menarche. Two studies (Rosenberg and Brinton) did not list a formal risk but it was calculated from the data in their paper.

**An example of a retrospective study is one in which women with breast cancer would be interviewed and asked questions about their risk factors such as family history, OCP use, induced abortion, etc.

Q-3J: Has anyone done a meta-analysis of retrospective studies that examined the question of risk to women under the age of 45 who had taken OCPs prior to their FFTP?

Yes. Two different researchers have addressed this question. Thomas et al, in 1991, found that women who took OCPs for extended periods of time prior to their FFTP had a 44% increased risk [RR=1.44 (1.23-1.69)] [20]. A more refined meta-analysis in 1990 by Romieu et al restricted her analysis to those studies done after 1980. The study showed that women under the age of 45 who had taken OCPs for 4 or more years prior to their FFTP had a 72% increased incidence [RR=1.72 (1.36-2.19)] of breast cancer [21].

Q-3K: Can you comment on why a recent large study published by researchers at Harvard claimed to show no increased risk of developing breast cancer in women who had taken OCPs for 5 years or more prior to their FFTP?

In 1997, a group of researchers at Harvard Medical School led by Dr. Hankinson published a study in *Cancer Causes and Control* [22]. It based its conclusions on data taken from the Nurses' Health Study and *claimed* to show that women who took oral contraceptive pills for 5 years or more prior to their FFTP had no increased risk of developing breast cancer compared to women who never took OCPs [RR=0.57 (0.24-1.31)]. The study's conclusions appear to have been based on a flawed analysis.

Q-3L: Can you describe the problems with the study?

Yes. The researchers compared women with breast cancer who took OCPs for 5 years or more prior to their FFTP [let's refer to these women as Group A] *to* women with breast cancer who never took OCPs [Group B].

It is known that women took OCPs *for longer periods of time and earlier in their reproductive lives* in the 1980s and 1990s than in the 1960s and 1970s as was clearly noted in the Oxford study [17, p.9S; Tables 14, 15]. So any group of women who had taken OCPs for 5 years or more prior to their FFTP (ie, Group A) *would have been more likely to have done so while in their late teens and 20s in the 1980s or 1990s,* whereas women in Group B (who never took OCPs) *would be more likely to contain a distribution of women who would have been in their late teens and 20s in either the 1960s, 1970s, 1980s or 1990s. But this strongly supports the contention that women in Group A would have a lower average age and a shorter follow-up time than the women in Group B, which would of course invalidate the study's conclusions.*

It is frightening to note that the Harvard team presented **no data** *on either the average age of women in the noted groups or their respective lengths of follow-up time. The research team instead chose to follow the noted groups in "person-years"* as their measure of follow-up time. This is the length of a follow-up period derived from the number of women followed, multiplied by the average number of years they were followed. For example, if group A had 100 women who were followed for 10 years, the total amount of follow-up time would be 100 x 10 = 1,000 person-years. But if group A had 250 women who were followed for 4 years it would also have 1,000 person-years of follow-up. This is totally inadequate because the measure of "person-years" gives no data on the length of follow-up time *in actual years* and without this information the study must remain suspect *because it was noted that women in group A most likely had both a younger average age and were followed for a shorter period of time than the women in group B.*

Q-3M: *Is there any way that the public will ever have access to the necessary data that was not presented in the Harvard study?*

I am not sure. This author tried in vain to obtain the answers to three basic questions over a 6 month period of time from three different researchers involved in the Harvard study via e-mail, phone calls and certified mail.

It is ironic that one cannot access data from these researchers especially because their study obtained its data from the Nurses' Health Study, *a study which was funded by citizen tax dollars through a grant via the NCI* (National Cancer Institute). The essential questions that need to be answered are presented at the end of this chapter. If the Harvard team had answered these questions the average age and follow-up time period for both Group A and Group B's women could have been easily calculated. Until the noted researchers at Harvard make their data available *for all* to see, the study's conclusions must remain suspect.

Q-3N: Have any other recent studies had methodological problems?

Yes, a large prospective study conducted in England by Beral et al [23] claimed that a "cohort" (ie, the group being examined in a prospective study) of 23,000 women who took the OCP had no greater risk of developing breast cancer than 23,000 women who did not take it. The main problem with the study is that women entered it from 1968 to 1969. But many of these women were taking OCPs *after* they had a FFTP because as we noted earlier, women took OCPs *for shorter periods of time and later in their reproductive lives* in the 1960s and 1970s than in the 1980s and 1990s [17]. The study's claim that OCP use had no long-term risk of increasing breast cancer cannot be applied to the subset of women who took (or currently take) OCPs for longer periods of time prior to their FFTP.

Q-3O: Can you give an overall statement regarding early OCP use and breast cancer?

Yes. If a woman takes the oral contraceptive pill before her FFTP, she suffers a 40% increased risk of developing breast cancer compared to women who do not take OCPs. If she takes OCPs for 4 years or more prior to her FFTP, she may have an even higher risk, as noted by Dr. Romieu earlier.

Q-3P: Are any other groups of women at high risk?

Yes. Women who take OCPs for *long periods of time* (ie, 4 years or more) [14,24,25], are at increased risk for developing breast cancer. Other women at risk are *those who use them after the age of 25* [26,27,28] and *nulliparous women* who use them for a long time (ie, 4 or more years) [14,29]. All three categories of women seem to be at increased risk, with individual studies ranging from 40% to over 200% increased risk. Women who took OCPs for longer time periods and started using them at an early age appear to be at an even greater risk. *For example, the Brinton study [15] is significant in that it allowed a longer latent period to pass and found a 210% increased risk of developing breast cancer in young women (ie, under the age of 35) who took OCPs for more than 10 years, if they began taking them before the age of 18 [RR=3.1 (1.4-6.7)].*

Q-3Q: The studies you cited involved women who were less than 45 years old from data taken after 1980. What will happen to the risk of developing breast cancer for these women as they grow older?

No one knows. It would be wise to learn from history. In the late 1940s an artificial female hormone named DES (Diethylstilbestrol) was given to women to prevent miscarriages. For more than 25 years researchers maintained that DES use did not increase the risk of breast cancer in women who took it. Finally, in the 1980s, it was discovered that DES use increased breast cancer risk by about 35% — especially in older women [30]. A similar phenomenon may be occurring with OCPs. The truth is, no one knows how dangerous OCP use will be for women as they grow older.

Q-3R: It has been noted that OCPs reduce the rate of uterine and ovarian cancer. Is this true?

Yes, it is true. However it must be noted that OCPs also increase the risk of cervical and liver cancer [31, 32, 33]. For example the largest study to date, performed by the World Health Organization, examined over 2,300 women and found that use of OCPs before the age of 25 increased the risk of invasive cervical cancer by 45% [34]. In addition, more women get breast cancer in the U.S. than all of the other alluded to cancers combined, making this the most dangerous risk in Western countries. Oral contraceptives may be particularly risky in *Asian and African countries where cervical and liver cancer are prevalent* [34, 35, 36].

Q-3S: Often women who have painful menstrual cycles are placed on OCPs. Are there medical alternatives with less risks than OCPs?

Menstrual cramps can be controlled by less harmful drugs than OCPs. For example, taking 1,000 mg of Calcium and 399 mg of Magnesium around the time of a woman's onset of menstrual bleeding appears to help with menstrual cramps and migraine headaches. In addition, taking high dose anti-inflammatory agents (eg, ibuprofen) *after* one's menstrual flow has started (and under a doctor's care) will often give relief. Also, the *Journal of Adolescent Medicine* published a case report of a young lady who experienced a 90% reduction in her cramping symptoms when taking Nicardipine *after* her menstrual cramps had begun [37]. Nicardipine is a type of calcium channel blocker that is used for treating hypertension.

Q-3T: What about the risk of "low dose" progestin containing contraceptives such as "the minipill," or long-acting progestins such as Norplant or Depo-Provera?

Skegg et al [38] pooled the data from the World Health Organization (WHO) and New Zealand studies, *the two largest studies that looked at women who took Depo-Provera* (active ingredient is DMPA: depot-medroxyprogesterone acetate) for long periods of time. He found that women who had taken DMPA for between 2 and 3 years before the age of 25 had a *310% statistically significant risk* of getting breast cancer [RR=4.1 (1.6-10.90)] whereas women who had taken DMPA for more than 3 years prior to the age of 25 had at least a *190% increased risk*, that was also significant [RR=2.9 (1.2-7.1)]. The risks for long-term Norplant use in young women could be just as high as for

Depo-Provera users, although widespread tests have not been done because Norplant was developed later than Depo-Provera. In regard to the progestin containing "minipill," the Oxford study noted an overall increased risk of 19% (ie, RR=1.19 [0.89-1.49]) in women who had taken minipills for 4 or more years, but they said nothing about extended use in young women, especially women who took them prior to their FFTP [17, p.98S]. The latter group of women might be at an especially increased risk.

Q-3U: How do the natural means of regulating birth compare to the artificial means?

Several well-designed trials by the World Health Organization have shown that Natural Family Planning (NFP) (ie, methods for determining when a woman is most fertile or infertile, based on qualitative observations of cervical mucus and, for some NFP methods, measuring basal body temperature) has had an effectiveness rate when used correctly that is better than OCPs, that is, less than a 3% rate of pregnancies per year. These trials have been done in both modern and less advanced countries and have shown low annual pregnancy rates: the United Kingdom — 2.7% [39], Germany — 2.3% [40], Belgium — 1.7% [41], and India — 2.0% [42]. *One of the largest trials (of 19,843 women performed by the World Health Organization in India) showed the failure rate to be 0.2 pregnancies per 100 women yearly* — a rate that is significantly better than almost all artificial methods of contraception [43]. (For more information regarding NFP see end of bibliography).

Q-3V: How can the above noted information be verified?

Go to the nearest medical library — nearly every hospital has one — and ask the librarian to help look up the medical references of interest.

Q-3W: What are the three questions never answered by the Harvard study?

The researchers at Harvard have never answered the following simple questions:

1) How many women were there in the group who were under the age of 45 and who used OCPs for 5 years or more prior to their first full-term pregnancy (FFTP) (see page 69, Table 3 of your paper [ie, the women who were followed for 9,741 person-years]). What was the mean age for the women in this group?

2) How many women were there in the group who were under the age of 45 and never used OCPs? (see Table 2 page 68, these women were followed for 176,306 person-years). What was their mean age?

3) How many women were in the group who were under the age of 45 and had used OCPs for 10 years or more of total duration? (see Table 2, p. 68, the group that had 21,760 person-years of follow-up)

References:

1. Kirschstein RL, et al. Infiltrating duct carcinoma of the mammary gland of a Rhesus monkey after administration of an oral contraceptive: a preliminary report. *J Natl Cancer Inst.* 1972; 48: 551-553.
2. Geil, et al. FDA studies of estrogen, progestogens, and estrogen/progesterone combinations in the dog and monkey. *J Toxicol Environ Health.* 3: 1979.
3. Shubik P. Oral contraceptives and breast cancer: laboratory evidence. In: Interpretation of Negative Epidemiological Evidence for Carcinogenicity. *IARC Sci Pub.* 1985; 65; 33.
4. Kahn RH, et al. Effect of long-term treatment with Norethynodrel on A/J and C3H/HeJ mice. *Endocrinology.* 1969; 84: 661.
5. Weisburger JH, et al. Reduction in Carcinogen Induced Breast Cancer in rats by an anti-fertility drug. *Life Sci.* 1968; 7: 259.
6. Welsch CW, et al. 17B-Oestradiol and enovid mammary tumorigenesis in C3H/HeJ female mice. *Br J Cancer.* 1977; 35: 322.
7. Anderson TJ, Battersby S, et al. Oral contraceptive use influences resting breast proliferation. *Hum Pathol.* 1989; 20: 1139-1144.
8. Alderson Reporting Company. Transcripts of oral arguments before court on abortion case. *New York Times.* April 27, 1989; B12.
9. Brind J, Chinchilli M, et al. Induced abortion as an independent risk factor for breast cancer: a comprehensive review and meta-analysis. *J Epidemiol Community Health.* 10/ 1996; 50: 481-496.
10. Stewart DR, Overstreet JW, et al. Enhanced ovarian steroid secretion before implantation in early human pregnancy. *J Clin Endocrinol Metab.* 1993; 76: 1470-1476.
11. Norman RJ et al. Inhibin and relaxin concentration in early singleton, multiple, and failing pregnancy: relationship to gonadotropin and steroid profiles. *Fertility and Sterility.* 1993; 59: 130-137.

12. Pike MC, Henderson BE, et al. Oral contraceptive use and early abortion as risk factors for breast cancer in young women. *Br J Cancer.* 1981; 43: 72-76.

13. Wingo PA, Lee NC, et al. Age-specific differences in the relationship between oral contraceptives use and breast cancer. *Cancer* (supplement). 1993; 71: 1506-1517.

14. Chilvers C, McPherson K, et al. Oral contraceptive use and breast cancer risk in young women (UK National Case-Control Study Group). *The Lancet.* May 6, 1989: 973-982.

15. Brinton LA, Daling JR, et al. Oral contraceptives and breast cancer risk among younger women. *J Natl Cancer Inst.* 6/7/1995; 87: 827-35.

16. Collaborative Group on Hormonal Factors in Breast Cancer. Breast cancer and hormonal contraceptives: collaborative reanalysis of individual data on 53,297 women with breast cancer and 100,239 women without breast cancer from 54 epidemiological studies. *The Lancet.* 1996; 347: 1713-1727.

17. Collaborative Group on Hormonal Factors in Breast Cancer. Breast cancer and hormonal contraceptives: further results. *Contraception.* 1996; 34: S1-S106.

18. Rosenberg L, Palmer JR, et al. A case-control study of the risk of breast cancer in relation to oral contraceptive use. *Am J Epidemiol.* 1992; 136: 1437-44.

19. White E, Malone K, Weiss N, Daling J. Breast cancer among young U.S. women in relation to oral contraceptive use. *J Natl Cancer Inst.* 1994; 86: 505-514.

20. Thomas DB. Oral contraceptives and breast cancer: review of the epidemiologic literature. *Contraception.* 1991; 43: 597-643.

21. Romieu I, Berlin J, et al. Oral contraceptives and breast cancer. Review and meta-Analysis. *Cancer.* 1990; 66: 2253-2263.

22. Hankinson SE, et al. A prospective study of oral contraceptive use and risk of breast cancer (Nurses Health Study, United States). *Cancer Causes and Control.* 1997; 8: 65-72.

23. Beral V, et al. Mortality associated with oral contraceptive use: 25 year follow up of cohort of 46,000 women from Royal College of General Practitioners' oral contraception study. *Br Med J.* 318. 1/1999: 96-99.

24. Rookus MA, Leeuwen FE. Oral contraceptives and risk of breast cancer in women ages 20-54 years. *The Lancet.* 1994; 344: 844-851.

25. Weinstein A, Mahoney M, et al. Breast cancer risk and oral contraceptive use: results from a large case-control study. *Epidemiology.* 1991; 2: 353-358.

26. Palmer J, Rosenberg L, et al. Oral contraceptives use and breast cancer risk among African-American women. *Cancer Causes and Control.* 1995; 6: 321-331.

27. Thomas DB, Noonan EA. Breast cancer and combined oral contraceptives: results from a multinational study [The WHO collaborative study of Neoplasia and steroid contraceptives]. *Br J Cancer.* 1990; 61: 110-119.

28. Wang Q, Ross R, et al. A case-control study of breast cancer in Tianjin, China. *Cancer Epidemiology.* 1992; 1: 435-439.

29. Miller D, Rosenberg L, et al Breast cancer before age 45 and oral contraceptive use: new findings. *Am J Epidemiol.* 1989; 129: 269-279.

30. Colton T, Greenberg ER, et al. Breast cancer in mothers prescribed diethylstilbestrol in pregnancy. *JAMA.* 1993; 269: 2096-3000.

31. Thomas DB, et al. Oral contraceptives and invasive adenocarcinomas and adenosquamos carcinomas of the uterine cervix. *Am J Epidemiol.* 1996; 144: 281-289.

32. Ebeling K, et al. Use of oral contraceptives and risk of invasive cervical cancer in previously screened women. *Int J Cancer.* 1987; 39: 427-430.

33. Kenya PR. Oral contraceptive use and liver tumours: a review. *East African Medical Journal.* 1990. 67:146-153.

34. Thomas DB, et al. Invasive squamos-cell cervical carcinoma and combined oral contraceptives: Results from a multinational study. *Int J Cancer.* 1993; 53: 228-236.

35. Parkin, et al. Estimates of the worldwide frequency of sixteen major cancers in1980. *Int J Cancer.* 1988; 41: 184-197.

36. Fauci AS, et al. *Harrison's: Principles of Internal Medicine.* 14th ed. New York: McGraw Hill; 1998.

37. Earl DT, et al. Calcium channel blockers and dysmenorrhea. *Journal of Adolescent Medicine.* 1992; 13: 107-108.

38. Skegg DCG, Noonan EA, et al. Depot medroxyprogesterone acetate and breast cancer (A pooled analysis of the World Health Organization and New Zealand studies). 1995; *JAMA:* 799-804.

39. Clubb EM, et al. A pilot study on teaching NFP in general practice: current knowledge and new strategies for the 1990s. Washington, D.C.: Georgetown University; 1990: 130-132.

40. Frank-Hermann P, et al. Effectiveness and acceptability of the symptothermal method of NFP in Germany. *Am J Obstet Gynecol.* 1991; 165: 2045-2052.

41. De Leizaola MA. De premiere d'une etude prospecive d'efficacite du planning famillial naturel realisee en Belgique francophone. *J Gyncol Obstet Biol Rev.* 1994; 23: 359-364.

42. DorairajK. The modification mucus method in India. *Am J Obstet Gynecol.* 1991; 165: 2066-2067.

43. Ryder RE. "Natural Family Planning": effective birth control supported by the Catholic Church. *Br Med J.* 1993; 307: 723-726.

For more information on NFP call or write to:

The Couple to Couple League	1-513-471-2000
Pope Paul VI Institute	1-402-390-6600
Family of the Americas	1-800-443-3395
Billings Ovulation Method Association	1-888-637-6371
The St. Augustine Foundation	1-877-554-4637
NW Family Services	1-503-215-6377
National Conference of Catholic Bishops	1-202-541-3240

Chapter 4:
Necessary Groundwork

Before starting this chapter the lay reader is again encouraged to be patient because it is slightly technical. The following groundwork will help one understand why certain studies are more important and/or better designed than others. By gaining an understanding of how these studies are constructed and analyzed, one will be able to decide what the data really show and mean. To do this some research vocabulary must be reviewed.

Q-4A: What is a <u>retrospective study?</u>

In the medical and/or scientific realm, researchers attempt to discover if a particular cause and effect are related. Does having an early induced abortion (*the suspected cause*) increase the risk of breast cancer (*the effect*)? The process is not simple, because there are many factors which increase or decrease the risk of breast cancer as noted in Chapter One. Furthermore, even if a particular factor is shown to be associated with a particular effect, one must be careful not to assume that the factor in question caused the effect. If one finds that women with breast cancer have a higher incidence of having induced abortions at a young age, does this prove that having an abortion causes breast cancer? No, although this certainly would make one suspicious that a "cause and effect" relationship could exist. Why is this so? Because having an early induced abortion *may be associated* with another factor which is the "real culprit." For example, suppose that one found that women who had an early abortion also tended to have children at a later age, or perhaps had used oral contraceptive pills (OCPs) more frequently than women who did not have an abortion at a young age. It then might be the case that these *"associated factors"* (ie, the late age at first birth or the early OCP use) were actually increasing the rate of breast cancer in women who had an abortion at a young age. Should this be the case, then having an abortion at a young age would simply be a factor which is associated with the "real causal factor(s)" and thus would not necessarily be a cause in itself.

In order to deal with this problem statisticians and researchers employ a type of study called a retrospective study. Such a study design is ideal for the situation in which there are many causes for a particular effect (ie, breast cancer). In this type of study, one works *"backwards"* or *"retrospectively"* by looking at the *effect* and going back to try to find the *cause* or *causes* of that effect. For example, in this book we will look at studies which looked at groups of women who had or have breast cancer (ie, women who experienced the effect) and go back to try to determine if a particular factor is a cause (eg, having an abortion at a young age, or using OCPs at an early age). The retrospective study has almost always been the preferred type of study when one wishes to measure the cause of an effect such as breast cancer in which the latter has a fairly small (overall) incidence in the general population. (The reason for this will be explained in the following section under prospective study.)

In a retrospective study researchers compare two groups of women — for example, women with breast cancer and women without breast cancer. The women with breast cancer are generally referred to as the "case group" or "cases,"* and those without the cancer are called the "control group" or "controls."* The researcher(s) will interview a large group of women ("cases" and "controls") — let us say 1,000 of each — and attempt to match them for age so that both groups have participants who have the same

* I write "cases" and "controls" with quotations to remind myself to avoid losing sight of the fact that behind the technical terms, are real women who have real problems (eg, breast cancer).

overall average age and distribution of age. The researcher can then ask the participants about any risk factor which he or she wishes to study. As a rule, a good researcher will ask about every possible factor that could cause breast cancer. Failure to do so could invalidate a study, because one might fail to account for a major risk factor. A typical retrospective study on breast cancer will ask the "cases" and "controls" such questions as: Do you have any family history of breast cancer? Do you have a history of any particular type of fibrocystic disease? What was your age at menarche (ie, the onset of a woman's monthly cycles) and/or menopause? Did you ever use oral contraceptive pills (OCPs)? At what age did you give birth to your first child (if you have children)? Did you ever breastfeed? Did you ever have an induced abortion?. . .

After obtaining responses from both groups, the researcher can then compare and look for any differences in trends between the two groups. For example, almost every study should find that the "case" group (ie, those women with breast cancer) had more women who answered affirmatively to the question: "Do you have any family history of breast cancer?" than the "control group." If 200 out of 1000 women in the "case" group had answered "yes," versus only 100 out of the "control" group, one would think that there is roughly a 2-fold risk of obtaining breast cancer if one were to have a positive family history, according to this study.

After collecting the data, the researcher(s) will enter it into a computer with a "particular statistical package" — this means a statistics software program that "analyzes the data." Modern-day statistics programs are so sophisticated that most researchers have little idea of the detailed manner in which they compute the data and usually work with a professional statistician to make sense of the results. The statistical program will compute what is called an "adjusted relative risk" for a particular risk factor. An adjusted relative risk is the risk of a particular factor after the statistics program has "adjusted for" or "factored out" the influence of the various other possible causes.

For example, if we note that in a particular study the "case group" had double the incidence of having an abortion at a young age compared to the "control group," but that the "case group" of women also tended to have a higher incidence of a positive family history of breast cancer, the computer would adjust for the influence of the family history and might show that instead of abortion conferring a 2-fold risk of breast cancer, it might, after adjusting for family history, actually confer only a 1.6 fold increased risk.

The classical paper that describes the advantages and background of the retrospective study was written by Mantel and Haenszel [1] and is consistently referred to by almost all researchers. Retrospective studies have many advantages over prospective studies when studying a subject such as "the causes of breast cancer." In general they are less expensive, require far fewer subjects, and take much less time.

Q-4B: What is a *prospective study*?

As its name implies, prospective studies attempt to find the "cause(s)" in a "cause and effect" relationship by going forward or "prospectively" through time. How would one perform a prospective study in order to see if early oral contraceptive pill (OCP) use increased a woman's risk of breast cancer? One would start with two large groups, namely, women who used OCPs at an early age (called the "cohort group"), and women who did not, called the "control group." These groups should be carefully matched for age as well as for other risk factors (eg, same country of birth, etc.) Both the "cohort" and "control" group would then be followed over many years and one would then note if there was any overall difference in the rate of development of breast cancer between the two groups over time.

There are many difficulties with a prospective study, especially as concerns breast cancer. First, it requires very large study groups. Because only a small percent of young women will develop breast cancer over 20 years, one usually needs to start out with a study group that contains thousands, if not tens of thousands, of women, in order to notice any appreciable difference between the "cohort" and "control group" through time. This is extremely expensive and often requires a "national effort" and the coordination of dozens of researchers. Even then, the results may not have much "*statistical power*" (defined shortly) because there may be very few women out of the original group who develop breast cancer.

Second, there is the "drop-out factor." Often prospective studies rely on women to complete an annual survey. Many subjects simply drop out with time for various reasons. It would not be uncommon to start out with a group of about 50,000 women, only to see it dwindle to 5,000 before 12 years had elapsed, as occurred in the Lindefors-Harris study [2]. This could obviously influence the results of the study.

Third, one can easily "fail to adjust" for a particular factor which certainly weakens a study's validity. For example, if one studies women during the 1970s or early 1980s, most researchers would not have asked them about their history of induced abortion because this factor was not widely discussed until the early 1990s. Unfortunately, one would then have a situation in which a major risk factor had never been inquired about in the original surveys, obviously limiting the usefulness of the study. An example of this occurred in a very large Danish prospective study conducted by Melbye et al [3]. Because the study was prospective in nature and obtained its information from governmental data banks, certain key variables were not adjusted for which include: 1) a family history of breast cancer; 2) a history of oral contraceptive use; 3) a history of alcohol use; 4) age of menarche, and 5) age of menopause. This weakness was even admitted by Patricia Hartge, the woman who wrote an editorial in the *New England Journal of Medicine* that was otherwise complementary to Melbye et al. Thus, although prospective studies offer certain advantages, these items as discussed can severely limit their usefulness.

A fourth concern is the length of the study. It may take 20 or 30 years for a risk factor (eg, smoking) to show up as a cause for a particular cancer (ie, lung cancer). Obviously this presents problems because so many variables may change after 20 to 30 years. Unfortunately, some studies such as Melbye's et al [3] claimed to be "definitive," but allowed less than 10 years of average follow-up time in their cohort groups.

Q-4C: What is a "relative risk" (RR)?

An author may conclude that women who had an abortion at a young age had a "1.5 relative risk" of getting breast cancer compared to women who did not have an abortion. What does one mean by a "1.5 relative risk?" It means that women who had an abortion at a young age have a 1.5-fold increased risk, or stated another way, they have a 50% increased risk of developing breast cancer compared to women who did not have an abortion at a young age. (A RR of 2.0 would mean a 100% increased risk, a 3.3 RR means a 230% increase etc.)

Q-4D: Can you demonstrate how to calculate a relative risk with an example?

Sure. Let us take a hypothetical example in which 1,000 women have breast cancer (the "cases") and 1,000 women do not have breast cancer (the "controls") where 100 of the "cases" had an abortion at a young age and 69 of the "controls" did. The data and estimated relative risk are shown in Table 4A.

Table 4A: A SAMPLE STUDY AND RELATIVE RISK

	Women with Breast Cancer ("Cases")	Women without Breast Cancer ("Controls")
Total Number in Group	100	1,000
Women who had an abortion prior to their first full-term pregnancy	10 = A	69 = C
Women who did not have an abortion prior to their first full-term pregnancy	90 = B	931 = D
Estimated Relative Risk	A/C divided by B/D = (A x D) / (B x C) =1.50	

The formula (A x D)/(B x C) = 1.50 is actually the definition of what is called the *odds ratio* (OR). Of note, the true definition of the relative risk is: [A/(A+C) divided by B/(B+D)] which equals 1.44 but may be *estimated as*: (A x D)/(B x C) in diseases with low incidences where (A + B) are small compared to (C + D) [4]. Here we see that the odds ratio is 1.50 but when fulfilling the stated conditions becomes an *estimate* for the relative risk. In general, this means that the "cases" have a 1.50-fold increased risk (ie, a 50% increase) of getting breast cancer than the "controls." How did we get this?

First, we took women who had an abortion at a young age and noted that 10 (A) of them had breast cancer and 69 (C) did not, for a ratio of 10/69 = 0.145.

Then we took women who did not have an abortion at a young age and noted that 90 (B) had breast cancer and 931 (D) did not, for a ratio of 90/931 = 0.0967.

Finally we divide 0.145 by 0.0967 to obtain an odds ratio or *estimated* RR of 1.50.

Now the question is, how much more likely are women who had an abortion at a young age, compared to those who did not, of developing breast cancer?

In layman's language, women who had an abortion at a young age in this example had about a 50% increased breast cancer rate compared to those who did not. Why is it so important to understand this term? Because, if you, the reader, ever browse through a paper and wish to "check the writer's conclusions," it is easy to calculate the odds ratio or estimated relative risk and compare your result to the authors. Another advantage of understanding the term "relative risk" and being able to calculate it is that often an author will present the raw data in a table but make no statement as to what the relative risk is. If in Table 4A, the author had simply said that women who have had an abortion at a young age are at "slightly increased risk," without telling the reader what the actual number was, the reader could calculate that "slightly increased risk" means a 1.50 estimated relative risk, that is, a 50% increased risk.

Q-4E: What is an "adjusted relative risk?"

An adjusted relative risk is simply a relative risk that has been adjusted for the various other factors which may influence breast cancer. For instance, in the example above, if one entered the data from a study into the statistics computer program, one might find that the adjusted RR (relative risk) might have been 1.40 instead of 1.50. The statistics program "adjusted for" or took the other breast cancer risk factors into account. In most studies the "case group" and the "control group" are carefully matched so that the adjusted RR is often very close to the RR. The reader can always go back and verify the veracity of the RR if the author has provided the data, but because only the researchers have access to their specific statistics program, the reader will not, in general, be able to verify an adjusted RR.

Q-4F: What is a "confidence interval" and what do researchers mean when they say a study's results are "statistically significant"? (This section is important to understand.)

The estimated relative risk of 1.50 calculated in Table 4A is an estimate of what the real-life relative risk is. If one entered data from the example cited above into the computer statistics program, it would "look at the data" and tell the researcher "how reliable" the 1.50 relative risk (RR) was, that is, how close the RR from the study is likely to be to the real or actual relative risk. For example, if the study is small, you may find a RR of 1.50 or more, but it may be difficult to tell whether the relative risk is "real" or whether it is simply a "fluke" or a "chance finding." That is, is having an abortion at a young age really linked to an increased risk of breast cancer, or was the study's statistical power so small that the results could be due to chance? In general, the larger the number of subjects in a study, the more likely that a RR accurately estimates the "real" relative risk and is less likely to be a "fluke."

Let us take the previous hypothetical example in which we found that having an abortion at a young age conferred a relative risk of 1.50 for breast cancer, that is, women who had an abortion at a young age sustained a 50% increased risk of obtaining breast cancer. In this example we might obtain the following results:

Relative Risk (RR) for having an abortion at a young age in the hypothetical example is:

[RR= 1.50 (1.11-1.90)]; 95% CI

The terms in the parenthesis, are called the 95% "confidence intervals" (CI).

When the statistical program analyzes the data it is able to make some statistical calculations based on the "variability of the data." *In other words, the computer can look at the data and tell the reader how likely it is that the results were due to chance versus a real effect.* A 95% confidence interval of 1.11–1.90 means that the computer is telling the reader that, based on the data from the study, there is a 95% chance that the real relative risk is between 1.11 and 1.90. (Conversely, this means that 5% of the time the real relative risk will be less than 1.11 or greater than 1.90. The 5% figure is called the "*p value.*" A p value of less than 0.05 (5%) is another way of stating that a researcher's relative risk lies within the 95% confidence intervals). The main thing a researcher looks for is to see if the lower number of the confidence interval is greater than 1.0. If it is not, then the relative risk cannot be said to be statistically different from 1.0. For example, if we had noted that the RR was 1.50 with 95% confidence intervals of (0.8–2.2), a researcher would *not* call this "statistically significant" because he or she could *not* say that 95% of the time he or she would expect the real RR to be greater than 1.0. *A calculated relative risk is only statistically significant if the lower number of the 95% confidence interval is greater than 1.0.*

Q-4G: What is "statistical power"?

This term refers to the strength of the statistical conclusions resulting from a particular study. In general, the larger a retrospective study is, the more "powerful" the results. For example, a study of 100 women with breast cancer compared to 100 "controls" might show that an abortion at a young age carries a relative risk of 1.5 with confidence intervals of 0.7-1.9 (95% CI). If the researchers increased the study size to 1000 "cases" versus 1,000 "controls," the new results might show a RR of 1.5 (1.2-1.7; 95% CI).

Note that by increasing the size of the study, the second result has become statistically significant whereas the first is not. *A larger study will almost always have more statistical power than a smaller one.*

Q-4H: What is "regression analysis?"

This is simply a fancy term that tells the reader that the statistics program in the computer has adjusted for the various other factors which are known to influence breast cancer risk. As noted previously, a good study will ask about all of the possible risk factors such as early first birth, parity (ie, the number of children a woman has), family history of breast cancer, early contraceptive use, induced abortion, etc.) The computer program uses regression analysis to "factor out" these variables. The process of adjusting for all of the other factors when calculating the adjusted relative risk is called regression analysis.

Addendum:

A simple overview of a medical research paper is presented which may aid the reader in analyzing a study more easily.

What is one to believe when he or she hears that "the most recent study says that X causes Y or that A prevents B?" From the body of this book, the reader will see that not all study results are of equal value. Often, the results of a particular study will be commented upon in national newspapers and magazines, but they may distort, amplify or diminish the actual findings of the original research paper. One way of avoiding this problem is for the interested reader to go to the nearest medical library, or even the public library, and speak with the librarian about how to obtain a copy of the journal article in which the study was published. Here again, the reader can now decide for him or herself how valid a study is and what its results really showed. To do this, an understanding of what to look for in a basic medical research paper would be helpful.

What are the basic parts of a medical research paper?

The Title Page:

In addition to the title, the title page lists the authors of the study. The first author is the one who ultimately takes responsibility for the study's findings although in practice, it is often the second, third or other authors who have done a great deal of the hands-on work behind the study. Either the title page or the final page of an article often lists two other key pieces of information. First, it tells where the study was done and usually gives an address where the reader may write to find out more about the study and to correspond with the author. Second, they often tell who funded the study. Sometimes the first page of the bibliography will state this. Obviously, this is a vital piece of information because a conflict of interest arises if the "payor" has a vital interest in a "certain outcome" of a study. An example is when a drug company which manufactures an oral contraceptive pill sponsors a study of their own contraceptive to see if it causes breast cancer.

Abstract or Summary:

The abstract gives the reader a summary of the entire article including the purpose, the main results, and the author's interpretation of them. For those with little time, this summary provides a rapid way to get the main points out of a long research paper. Often, however, the abstract may fail to mention important findings contained within the paper if those findings are "too controversial."

Material and Methods:

This section gives the details on how the study was actually conducted. A thorough material and methods section will list such things as when the study was done, the characteristics of the women who were studied, how the data were collected, who interviewed the subjects, how many subjects dropped out of the study, and especially, the various risk factors that were discussed in the questionnaire or interview. It will also usually tell which type of statistical testing was used and which factors were adjusted for in the regression analysis.

Results:

As its name implies, this section presents the results of the study. Perhaps the best and quickest way to understand this section is to simply look at the graphs, charts and tables. Many authors spend pages discussing the results when, in fact, they are commenting on the data contained within the graphs and tables. It is important to note that often under each table a comment will state which factors the authors have adjusted for.

Discussion:

In this section the authors discuss the relevance and implications of their various findings. Unfortunately, when an author discovers "medically incorrect" findings, there is often a paucity of discussion on those specific results.

References or Bibliography:

This is the last section of a typical research paper and lists the references to all of the footnotes of the general text. Often the reference section is preceded by a list of participants or organizations who helped take part in the study (eg, those who aided financially or allowed their services to be used).

References:

1. Mantel N, Haenszel. Statistical Aspects of the analysis of data from retrospective studies of disease. *J Natl Cancer Inst.* 1959; 22: 719-748.
2. Lindefors-Harris BM, Edlund G, et al. Risk of cancer of the breast after legal abortion during the first trimester: a Swedish register study. *Br Med J.* 1989; 299: 1430-1432.
3. Melbye M, Wohlfahrt J, et al. Induced abortion and the risk of breast cancer. *N Engl J Med.* 1997; 336: 81-85.

Chapter 5:
Learning to Analyze the Data

A basic understanding of this challenging chapter will greatly help one comprehend the data and arguments in the remaining chapters. The more technical sections are at the end of the chapter.

Often when a large new research study is performed, the public reads or hears about it. The "experts" frequently comment on their findings in public. In order to assess the credibility of these experts and their conclusions, it is important to understand which things to look for when analyzing a study. Once the following basic principles are understood, one will be able to decide for oneself as to the validity of a certain "expert's" commentary.

Q-5A: What are the basic items that one should understand regarding the analysis of medical research studies? The critical items are the following:

The reverse "file-drawer" problem:

The "file-drawer" problem has been described as the tendency to file away negative data [1] but its converse, that is the failure to present positive data (ie, the "reverse file-drawer" problem), may be a more serious problem. It is discouraging to think that a researcher, after conducting a research project, might be so biased or may be under so much financial or political pressure that he or she might choose to discard or "file away" those results which do not fit his or her agenda. Although this problem is difficult to prove, it is hard to be confident that all researchers present their more controversial findings because of the "medically correct" atmosphere which currently exists. It is not difficult to believe that pressure from drug companies and organizations that benefit from the sale of contraception or abortion, can influence a researcher enough to cause him or her to "water down" important findings or place controversial results in the "file-drawer."

One example comes from a researcher (ie, Dr. Brind) who analyzed the work of an Australian researcher (Rohan) [2]. In 1988, Rohan et al [3] performed a study that was published in the *American Journal of Epidemiology* regarding dietary risk factors for breast cancer. No information was published concerning induced abortion and breast cancer in that study. In 1995, a study by Andrieu et al was noted to contain data from the Australian study which noted that it actually had shown a 160% increased risk for induced abortion! Dr. Brind noted: "The obvious question, of course, is why these findings concerning an eminently avoidable risk factor were suppressed for seven years." [2, p.7]

An example of a slightly different type of "file drawer" problem is displayed in a remarkable admission from Mitchell Creinin, a man noted for his advocacy of the chemical abortion involving methotrexate and misoprostol (brand name is Cytotec®). He stated: "The entire field of early abortion is changing. In the seventies physicians tried to perform them, but we didn't have sensitive pregnancy tests so we sometimes did them (ie, abortions) on women who weren't pregnant" [4, p.26]. *This stunning admission* ought to shock the medical world, but instead the alluded to information was "filed away" so that few in the medical field and/or the laity even realize this deception occurred. In addition to its ethical violations (ie, *among other things it admits that some of today's women underwent an "abortion procedure" when they were not pregnant*), it should be noted that "controls" who said they had an early abortion, may never have had an actual abortion because they may never have been pregnant. By "filing away" this type of information, this segment of the medical community may have artificially decreased the relative risks that today's papers are able to detect in regard to the risks of early abortion.

The funding conflict:

Money has the ability to corrupt almost every known field and/or organization and the research arena is no exception. Unless a researcher is independently wealthy, he or she must rely on financial grants to fund his or her lab and ongoing area of study. Most grants come from agencies of the Federal Government which include some of the following in descending hierarchical order: the Department of Health and Human Services, the Public Health Service, the National Institute of Health (NIH), the National Cancer Institute (NCI), and the National Institute of Child Health and Human Development (NICHHD) as well as others. Grants from the government may at first appear to be "clean grants," but one must remember that the U.S. Government spends millions of dollars for hormonal contraception in "foreign aid" (eg, via USAID) as well as giving millions annually to the largest single abortion provider in the U.S. (ie, Planned Parenthood). These examples of government funding certainly create a scenario that provides ample opportunity for conflict of interest to present itself as concerns honest research on abortion, hormonal contraceptives, and their link to breast cancer.

Grants may also come from trusts or foundations or drug companies. Obviously, if the grantor of the funds has a particular bias, the grantee (ie, the researcher) will have a difficult time publishing results that conflict with the grantor's interest or philosophy. A good medical example concerns that of the chickenpox vaccine produced by Merck, a huge drug company (see Appendix 3 for a detailed account of how the funding conflict may influence the medical literature in regard to the chickenpox vaccine). The *Journal of Pediatrics* published a highly favorable article, written by Daniel Huse, on the benefits and costs of the chickenpox vaccine [5], *however, the article was funded by Merck*. This hardly leaves room for an unbiased analysis. This type of event, however, is not atypical, and occurs in the realm of breast cancer research also. For example, many authors have accepted grant money for their studies on oral contraceptives from pharmaceutical companies who produce oral contraceptives. Rosenberg [6, 7, 8], Miller [9], Palmer [8], Jick [10], La Vecchia and Parrazini et al [11], and Kay [12] are among some of the top researchers who have accepted funds from drug companies in their research efforts.

Another type of funding conflict occurs when the grantor has demonstrated a particular bias which would leave any receiver of funds from that source in a questionable position. For example, the World Health Organization (WHO) has openly funded research on a vaccine which works by causing an early abortion [13]. They also funded an experiment on human subjects with a controversial injectable contraceptive which at the time even the FDA had rejected because of its propensity to cause breast tumors in beagles [14]. The International Planned Parenthood Federation (IPPF), the Family Planning International Assistance (FPIA), and the U.S. Agency for International Development (USAID) are organizations which spend millions of U.S. taxpayer dollars for contraceptives in third world countries. For example, *Population Reports* noted that from the years between 1978 and 1981 alone, these three agencies donated a total of over 38 million prescriptions of oral contraceptive pills (OCPs), which translates to about 10 million prescriptions per year. U.S. taxpayers have literally been donating hundreds of millions of dollars to foreign countries — money which was given to drug companies and family planning agencies. In spite of this conflict of interest, researchers studying oral contraceptives have consistently accepted funds for their work from these controversial sources. Some examples include: Paul et al [15], Thomas et al [16], Lee et al [17], Lindefors-Harris and Meirik [18, 19], and Ellery [20].

The size of the study:

Many studies claim to show a cause/effect relationship but are often so small that the results mean very little. Because breast cancer has so many risk factors, it is usually necessary to obtain a fairly large group of "cases" to study. One must be careful to note that although the study's authors may claim that their study is large, the actual number of "cases" that might be affected by a particular risk factor may be small. For example, one study may interview 1,000 women and another 10,000 women. One might assume that the second study is larger but this may be deceiving. If the first study's authors interviewed women under the age of 45 and the second group interviewed women aged 40 to 90 years old, the first group might actually have more women under the age of 45. Because these are the women who are more likely to have been exposed to having an abortion at a young age and/or early OCP use, the first study may actually be more powerful than the second. (Note: Women who were under the age of 45 as of 1990 would have been more likely to have been exposed to early OCP use than women over the age of 45 as of 1990 because OCPs began to be used more often at an earlier age in the 1970s and 1980s [21, p.9S].)

A proper latent period:

The time between the influence of a breast cancer risk factor such as radiation, having an abortion at a young age, or early OCP use, and the subsequent clinical manifestation of a breast cancer growth, is called the latent period. Many studies concerning both abortion at a young age and early oral contraceptive pill use claim to show little increase in the rate of breast cancer, but these studies often fail to allow a proper latent period to pass between cause and effect. Why is this important? We noted earlier that a cancerous growth starts when one breast cancer cell starts growing abnormally and that it often takes 15 to 25 years or more to discover that certain factors are indeed true risk factors for breast cancer or other cancers. *For example, most people are well aware that it often takes decades for "the cause" of cigarette smoking to result in "the effect" of lung cancer.*

In the realm of breast cancer, it was noted that "very young women, survivors of the bombs of Hiroshima and

Nagasaki, experienced a radiation dose-related increase in breast cancer incidence, but not until 15 years after exposure." [22, p.985] Another example is that of DES (diethylstilbestrol) — a synthetic estrogen which was given to pregnant women from the late 1940s through the 1960s to prevent miscarriage and/or premature labor. It took more than 25 years before researchers discovered that DES results in a 35% increased risk in breast cancer, a risk that was even noted to affect women older than 60 years of age, when the prevalence rates of breast cancer are especially high [23]. Dr. McPherson, a researcher from England, noted both of these effects in his research paper in 1987 [24].

Unfortunately many researchers have claimed to "find no effect" from either induced abortion in young women, or early OCP use, in spite of the fact that the researchers often allowed fewer than 10 or 15 years to pass between the suspected cause and the effect (breast cancer). An editorial in the British journal, *The Lancet*, commented directly upon this. "If long-term OCP use in early life does affect the risk, it might show itself in terms of excess cases 10 or 20 years after exposure." [22, p.985]. A Swedish researcher, Dr. Olsson, wrote: "If latency time is required, it will take another 15 to 20 years to know if the presently used pills affect the risk (of breast cancer)" [25, p.269]. Finally, Dr. Hulka, commenting on latency wrote: "More commonly, 15 to 20 years are required, and for a few carcinogens, it may require 30 years to demonstrate their peak effects." [26, p.1624] *Thus, studies published from the 1960s until even the late 1970s will have little possibility of picking up the effects of induced abortion and/or early OCP use on the increased risk of developing breast cancer.* Authors who claimed to "show no effect" when publishing studies in the 1960s or early 1970s often failed to take the latent effect into account. An example of this occurred in the Melbye study [27] in which he followed women who had abortions for fewer than 10 years and rashly proclaimed his study as "definitely" showing that abortion does not cause breast cancer.

Even a large meta-analysis may fail to give an accurate result if it takes data from studies that were too old (ie, studies from the 1960s and 1970s). For example, a famous meta-analysis performed in Oxford, regarding the risk of OCPs and breast cancer, took more than 50% of its data from women who developed breast cancer before 1985 [21, Table 1]. But researchers Malone and Daling pointed out that "Studies conducted in the latter half of the 1980s may be the first studies conducted in women born recently enough to have used oral contraceptives at a young age and for a long duration followed by a sufficient amount of time to be consistent with the possible induction period for breast carcinogenesis suggested by studies of other risk factors" [28, p.93]. As we shall see shortly, it is indeed the studies of the late 1980s and 1990s that show the largest effects from induced abortion/OCP use and it may well be that, as occurred with DES, the studies showing the highest risks will be those that have allowed a latent period of at least 20 years to pass.

Bias:

(This topic is so important that it merits a separate appendix. For those who wish to gain a more complete understanding, see Appendix 2).

In general, there are two major types of bias. The first type concerns the opinion(s) of the author which he or she may at times fail to separate from true scientific analysis and may thereby influence the data and results. The second type concerns the patient's own bias, that is, his or her truthfulness in answering a questionnaire or interview question. This has been referred to as "recall bias." Some researchers have hypothesized that women who have breast cancer answer more honestly than women who do not have breast cancer, to the following question: "Did you ever have an induced abortion?" This is the so-called "recall bias."

The main study which claims to show evidence of recall bias concerning the issue of having an abortion at a young age is a study in 1991, which was funded by Family

Health International and conducted by researchers Britt-Marie Lindefors-Harris and Olav Meirik from Sweden. Here are their thoughts on recall bias: "We hypothesized that a woman who had recently been given a diagnosis of a malignant disease, contemplating causes of her illness, would remember and report an induced abortion more consistently than would a healthy control" [19, p.1003]. The immediate question which may enter the mind is: "Why was this the working hypothesis instead of its direct counterpart?" *That is, why did these authors not originally hypothesize that a woman who has breast cancer might be less candid about her recall of abortion?* After all, "*denial*" is one of the first reactions that patients have. When a woman is told that she has breast cancer it is not uncommon to deny to herself that she really has it. *It would seem just as logical to think that such women would be more likely to deny factors that may have contributed to the breast cancer such as abortion and/or early oral contraceptive use.*

Q-5B: What did Lindefors-Harris' study show?

The study *claimed* to show that women who had breast cancer were about 50% more likely to tell that they had an abortion, if they indeed had had one in the past, than women who did not have breast cancer. The study, however has been criticized by Daling, a prominent epidemiologist, who noted that the study actually showed only a 16% "recall bias" when analyzed properly. In this Swedish study, in the group of women who had breast cancer and stated that they had had an induced abortion, the government's national registry bank recorded 27% of these women as never having had an abortion. *Few people would believe that 27% of a group of women would lie, and state that they had an abortion, when in fact they never had one.* Because of this, the study's credibility was called into question in separate publications [1, 29] by two different researchers (Daling, Brind).

In addition, if Lindefors-Harris' hypothesis was correct, it would mean that thousands of other studies in medicine might now be deemed "questionable." Every time one had a disease or "effect" that was caused by a controversial risk factor (ie, one of the causes), the study might be considered invalid because of "recall bias." Studies on "liver cancer and a history of alcoholism" or "cervical cancer and the number of sexual partners a woman has had" or "the diagnosis of AIDS and the number of homosexual encounters a man has had," are all examples of an *effect that is associated with a controversial cause.* Accepting the Lindefors-Harris hypothesis, implies that all these studies, and thousands of others, are possibly compromised because they all could suffer from recall bias due to a controversial risk factor.

Q-5C: Is there a way to adjust for recall bias, if it exists?

Yes. Actually there is a fairly direct way to adjust for it and that is to *measure it.* Researchers did this already in the oral contraceptive and breast cancer debate in which some researchers claimed that women with breast cancer would be more honest about their history of oral contraceptive use. A number of studies refuted this claim by going back to a woman's medical records and comparing the results of her interview response to that of the written record. All three of the studies that did this found less than a 2% difference between the "case" and "control" responses [30,31]. But the same technique can be used in the studies involving abortion and breast cancer. *Most good obstetricians and gynecologists obtain a thorough medical history of their patients especially on their initial visit. A standard question would be to ask a woman how many miscarriages and/or induced abortions she had. If one wished to measure the degree of "recall bias" between "cases" and "controls," one would simply have to compare their oral responses given in a study's interview, to those of the written medical record* — any degree of bias could be recorded and accounted for.

The age factor:

The "age factor" is the most critical factor to be aware of in the studies concerning breast cancer, so Appendix 1 has been set aside for the reader who wishes to gain a deeper understanding of this important factor. Even the following abbreviated explanation is a bit challenging, but it is important to understand so please be patient and try to work through it.

When one performs a retrospective study it is *crucial* that the "case group" and the "control group" *be matched* for *average age* as well as *distribution of age*. This means that not only should both groups have the same overall average age, they should also have the same *distribution of age*. Obviously, if two groups have women with very different average ages, the younger group may well be exposed to different risk factors than the older group. For example, if one would compare a group of 65-year-old women to a group of 40-year-old women in the year 1998, one might expect the younger group to have experienced more abortions and early oral contraceptive use, simply because these two risk factors were not generally available to the older women.

McPherson et al noted this in 1987 when he wrote that OCP (oral contraceptive pill) use before a <u>first full-term pregnancy</u> (FFTP) was markedly different in the groups of women who were over the age 45 compared to those under 45. "Among the older group, barely 3% had any OCP use before first term pregnancy, while in the younger group around 25% reported such use" [24]. It is obvious that when comparing the two groups, namely, women with and without breast cancer, the latter (ie, the "controls") may have had significantly more early OCP use and/or abortions if they are even 1 or 2 years younger than the "case group." This effect could easily be responsible for the Bostonian researcher Lynn Rosenberg's "statistically borderline" finding of an increased relative risk of 40% for developing breast cancer from having an induced abortion at a young age: [RR=1.4 (1.0-1.9)]. In her study [8], the mean age for the *"cases" was 52 years old*, whereas that of the *"controls" was 40!* In another example concerning the area of OCPs and breast cancer, Paul's New Zealand study suffered from a large age difference with the "cases" being almost 4 years older than the "controls." [15]. This study may well have shown a larger relative risk, which might have been statistically significant, had she matched the "cases" and the "controls" properly. Unfortunately, the researcher who claims to find "no difference" between two groups when failing to match subjects for age at the beginning of the study may well be masking the real cause/effect relationship.

The Stack Effect:
This section is technically challenging but important to understand.

As concerns the "*distribution of age,*" two groups of women may have the same average age, such as age 40 as noted in Figure 5A, but one group may have many more women around age 40 (the "cases"), whereas the other group may have a number of women who are very young and very old, and fewer women who are near age 40 (the "controls"). If the "controls" had many women in their 20s as well as their 50s, then the two groups would have totally different distributions of ages. Another way of saying this is that the "control group" is "*stacked*"; that is, the researcher has "weighted" or "stacked" women at both the young and old ends of the age scale. *When two groups have the same average age but a different distribution of age, they will almost always have been exposed to different breast cancer risk factors (eg, having an abortion at a young age and/or early OCP use) and this may well reduce the credibility of an entire study. In many research studies the "control group" has a stacked distribution of its women. Because this group has disproportionately more younger women, it has the effect of reducing the relative risks that a study finds, because younger women usually have a greater participation in early OCP use and abortion than older women.* Appendix 1 examines this critical effect in detail.

Figure 5A:

THE STACK EFFECT

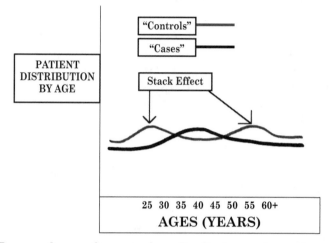

Researchers often study a limited number of younger women with breast cancer (eg, the "cases" less than the age of 35), because of the low prevalence of this cancer in younger women. *Often they "overmatch" or "oversample" (ie, put more women in one group than another group) these younger groups with excessive young "controls" of the same age in an attempt to "increase the statistical stability" of any findings in these lower age groups.* Dr. Newcomb noted this in her 1996 study on the risks of OCPs in the U.S.: "The controls were selected at random to have an age distribution similar to that of the cases, but were oversampled in younger age strata in the New England states to increase statistical power" [32, p.526]. Unfortunately, this attempt to "oversample" or "overmatch" young "cases" among "the controls" *has led to one of the largest and most unacknowledged flaws in many major research studies* and has been recognized by only a few discerning researchers, such as Pike and Bernstein [33, 34], and Olsson [35].

What effect does "stacking the data" (ie, the *stack effect*) have on the relative risks of a particular risk factor such as having an abortion at a young age and/or early OCP use? *When researchers "stack" a study by oversampling* the "controls" in the younger age groups, they end up underestimating the relative risk for early OCP use and/or having an abortion at a young age. Why? Women in the late 1970s and the 1980s used OCPs far earlier and longer and had more abortions at young ages than women did in the late 1960s and early 1970s [21, p.9S]. *Thus, if the younger aged "controls" (eg, those women under the age of 35) are oversampled compared to the younger "cases," the "control group" will be much more likely to have more women in it who had early OCP use and/or an abortion at a young age, and this will artificially inflate the risk of this group.* But artificially inflating the "control group's" risk is another way of saying that one has artificially deflated the "case group's" risks. *In other words, when the control group is stacked, one ends up underestimating the risks of developing breast cancer from abortion performed at a young age and/or early OCP use.*

Obviously the "stack effect" is critical if the "control group" has a larger percentage of subjects in the lowest aged brackets as noted again in Figure 5A. A difference of 1% or 2% between two different group's population distribution in the younger age brackets can alter the outcome of an entire study. It means that a study whose results claimed to show "no real risk" may in fact "have a real risk" (this is referred to as a "false negative") and those studies which showed a real risk may well have shown a greater risk if the stack effect had been compensated for when the study was designed. *In other words, when the "control group" is stacked it generally means that the risks of early OCP and/or having an abortion at a young age are even greater than those stated in the paper.* Unfortunately, some of the best known studies in both the fields of breast cancer/abortion, and breast cancer/early OCP use, are riddled with this effect.

In regard to the abortion/breast cancer studies, we find this effect in Janet Daling's 1994 study in which a larger percentage of women were concentrated in the younger age bracket in the "control" group than the "case" group (17% "controls" vs. 8% "cases" in the 21-30 year-old age bracket) and again in the 1996 study (19.7% "controls" vs. 14.6% "cases" in the 20-34 year-old age bracket). Both show a large stack effect. In spite of the noted positive findings for abortion as a risk factor in these studies, the results may well have shown abortion at a young age to be even riskier and with stronger statistical significance, had this effect been eliminated by proper age distribution matching from the onset.

The stack effect is even more prevalent in the OCP/ breast cancer literature. Some of the most prominent studies show this: The CASH study (Cancer and Steroid Hormone Study) [36] noted that 3.9% of the "controls" versus 0.5% of the "cases" were in the youngest age bracket of 20 to 24 year-olds, and 24.8% of "controls" versus 16.2% of "cases" were less than 35 years old; the WHO (World Health Organization) study by Thomas [37] showed that 35.8% of the "controls" were less than the age of 35 whereas only 14.2% of the "cases" were; Paul's New Zealand study [15] had 21.7% of the "controls" in the youngest age bracket of 25 to 34 year-olds, versus only 7.2% of the "cases"; and Emily White's large study [38] in the 1994 *Journal of the National Cancer Institute* showed that "controls" comprised 17% of the 21 to 30 year-old age bracket versus 9% of the "cases."

Fortunately, as noted earlier, some researchers have commented on this effect, especially in regard to the CASH study. For example, Pike and Bernstein wrote: "But in the CASH study, where the age distributions of cases and controls differ so much, adjustments are important. . . In neither of the CASH papers are the adjustments for age or the rationale for lack of adjustment for region described in detail, but it does not seem that the required finely stratified age-adjusted analyses were made." [34, p.615]. In a later article, in the July 15, 1989 issue of *The Lancet*, Pike and Bernstein again took issue with the stack effect in CASH: "In the footnote to their Table 1, however, they (ie, the authors of CASH) state that, in a logistic regression analysis, age (and hence cohort) is adjusted for as a continuous variable. This is inadequate; as we stated previously, 'in data on OCP use where there are striking changes by birth cohort and by single years of age, adjustment needs to be made in single years for both birth cohort and age."' [33, p.158] Last, *Olsson summarized the stack effect most concisely* in his response to the CASH study (commenting on Dr. Stadel's work, who was involved with the CASH study): "Sir, — In view of the high relative risks found in our study of oral contraceptives (OC) and breast cancer, we were surprised by the negative findings of Dr. Stadel and colleagues. The seemingly contradictory results between the two studies may be explicable by a flaw in Stadel's statistical analysis. As your Nov. 2 editorial notes, *there is a strong time trend in the exposure to OC in young ages. The Stadel study design does not seem to take this effect into account. This could imply that the young OC starters among the controls represent women born recently and thus having short latency times. The relative risk would be biased downward because of interactions bias from the shorter latency times for this young group. Adjusting for age alone will (not) thus eliminate such a bias."* (emphasis added) [35, p.1181]

In short, the widespread inclusion of the stack effect in many prominent studies certainly has the effect of underestimating the real risk of early OCP use and/or having an abortion at a young age. Hopefully, future studies will avoid this subtle but critical effect.

Journal bias:

Is there really a "medical correctness" in the medical literature? It would appear that many of the prominent journals, especially those published in the U.S., have perhaps become more ideological than idealistic. They seem to have embraced a certain type of "medical correctness" instead of letting the data speak for itself. For example, in 1992 the *New England Journal of Medicine* [39] published a review on breast cancer and never mentioned abortion as a possible risk factor. In addition, the authors stated that "The use of oral contraceptives appears to increase the risk of breast cancer by 50%, but the excess risk drops rapidly after the drug is stopped, suggesting a late-stage tumor promoting effect." [39, p.322]. As Chapters 9, 10, 11, and 12 will show, their statements and/or omissions are imprecise at best.

Unfortunately, three of the most prominent journals published in the U.S. are closely tied to major medical groups such as the AMA (American Medical Association) which publishes *JAMA*, the ACOG (American College of Obstetricians and Gynecologists) which publishes *Obstetrics and Gynecology,* and the AAP (American Academy of Pediatrics) which publishes the journal of *Pediatrics.* All three have endorsed early contraceptive use as well as induced abortion [40], with the ACOG going so far as to oppose a federal ban on partial birth abortion (October 9, 1997; *The New York Times*). It is therefore no surprise that certain American authors (eg, Brind et al [1] and Howe et al [41, 13]) have ended up publishing their findings in the British literature. Apparently, the British have more "tolerance" to an open presentation of the controversial findings. *The irony is that, although women in the U.S. are at higher risk for breast cancer due to their higher rates of abortion at a young age and early OCP use, their own country's medical establishment appears to be muzzling an open discussion of these very factors.*

A measurable risk factor:

As noted previously, breast cancer is a complicated cancer that is multifactorial in origin. There are at least ten different factors that influence a woman's risk of developing breast cancer. In order to pick up the influence of a particular risk factor in a significant way, it must have a certain prevalence in the group of women that is being studied or it could be missed. What does this mean, and why is this important? It means that if a factor is a true risk factor for a disease, one may miss this fact if one were to study a population in which that factor was very uncommon.

It is known that men with AIDS develop non-Hodgkin's lymphoma (NHL) almost one hundred times more frequently than the general population [42]. If one studies people who had lymphoma from two different populations

— one in which AIDS is common and one in which it is not, one may very well miss the fact that AIDS is a real risk factor for lymphoma. For example, if one studied men who had lymphoma in San Francisco, one would expect that out of a group of 1000 men in the population, a number would have AIDS, and it would be easy to see that AIDS predisposed men to the development of non-Hodgkin's lymphoma. But what if one had studied a group of people in whom AIDS is far less common? If one performed the same study in a group of 1000 people with lymphoma in Kansas — where the rate of AIDS is far lower than in San Francisco — one might find that one cannot measure the risk of AIDS simply because so few of the population have it.

This phenomenon is quite important when one wishes to determine if a factor such as having an abortion at a young age and/or contraceptive use is a significant risk. Why? Because the rates of early contraceptive use and/or abortion vary widely depending on which group of women one is studying, as well as the country and period of time in history one studies. For example, women in the U.S. and other countries around the world are using OCPs more frequently at younger ages today than they did in the 1960s and 1970s [28, p.81; 43, p.709; 21, Table 14]. This means that if one were to compare women from the late 1960s and early 1970s to those of the 1980s and 1990s, the latter would have used OCPs far more frequently before a first full-term pregnancy (FFTP) than the former. Studies which were conducted in the 1960s or 1970s could have failed to pick up the risk of early OCP use, because it was less prevalent in those decades. The converse is that future studies may demonstrate more accurately how big a risk factor early OCP use actually is.

Another important consideration in regard to the prevalence of a factor is the place in which a study is being conducted. The U.S. has one of the highest rates of women who have an abortion at a young age and have used OCPs. Tietze pointed out that although every other country in the world had an abortion rate of less than 30 per 1,000 in women under the age of 19 in the early 1980s, the U.S.

had a rate of 44.4 per 1,000 [44, p.46]. In addition, the U.S. has the "distinction" of having more than three times the rate of abortions compared to any other country in the world in young women aged 13 or 14 years old [45, p.252]. The U.S. also has the highest cumulative amount of OCP use when measured in total number of prescriptions used in a given country [46]. Even in the early 1980s, more than 84% of women born after 1950 had taken OCPs (CASH study [21, p.36S]). *Because the U.S. unfortunately leads the world in the prevalence of these risk factors — especially in young women — studies of its population carry more weight than almost any other country in the world.*

Another example of this phenomenon is pointed out in a study from Sweden [47]. Olsson et al noted that although their study had only 174 premenopausal women with breast cancer — compared to the CASH study which had 2089 women less than the age of 45 or the New Zealand study which had 388 women younger than the age of 45 — the Swedish study may have had far more statistical power because Sweden has had a high rate of early OCP use for many years: "Thus, one possible reason for the discrepancies between our results and those of the CASH study and the New Zealand study is the higher rate of OCP use among women at an early age in southern Sweden. Use of OCPs before the age of 21, in combination with a minimum of 15 years latency after the age of 25, was 12 times more common (6% vs. 0.5%) among controls in this study than those in the CASH study [47, p.1003].

High prevalence rate of a risk factor:

In some areas in the world, for example in the U.S., Australia, New Zealand, England, France, Sweden, and the Netherlands, a very high percentage of women born after 1950 have taken OCPs (ie, between 80-95%) [21]. Will this affect the results of future studies? It can. If a very high percentage of the female population used OCPs, one may "fail to find" a significant difference between "cases" and "controls." It was noted above that if a factor was rarely found in a society, it would be difficult to measure and assess its risk. In a similar manner, if a factor is almost universally prevalent, it again becomes difficult to assess that factor's true risk. An easy way of conceptualizing this is to consider what would happen if every woman in the population used OCPs in her life. Obviously, both "cases" and "controls" would have a 100% usage rate and it would be impossible to tell the difference between them. It is ironic to note that as more information continues to document the strong risk of early OCP use (Chapters 8 and 9), the population of young women in some countries (eg, Australia) who have used the OCP is approaching 100% [21, p.36S].

Mixing older and younger women in the database:

Mixing women of various ages in a study may artificially reduce the risk of certain factors such as an abortion at a young age or early OCP use, if the older women never experienced "accessibility" to that factor. Let us illustrate by comparing two studies. In the first, we study 100 "cases" and 100 "controls" ages 20 to 40 years old at the time of interview, assuming they were all interviewed in 1990. This is illustrated in Table 5A. ("first full-term pregnancy" is abbreviated as FFTP).

Table 5A:

EXAMPLE DEMONSTRATING
THE "MIXING OF DATA" EFFECT

	"CASES"	"CONTROLS"
Total Number in Group→	100	100
Women age 20-40 who had an abortion prior to their FFTP	50	40
Women age 20-40 who had no abortions	50	60

Here one can see that the estimated relative risk (RR) is 50/50 divided by 40/60 = 1.50. That is, this study shows that young women 20 to 40 years old who had an abortion prior to their FFTP, suffered a 1.50 or 50% increased risk of breast cancer. Now what would happen if we expanded the study and added 100 "cases" and 100 "controls" who were ages 40 to 45 years old to each group? These women would have been very unlikely to have had an abortion prior to their FFTP because they would have been 23 to 28 years old in 1973 — the year that the U.S. Supreme Court decriminalized abortion. If none of these women had an abortion prior to their FFTP, our second study would contain data as noted in Table 5B.

Table 5B:
EXAMPLE DEMONSTRATING
THE "MIXING OF DATA" EFFECT

	"CASES"	"CONTROLS"
Total Number in Group→	200	200
Women who had an abortion prior to their FFTP	50	40
Women who had no abortions	150	160

Note that the estimated relative risk is now: 50/150 divided by 40/160 = 1.33. *We can see that by adding older women to the database, who had little chance of having an abortion at a young age, the estimated relative risk has been artificially decreased.* This is an important point because many studies mix older women with younger women and then erroneously claim that abortion at a young age or OCP use has no effect.

The "real risk factor":

Certain studies have concluded that there is "no link" between early induced abortion and/or early OCP use and breast cancer in spite of failing to ask the proper question. For example, Dr. Brind et al in their meticulous meta-analysis published in October 1996 [1], noted 33 studies that reported on the risk of abortion and breast cancer but failed to distinguish between induced and spontaneous abortion (miscarriage). Often the authors of these studies would conclude that abortion either is or is not a risk factor for breast cancer without distinguishing between the two different types of abortion. This is critical as will be noted in detail in Chapter 6, because both estradiol, progesterone and hCG levels are far lower in pregnancies which eventually miscarry than in healthy pregnancies which are unnaturally aborted (ie, induced abortion). Because of this phenomenon, induced abortion carries a higher risk than does miscarriage, and failure to distinguish between them can easily result in failure to pick up the real risk of induced abortion.

Other studies claim to measure the risk of induced abortion and breast cancer but have failed to ask the women in the study whether their particular induced abortion was before or after their first full-term pregnancy (FFTP). This is important also, because Dr. Brind et al found that having an induced abortion before a FFTP was associated with a 50% increased risk, whereas having an induced abortion after a FFTP resulted in a 30% increased risk. Any study that claims either to show or deny a link between abortion and breast cancer must specifically examine the risk of abortion performed at a young age (ie, before a FFTP) and should also distinguish induced from spontaneous abortions.

A similar phenomenon exists in the literature regarding OCPs. In the largest meta-analysis ever performed concerning OCPs, the authors of the Oxford study concluded: "Women who are currently using combined contraceptives or have used them in the past 10 years are at a slightly increased risk of having breast cancer diagnosed. . . There is no evidence of an increase in the risk of having breast cancer diagnosed 10 or more years after cessation of use. . ." (*The Lancet* [48]). *The study, however, failed to study the real risk factor, namely, OCP use prior to a first full-term pregnancy (FFTP) in premenopausal women.* This is extremely important, because women today are using oral contraceptives more often and for longer periods of time prior to their FFTP, than they did in the 1960s and 1970s. Thus, millions of women may be at risk [21, Table 14]. Unfortunately, when a study of this magnitude reaches the medical community and the public it often gets translated into the message that "oral contraceptives pose no long-term risk." If the authors of the Oxford study had pursued the real question, namely, "Does OCP use prior to a FFTP cause breast cancer in premenopausal women?" They may have found their results to correspond closely with those of another author's meta-analysis in which she accounted for OCP use before a woman's FFTP and found that women who had taken OCPs for 4 or more years prior to their FFTP had a 72% increased risk in breast cancer [49]. Clearly, one must ask about and measure the real risk factor (ie, OCP use prior to a FFTP) if one is to honestly study this issue.

The death factor:

In most retrospective studies the researcher(s) will choose a number of women who have breast cancer, from a certain database, and then go on to interview them at a later date. If there is a period of even a few months (eg, 6 months) between the choosing of subjects and the subsequent interview, some of them, especially those with more aggressive breast cancer, may already have died, and thus cannot be interviewed. This is referred to as "the death factor." A good example of this is found in the example of a study performed in Oxford called the United Kingdom National Case-Control Study by Chilvers et al. All women in the study who had breast cancer were diagnosed with it between the dates of January 1, 1982 and December 31, 1985, but they were interviewed between the dates of January, 1984 and February, 1988. *During this time 16% of the "cases" died* [30, p.974]. This factor becomes critical when one notes that several papers have noted that women who have had an abortion at a young age or had taken OCPs early in life, developed a more aggressive type of cancer ([25, p. 267; 50, 51]. *If this is true, then the women with breast cancer who died during the 6 months between identification and interview may well be disproportionately represented by those women who had an abortion at a young age and/ or used OCPs early in life.* In other words, studies in which a significant number of women have died before they were interviewed may well be giving results which we refer to as "false negatives." These studies may well claim that there is no relationship between abortion at a young age/OCP use, and an increased risk in breast cancer, when in reality the study could fail to pick up the risk factor(s) because the women who died were more likely to be those who had an abortion at a young age and/or had early OCP use.

Let us look at an example. Suppose a researcher interviewed two groups of women, 1,010 women with breast cancer and 1,000 without. Here 65 of the "cases" had an abortion at a young age versus 40 of the "controls." The estimated relative risk (RR) can be calculated below as:

Table 5C:
SAMPLE STUDY OF THE DEATH FACTOR

	1010 women with breast cancer	1000 without breast cancer
had an abortion pFFTP	65 (A)	40 (C)
no abortion pFFTP	945 (B)	960 (D)

The estimated relative risk (RR), as noted earlier, would be A/C divided by B/D = (65) (960)/(945) (40)= 1.65 RR.

Now let us see what would happen if only 1% (10 "cases") had died before the scheduled interview and if 5 out of those 10 women had had an abortion at a young age. The table would now look as follows:

Table 5D:
SAMPLE STUDY OF THE DEATH FACTOR

	1010 women with breast cancer	1000 without breast cancer
had an abortion pFFTP	60 (A)	40 (C)
no abortion pFFTP	940 (B)	960 (D)

The estimated relative risk (RR) now becomes: (60) (960)/(940) (40)= 1.53, which is about a 7% decrease from 1.65. In statistical terms, this difference could be the difference between a statistically significant or insignificant result. Janet Daling, a prominent researcher from the Fred Hutchinson Cancer Research Center in Seattle, Washington, is one of the few researchers to acknowledge this effect*: ". . .it could be argued that those women with breast cancer whom we were unable to interview because of serious illness or death may have been more likely to

*This author knows of no researcher who has pointed out this effect, except Daling.

have had an induced abortion than the women we did interview. If this bias were present, we would have underestimated the risk of breast cancer that is associated with induced abortion." [29, p.1589].

Unfortunately, even some of the larger studies which have studied early OCP use have had huge "death factors" in which the "cases" have had a far higher incidence of death or serious illness than the "controls" and thus could not be interviewed. Some examples include: the CASH study [52], 9% of "cases too ill" before interview (BI); the New Zealand study [15], 1.9% of "cases" died versus 0.5% of "controls"; the United Kingdom study [30] by Chilvers, 16%"cases" died BI; and White's study [38] in the *Journal of the National Cancer Institute,* 6.5% "cases" died BI. All of these studies have had large percentages of "cases" who either died or were too ill and so could not be interviewed.

A similar phenomenon has occurred in the studies concerning abortion at a young age. In her well-known study, Janet Daling [29] noted that 5.7% of the "cases" died before interview (BI); Newcomb [53] noted that 5.4% died BI; and Pike [54] noted that about 15% had died BI. This effect, which has rarely even been acknowledged, may well be responsible for underestimating the real risk of both having an abortion at a young age and OCP use. Hopefully in the future, researchers will compensate for this effect by interviewing women soon after they are chosen to be in a study or by obtaining the medical histories from the women who have died before interview by looking at their medical records.

References:

1. Brind J, Chinchilli M, et al. Induced abortion as an independent risk factor for breast cancer: a comprehensive review and meta-analysis. *J Epidemiol Community Health.* 10/ 1996; 50: 481-496.

2. Brind J. ABC down under. *Abortion Breast Cancer Quarterly Update.* Summer, 1997.

3. Rohan, et al. *Am J Epidemiol.*1988; 128: 478-489.

4. Leishman K. On the abortion front line. *Health and Medicine for Physicians.* March 1997: 22-26.

5. Huse D. Childhood Vaccination Against Chickenpox: An Analysis of Benefits and Costs, *Pediatrics.* June, 1994; 124: 869-873.

6. Rosenberg L, Palmer JR, et al. Case-control study of oral contraceptive use and risk of breast cancer. *Am J Epidemiol.* 1996; 143: 25-37.

7. Rosenberg L, Palmer JR, et al. A case-control study of the risk of breast cancer in relation to oral contraceptive use. *Am J Epidemiol.* 1992; 136: 1437-1444.

8. Rosenberg L, Palmer JR, et al. Breast cancer in relation to the occurrence and time of induced and spontaneous abortion. *Am J Epidemiol.* 1988; 127: 981-989.

9. Miller D, Rosenberg L, et al. Breast cancer before age 45 and oral contraceptive use: new findings. *Am J Epidemiol.* 1989; 129: 269-279.

10. Jick SS, Walker AM, et al. Oral contraceptives and breast cancer. *Br J Cancer.* 1989; 59: 618-621.

11. La Vecchia C, Decarli A, et al. Oral contraceptives and cancers of the breast and of the female genital tract. Interim results from a case-control study. *Br J Cancer.* 1986; 54: 311-317.

12. Kay CR, Hannaford PC. Breast cancer and the pill-A further report from the Royal College of General Practitioners' oral contraception study. *Br J Cancer.* 1988; 58: 675-680.

13. Somerville S. Before you choose: The link between abortion and breast cancer. Purcellville, VA. *Ann Intern Med.* 1993.

14. Laarsson KS, et al. Predictability of the Safety of Hormonal Contraceptives from Canine Toxicology Studies. In: Michal, F. ed. *Safety Requirements for Contraceptive Steroids.* Cambridge: Cambridge University Press; 1989: 203-269.

15. Paul C, Skegg DC, et al. Oral contraceptives and risk of breast cancer. *Int J Cancer.* 1990; 46: 366-373.

16. Thomas DB, Noonan EA. Breast cancer and combined oral contraceptives: results from a multinational study [The WHO collaborative study of Neoplasia and steroid contraceptives]. *Br J Cancer.* 1990; 61: 110-119.

17. Lee NC, Rosero-Bixby L, et al. A case-control study of breast cancer and hormonal Contraception in Costa Rica. *J Natl Cancer Inst.* 1987; 6: 1247-1254.

18. Lindefors-Harris BM, Edlund G, et al. Risk of cancer of the breast after legal abortion during the first trimester: a Swedish register study. *Br Med J.* 1989; 299: 1430-1432.

19. Lindefors-Harris BM, Eklund G, et al. Response bias in a case-control study: analysis utilizing comparative data concerning legal abortions from two independent Swedish studies. *Am J Epidemiol.* 1991; 134: 1003-1008.

20. Ellery C, MacLennan R, et al. A case-control study of breast cancer in relation to the use of steroid contraceptive agents. *The Medical Journal of Australia.* 1986; 144: 173-176.

21. Collaborative Group on Hormonal Factors in Breast Cancer. Breast cancer and hormonal contraceptives: further results. *Contraception.* 1996; 34: S1-S106.

22. Anonymous. Another look at the pill and breast cancer. *The Lancet.* November 2, 1985: 985-987.

23. Colton T, Greenberg ER, et al. Breast cancer in mothers prescribed diethylstilbestrol in pregnancy. *JAMA.* 1993; 269: 2096-3000.

24. McPherson K, Vessey MP, et al. Early oral contraceptive use and breast cancer: Results of another case-control study. *Br J Cancer.* 1987; 56: 653-660.

25. Olsson H, Borg A, et al. Early oral contraceptive use and premenopausal breast cancer-A review of studies performed in southern Sweden. *Cancer Detection and Prevention.* 1991; 15: 265-271.

26. Hulka BS. Oral contraceptives, the good news. *JAMA.* 1983; 249: 1624-1625.

27. Melbye M, Wohlfahrt J, et al. Induced abortion and the risk of breast cancer. *N Engl J Med.* 1997; 336: 81-85.

28. Malone K, Daling J, et al. Oral contraceptives in relation to breast cancer. *Epidemiologic Reviews.* 1993; 15: 80-94.

29. Daling J, Malone K, et al. Risk of breast cancer among young women: relationship to induced abortion. *J Natl Cancer Inst.* 1994; 86: 1584-1592.

30. Chilvers C, McPherson K, et al. Oral contraceptive use and breast cancer risk in young women (UK National Case-Control Study Group). *The Lancet.* May 6, 1989: 973-982.

31. Rookus MA, Leeuwen FE. Oral contraceptives and risk of breast cancer in women ages 20-54 years. *The Lancet.* 1994; 344: 844-851.

32. Newcomb PA, Longnecker MP, et al. Recent oral contraceptive use and risk of breast cancer (United States). *Cancer Causes and Control.* 1996; 7: 525-532.

33. Pike MC, Bernstein L. Oral contraceptives and breast cancer. *The Lancet.* July 15, 1989: 158.

34. Pike MC, Bernstein L. Oral contraceptives and breast cancer. *The Lancet.* March 18, 1989: 615-616.

35. Olsson H, Ranstam J, et al. (Letter on CASH) *The Lancet.* November 23, 1985; 1181.

36. Stadel BV, Lai S, et al. Oral contraceptives and premenopausal breast cancer in nulliparous women. *Contraception.* 1988; 38: 287-299.

37. Thomas DB. Oral contraceptives and breast cancer. *J Natl Cancer Inst.* 1993; 85: 359-364.

38. White E, Malone K, Weiss N, Daling J. Breast cancer among young U.S. women in relation to oral contraceptive use. *J Natl Cancer Inst.* 1994; 86: 505-514.

39. Harris JR, Lippman ME, et al. Breast cancer. *N Engl J Med.* 1992; 327: 319-328.

40. American Academy of Pediatrics. The adolescent's right to confidential care when considering abortion. *Pediatrics.* 1996; 97: 746-751.

41. Howe H, et al. Early abortion and breast cancer risk among women under age 40. *Int J Epidemiol.* 1989; 18: 300-304.

42. Gabutti G, et al. AIDS related neoplasms in Genoa, Italy. *Eur J Epidemiol*. 1995; 11: 609-614.

43. McPherson K. The pill and breast cancer: why the uncertainty? *Br Med J*. Sept. 20, 1986; 293: 709-710.

44. Tietze C. *Induced Abortion: A World Review*. 1983. 5th ed. Population Council.

45. Henshaw SK. Induced abortion: a worldwide perspective. *Family Planning Perspectives*. 1986; 18: 250-254.

46. Anonymous. Oral contraceptives in the 1980s. *Population Reports*. May-June 1982; X: A189-A222.

47. Olsson H, Moller TR, Ranstam J. Early contraceptive use and breast cancer among premenopausal women: Final report from a study in southern Sweden. *J Natl Cancer Inst*. 1989; 81: 1000-1004.

48. Collaborative Group on Hormonal Factors in Breast Cancer. Breast cancer and hormonal contraceptives: collaborative reanalysis of individual data on 53,297 women with breast cancer and 100,239 women without breast cancer from 54 epidemiological studies. *The Lancet*. 1996; 347: 1713-1727.

49. Romieu I, Berlin J, et al. Oral contraceptives and breast cancer. Review and meta-Analysis. *Cancer*. 1990; 66: 2253-2263.

50. Olsson H, et al. Her-2/neu and INT2 prot-oncogene amplification in malignant breast tumors in relation to reproductive factors and exposure to exogenous hormones. *J Natl Cancer Inst*. 1991; 83: 1483-1487.

51. Olsson H, Ranstam J, et al. Proliferation and DNA ploidy in malignant breast tumors in relation to early contraceptive use and early abortions. *Cancer*. 1991; 67: 1285-1290.

52. Ory HW, et al. Long-term oral contraceptive use and the risk of breast cancer (CASH Study). *JAMA*. 1983; 249: 1591-1595.

53. Newcomb PA, Storer BE, et al. Pregnancy termination in relation to risk of breast cancer. *JAMA*. 1996; 275: 283-322.

54. Pike MC, Henderson BE, et al. Oral contraceptive use and early abortion as risk factors for breast cancer in young women. *Br J Cancer*. 1981; 43: 72-76.

Chapter 6:
Breast Cancer and Abortion

The most difficult parts of the material have now been covered. The remainder of the book addresses specific questions in greater detail.

Does an induced abortion prior to a woman's <u>first full-term pregnancy</u> (FFTP) increase her risk of developing breast cancer? This central question will be addressed here, but first it would be helpful to review the history of this issue.

One of the main questions that people have when they hear or read that having an abortion at a young age increases a woman's risk of breast cancer is: Why? That is, what link could there be between abortion and cancer of the breast?

Two renowned researchers, Jose and Irma Russo, were among the first prominent scientists to offer a possible explanation of this phenomenon in their work with rats in the 1980s and 1990s. The Russos took a number of rats and divided them into different groups. One of the groups were rats that had one pregnancy in the past, the second group were virgin rats, and the third group were pregnant rats who underwent an abortion at a young age. Each of these three groups was then subjected to a cancer producing agent called DMBA (7,12 dimethylbenz(a)anthracene). *They found that none of the 9 rats that had a full-term pregnancy developed breast cancer, 15 out of 22 of the virgin rats (ie, 68%) developed breast cancer, and 7 out of 9*

(77.7%) of the rats that had an abortion developed breast cancer. It was further noted that when one looked microscopically at the breast tissue of each of the aforementioned groups, the full-term pregnancy group had many more mature (*differentiated*) breast cells than did the rats that had an abortion. "Therefore, while pregnancy and lactation protected the mammary gland from developing carcinomas and benign lesions by induction of full differentiation, pregnancy interruption did not elicit sufficient differentiation in the gland to be protective. . ." [1, p.497]. The correlation between the rat model and the human breast could not be ignored. The Russos continued: "In women, protection against breast cancer is provided when pregnancy occurs before age 24. In contrast, abortion is associated with increased risk of breast cancer. The explanation for these epidemiologic findings is not known, but the parallelism between the DMBA-induced rat mammary carcinoma model and the human situation is striking." [2, p.27] These words, written in 1980, led a number of researchers to study the link between induced abortion and breast cancer in women.

The next question was: What is it about an abortion at a young age that leaves the human breast especially vulnerable to carcinogens (ie, an agent that causes cancer)? That is, why would a woman's breast cells be left in a more vulnerable state if she were to have an induced abortion early in her life, instead of completing her pregnancy?

Figure 6A offers a visual explanation. Here we see that the levels of both of the sexual hormones, estradiol and progesterone, as well as hCG (human Chorionic Gonadotropin), all rise rapidly in early pregnancy. These hormones trigger the breast cells to begin dividing and maturing. The combination of these hormones, as well as others, causes the cells of the breast to divide rapidly and start a maturing process that will continue over the next 9 months, after which the breast cells will be matured or differentiated. What happens to the woman who has an abortion early in her life? Russo and Russo again provide an insight into this puzzle in their work on the rat. They found that the group of virgin rats who received the carcinogen DMBA and the pheromone hCG, developed breast cancer far less often than those that received the DMBA alone [3]. The implication is that in the human, a woman needs to complete her pregnancy in order for the breast cells to receive the full protective effect of the pheromone hCG.

Figure 6A: HORMONE LEVELS DURING PREGNANCY AND AFTER AN INDUCED ABORTION

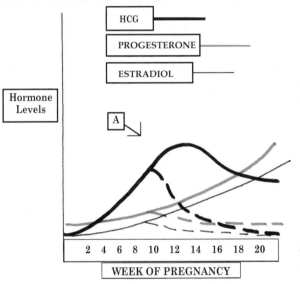

In Figure 6A we see that if a woman has an induced abortion — at about the 10th week of pregnancy (point A) — her estrogen, progesterone and HCG levels plummet to baseline levels (ie, the levels of a woman in the non-pregnant state). These hormones, among others, are critical for the full development and maturation of a woman's breast cells, especially in her first pregnancy. Once the levels drop, the process of breast cell differentiation is in a sense "frozen." This state, in which a breast cell has started to divide but has never completed the differentiation process, leaves the cell far more susceptible to becoming cancerous than breast cells which have completed their differentiation. Now one can see why a woman's first pregnancy is so important. If the pregnancy goes to term, her breast cells will have undergone the natural maturation process and be less likely to become cancerous. If the natural process in a woman's first pregnancy is interrupted via an induced abortion, those same cells are left in a vulnerable state.

What about miscarriages, also called spontaneous abortions. Do they increase the risk of breast cancer if a woman experiences one in her first pregnancy? Most authors have found that miscarriages increase the risk of breast cancer less than an induced abortion does (see Chapter 7 for details). Why is this so?

Table 6A:
Comparison of Hormone Levels in Women with
Healthy Pregnancy Vs. Miscarriage

Hormone Level➜	Progesterone(ng/ml)	Estradiol (pg/ml)	hCG (mIU/ml)
Healthy Pregnancy	25.3	766	65,717
Miscarriage	5.2	117	10,643

If we look at Table 6A [data from Witt et al, 4], we note that women who experience a healthy pregnancy (eg, women considering induced abortion) have far higher hormone levels than women who are about to miscarry. Because hormone levels drop rapidly after an abortion or miscarriage, women who choose abortion will experience a greater change in hormone levels than women who miscarry. Their breast cells essentially experience a greater "hormonal blow" (ie, a rapid drop in hormone levels) which leaves their breast cells more vulnerable to carcinogens. Thus, we would expect that women who miscarry would have less risk than women who have induced abortions, although as Chapter 7 will show, women who miscarry *before* their first full-term pregnancy (FFTP) still appear to be at increased risk.

Q-6A: What has the history of various research studies shown?

As early as 1957, the first research study to formally show a link between abortion and breast cancer was published by a Japanese researcher named Segi. During the years of 1953 to 1955 he and his group pooled most of the cancer patients from nearly all of Japan's major hospitals; 644 of the women had breast cancer. He noted that the women who had "an artificial interruption of pregnancy" experienced at least a 2-fold statistically significant increased risk in breast cancer rates compared to "controls" (ie, those who did not have an abortion [5, p.43]). Segi et al also noted a number of other important findings: 1) women who had an early pregnancy, 2) those who had a later age of the menarche (ie, the onset of a woman's menstrual cycles), and 3) those who had more children, all had lower rates of breast cancer than the norm. Unfortunately, this remarkable study went largely unheeded.

The next major breakthrough came with a stunning study [6] published in 1981 by M.C. Pike and B.E. Henderson et al from the University of California, entitled: "Oral contraceptive use and early abortion as risk factors for breast cancer in young women." Pike studied 163 women, all of whom were under the age of 32 when they discovered that they had breast cancer. He made two important discoveries. First, women who had a first trimester abortion before their first full-term pregnancy (FFTP) had a 2.4-fold significantly increased risk of breast cancer compared to "controls." Second, the risk from early oral contraceptive use — specifically, the use of OCPs for at least 4 years before a FFTP — resulted in a 2.25-fold statistically significant risk (125% increased risk). This result sparked the medical world's continued study of both of these findings until the current time.

Since 1981 a number of studies from around the world, have continued to show that having an abortion at a young age is a significant risk factor for breast cancer [7, 8, 9, 10, 11, 12]. A major development occurred in late 1994, after Janet Daling et al [9] revealed the results of a study which commanded the attention of both the medical and the lay realms. In her study of 845 women who had breast cancer and were under the age of 45, she noted a number of significant findings: 1) In general, women who had an abortion experienced a 50% increased risk of breast cancer; 2) Women who had an abortion before the age of 18 had a 150% increased risk of developing breast cancer; 3) Women who were over the age of 30 at the time of their abortion had a 110% increased risk; and 4) Women who were less than the age of 18 at the time of their abortion and had a later abortion (ie, after 8 weeks of pregnancy) experienced an 800% increased risk of breast cancer! In addition, Daling noted that women who had an abortion at a young age (before the age of 18) and who also had a positive family history for breast cancer, were at infinitely increased risk compared to young women who had no abortion and a positive family history for breast cancer (confidence intervals 1.8 to infinity)! Daling was paraphrased by another writer in the *Journal of the National Cancer Institute* as saying: "Daling indicated that abortion should be included as a risk factor if the cohort — women who had abortions prior to the age of 18 — is specified" [13].

These stunning findings led to an abrupt criticism of Daling's study. In fact, the very same issue of the journal which published the study — The *Journal of the National Cancer Institute* — printed an editorial by Lynn Rosenberg which severely criticized the study. Rosenberg argued that Daling's study might be limited by recall bias, as was discussed in Chapter 5. This was a remarkable claim, because Daling et al had taken great pains to address this issue, even going so far as performing a side study comparing abortion and cervical cancer, which would have specifically identified reporting bias [9, p.1590]. Rosenberg also made the bizarre claim that "While the findings of Daling et al add to the limited evidence that induced abortion increases the risk of breast cancer, neither a coherent body of knowledge nor a convincing biologic mechanism has been established." She wrote this comment despite the work by Russo and Russo, done more than a decade earlier, which implied a clear biological mechanism.

Finally, in the Fall of 1996, a group of researchers led by Dr. Joel Brind published the most comprehensive and meticulous meta-analysis of all the abortion/breast cancer related studies performed until that time [14]. In their analysis, they reviewed 61 different studies ranging between the years 1957 to 1996. From those 61, they selected out the studies which did not adequately distinguish between induced and spontaneous abortion, leaving 28 studies, which were further reduced to 23 studies after combining the results of the studies that overlapped. He and his group also reviewed studies from around the world, including Japan, Russia, Yugoslavia, France, Denmark, Sweden, Norway, Greece, and many others including the U.S.

The paper by Brind and colleagues provided an extensive commentary on many of the previous studies and included a thorough historical review of the entire field. One conclusion stood out clearly:

Women who had an induced abortion had a 30% increased risk of developing breast cancer, whereas parous women who had an induced abortion prior to their FFTP had a 50% increased risk of developing breast cancer, compared to women who did not have an induced abortion. The meta-analysis led to a flurry of discussion but left few able to argue with its methods or results. Janet Daling, an epidemiologist at the Fred Hutchinson Cancer Research Center in Seattle, defended Dr. Brind's paper as "very objective and statistically beyond reproach. (The authors did) a fair job of compiling the data, having taken pains to include studies of every point of view." [15]

What did Dr. Brind's paper state regarding the major studies which examined the effect of an early induced abortion and the consequent risk of developing breast cancer? The studies are noted in Table 6B:

Table 6B:
FINDINGS OF STUDIES WHICH EXAMINED BREAST CANCER RISK FROM INDUCED ABORTION PRIOR TO A WOMAN'S FIRST FULL-TERM PREGNANCY (FFTP)

RESEARCHER	PERCENT CHANGE	YEAR	COUNTRY	RELATIVE RISK
Brinton [8]	34% increase*	1983	USA	1.34 (0.3-5.6)
Rosenberg [12]	10% decrease*	1988	USA	0.9 (0.5-1.4)
Harris [10]	18% decrease*	1989-90	Sweden/Norway	0.82 (0.44-1.51)
Daling [9]	40% increase*	1994	USA	1.4 (1.0-2.0)
Lipworth [11]	106% increase	1995	Netherlands	2.06 (1.45-2.90)
Rookus [16]	160% increase*	1996	USA	2.6 (1.0-6.8)
Totals→	50% increase			1.5 (1.2-1.8)

* This result reflects a trend toward an increased or decreased risk but does not attain statistical significance.

Table 6B, whose data comes from Table 2 in the Brind meta-analysis, clearly shows that when data from all the major studies from around the world were pooled and conservatively analyzed via a meta-analysis, it indicated that women had a 50% increased risk of developing breast cancer from an abortion performed before a woman's first full-term pregnancy. Why does this author refer to it as a "conservative" estimate? Because, a closer look at each of the individual studies would have yielded an even higher risk, had they adjusted for the many factors which could affect the results. A comprehensive review of those factors is presented at the end of this chapter but two of them stand out.

Lynn Rosenberg's 1988 study suffers profusely from the "age factor" problem. Ms. Rosenberg compares "cases" with a mean age of 52 years old to "controls" with a mean age of 40 years old. As noted in Chapter 5, this is a serious error and one that results in a lower reported risk from abortion at a young age than would have been, had she designed the study properly.

The second example comes from the Daling study in 1994. Although it was one of the best-designed studies, it still had a huge "stack effect." The researchers ended up "stacking" the younger spectrum of the data. They had 8% of the "cases" in the 21 to 30 year-old age group, whereas

17% of the "controls" were in this age group. If the study had distributed the "case" and "control" populations proportionally among the various age groups (ie, have the same percent of each population in each of the various age brackets), the "stack effect" would have been averted, most likely yielding a higher relative risk from abortion at a young age, because young women who are disproportionately represented in the "control group" will most likely report having had more abortions prior to their FFTP, given that the percentage of young women who have had abortions in their early reproductive years has increased dramatically since 1973.

In short, almost every study noted in Table 6B has a factor or factors (these factors are all reviewed in Chapter 5) which would have served to increase the relative risk markedly, had they been accounted for. These include: 1) the "death factor" [8, 9;], 2) the "stack effect" and/or "age mismatching" [9, 12], 3) too short of a latent period [8, 12], and/or 4) a financial bias from a sponsor of one of the studies [10, 12]. What does all this mean? The short answer, is that the 50% increased risk which Dr. Brind et al reported from induced abortion prior to a FFTP is a *very conservative estimate. Had the above-mentioned factors been properly adjusted for, the real risk from an abortion before a FFTP would almost certainly have been significantly higher.* It should again be emphasized that many of the studies that evaluated the risk of an abortion in young women took their data from the late 1970s or early 1980s. We noted earlier that the latent period for risk factors in breast cancer (eg, DES or radiation) could be 20 to 30 years or longer. This implies that the full impact of having an abortion at a young age upon a woman's risk of developing breast cancer may only be fully appreciated in studies from the late 1990s and the first decade of the next century.

Q-6B: What has transpired since Dr. Brind's meta-analysis was published?

A number of studies have been published since Dr. Brind's study so that by January, 1999 a U.S. Congressman familiar with Dr. Brind's work noted that: "Fully 25 out of 31 epidemiological studies worldwide and 11 out of 12 studies in the U.S. . . . show that women who elect to have even one induced abortion show an elevated risk of subsequent breast cancer." [17, 18]. What were some of the recent studies?

First, Dr. Janet Daling came out with a "repeat study" which was designed similar to the one she wrote in 1994. The 1996 study did not show abortion to be as great a risk factor as her previous study, but several weaknesses appear in this latter study, as noted in the Addendum 6A at the end of this chapter. In addition, Daling's second study would have done little to change the results of Brind's meta-analysis because it would have been just one more study that would have been averaged into many. The second study by Rookus et al came out in the *Journal of the National Cancer Institute* and reported on bias. The authors concluded that "Reporting bias is a real problem in case-control studies of induced abortion and breast cancer risk if these studies are based on information from study subjects only." [16, p.1759]. (Reporting bias is another name for recall bias, which was discussed in Chapter 5. Remember that researchers who cite recall bias as a factor are hypothesizing that women who have breast cancer will be more truthful about their abortion history if asked about it in an interview than women who did not have breast cancer). The Rookus study is discussed at length in Appendix 2. *The main problem with the "bias argument" is that it can easily be measured and accounted for in the same way that the studies involving oral* contraception *and breast cancer accounted for its effect* (or lack thereof). As noted previously in Chapter 5, researchers such as Rookus and others simply need to obtain permission from both the "case" and the "control" patients to review their current medical charts from their current or previous gynecologist or obstetrician. Well trained obstetricians and/or gynecologists ask their young patients (ie, usually if under the age of 45) if they have had any induced or spontaneous abortions (miscarriages) when conducting a complete history and physical examination. *It is critical to note that the gynecologist's records would thus give the information concerning a woman's abortion history before she would have developed breast cancer.* Thus, one has an excellent tool to measure what the "case" and "control" patients' responses were, both before and after developing breast cancer, and one can easily compare the amount or degree of "reporting bias" between the "case" and "control" groups. Any author who wishes to measure the degree of reporting bias in studies that have been done recently or will be done in the future, can perform this exercise by taking the time to obtain permission and access to a patient's medical records. *In short, there is no longer any reason to "speculate" about reporting bias. It can be measured.*

A third study received little attention. It originated from an Australian researcher named Rohan [19]. His study was published in the *American Journal of Epidemiology* in 1988 but no information was presented concerning induced abortion and its risk for breast cancer. But in 1995 Andrieu et al noted that data from the Australian study actually had shown a 160% increased risk for induced abortion. Dr. Brind noted: "The obvious question, of course, is why these findings concerning an eminently avoidable risk factor were suppressed for seven years." [20, p.7]

The fourth major event since Dr. Brind's publication concerns the study from Denmark by Dr. Mads Melbye et al. This prospective study — one of the largest studies ever done — looked at a "cohort" of 1.5 million women, 10,246 of whom had breast cancer. The study had a number of serious flaws, however, and was meticulously critiqued in the *New England Journal of Medicine* [21]. A complete analysis of this study is provided at the end of this chapter for the interested reader but the most egregious flaws must be pointed out here.

The study claimed that "induced abortions have no overall effect on the risk of breast cancer." [22, p.81]. This is not what the authors' data showed. The authors noted that 1338 "cases" (A) of breast cancer developed in the group of women who did have abortions (2,697,000 person-years) (B), and that 8,908 "cases" (C) of breast cancer developed in the group who did not have abortions (25,850,000 person-years) (D). This simple calculation (ie, A/B divided by C/D) yields a 1.44 relative risk or a 44% increased risk for those women who had an abortion. The question of how and/or why the *New England Journal of Medicine* could allow a study to purport that abortion caused no risk of breast cancer, when the study's own figures give evidence that such a risk does exist, is an interesting one.

Second, Melbye's study suffered from a marked "follow-up differential." (see Appendix 1 for details). They allowed less than a 10 year average follow-up time for the "cohort population" (ie, women who had abortions) whereas the "control group" had a follow-up period of over 20 years. In addition to the huge difference between the two groups, allowing less than 10 years follow up after an induced abortion does not yield an adequate latent period to observe the increased risk of breast cancer.

The third problem is that Melbye et al noted that the breast cancer risk for later term abortions was significant. But this received far less attention than Dr. Melbye's rash statement recorded in the *Wall Street Journal*: "I think this settles it. Definitely — there is no overall risk of breast cancer for the average woman who has had an abortion." [23]. Most of the public never heard that Melbye found that women who had an abortion after the 12th week of pregnancy sustained a 38% increased risk, and women who had late-term abortions past 18 weeks sustained an 89% statistically significant risk [1.89 (1.11-3.22)]. It should be noted that in the U.S. in the 1970s and early 1980s, more than 100,000 women annually had abortions after the 12th week of pregnancy [24, p.10].

In conclusion, the beginning of this chapter asked the central question: Does an induced abortion before a woman's first full-term pregnancy (FFTP) increase her risk of developing breast cancer? The most honest answer that this author can conclude based on the research known to date and presented in this book is the following:

All of the evidence to date points to at least a 50% increased risk of developing breast cancer in parous women who have had an induced abortion prior to their first full-term pregnancy.

It is now time to let the reader decide what to think.

Addendum 6A:

Daling et al came out with a "repeat study" in 1996 [25] which revealed less dramatic risks than her original study in 1994 [9]. What were this study's weaknesses and why did it show less risk?

[The answer to this question is slightly technical and can be skipped without a loss of continuity].

Daling et al [9] published a landmark study in the November 4, 1994 issue of the *Journal of the National Cancer Institute*; it received intense publicity and scrutiny. Surprisingly, two years later she published a similar study in conjunction with another researcher named Louise Brinton in the *American Journal of Epidemiology*, which produced less dramatic results. For example, the second study reported the risk of abortion prior to a FFTP to be only 10%. The first study found a 40% risk. The second study also found only a 20% increased risk for abortion in general. The first study found a 50% risk. Why were the results so different?

Both of Daling's studies looked only at white women, but in Daling's first study about 5% of the population was black, whereas the second study had a base population of about 15% of black women who were excluded. By excluding a significant percent of its study population, the second study left out a particularly high risk group — namely young black women; this weakens the strength and impact of the study.

Another possible weakness is that the second study had a far higher percent of "cases" and "controls" in the 40 to 44 year-old age group than the first study (55% vs.

23%). Because the second study had a higher percentage of women in an older age group, it could reduce the reliability of the study because these women would be less likely to have had an abortion prior to a FFTP. (This type of phenomenon — *mixing "relatively" older women into the database*, was discussed in Chapter 5 and may have the effect of artificially reducing the relative risk for having an abortion at a young age or OCP use).

A third phenomenon concerns the political climate in which the 1996 study was published. It is no secret that Daling received widespread criticism after her initial study was published. Her own study was severely critiqued in the same issue of the *Journal of the National Cancer Institute* in which it appeared [26]. The environment at the National Cancer Institute (NCI) and among the editors of its journal (ie, the *Journal of the National Cancer Institute*) grew so controversial that Douglas Weed, editor of the journal, found the need to defend himself in the lay press against accusations of bias [27] after he was criticized in the *Wall Street Journal* [28] for showing partiality. Could the intense political pressure have affected the tone of the second article? That is a question that Dr. Weed might wish to answer.

Despite the fact that her second study found less dramatic results than her first, there is little doubt that it would have had an insignificant effect on Dr. Brind's meta-analysis because it would have been one more study added to the current "pool of several studies."

Addendum 6B:
Analysis of weaknesses of studies which looked at risk of abortion prior to first full-term pregnancy (FFTP):

It was stated that 4 out of the 6 studies which were used in Dr. Brind's meta-analysis were analyzed in a "conservative manner." In other words, if there was a possibility of looking at the data or results of a study in two different ways, Dr. Brind always chose to analyze the data in a way that would yield the lowest increased risk in breast cancer, that is, the most conservative estimate.

There are a number of factors in many of the studies that would probably have yielded significantly higher risks of breast cancer from having an abortion at a young age had they been accounted for. What are those factors, and in which of the quoted six studies can they be found?

A) Brinton's study [8] suffers from: 1) A short latent period. Subjects were interviewed from the years 1973 to 1977. This is inadequate, considering that the latent period for certain risk factors is more than 20 years; 2) The analysis was restricted to white women only, which would serve to underestimate any risk because black women are known to be at especially high risk (see Chapter 11). By cutting them out of the study, Brinton's study is more likely to yield risks that will be underestimated; and 3) The "death effect" (4.3% of "cases" vs. 2.4% of "controls" died). All three weaknesses serve to underestimate her study's risk of breast cancer due to having an abortion at a young age.

B) Daling et al's study [9] suffers from: 1) the stack effect because a total of 17% of "controls" versus 8% of "cases" were in the 21 to 30 year-old age bracket. It also suffers from the "death factor" — 5.7% of "cases" died before they could be interviewed. Although Daling acknowledged the possibility of the "death factor" playing a role, both weaknesses serve to underestimate the relative risks. This study did have the longest latent period with women being diagnosed from 1983-1990.

C) Rosenberg et al's study [12] suffers from multiple weaknesses: 1) a huge age mismatch: "cases" had a mean age of 52, whereas "controls" had a mean age of 40; 2) a short latent period. Interviews were held from 1978 to 1982 (ie, not even 10 years after the *Roe v. Wade* decision); and 3) the study was partially funded by Hoechst, a pharmaceutical company that is responsible for producing RU-486, the drug that causes a chemical abortion.

D) The Lindefors-Harris et al study [10] was funded by Family Health International. In addition, although she started out with 49,000 subjects, after 11 years she had fewer than 5,000. Only 10.2% of the original group of women stayed in the study and even these women would have had a latent period that may not have been long enough to detect the full impact of having an abortion at a young age (latent period of only 12-14 years). Last, as the investigators of the study admit, they made no adjustment for such basic variables as family history of breast cancer and OCP use [10, p.1432].

In conclusion, four out of six of the studies which Brind et al used in their meta-analysis would most likely have resulted in significantly higher risks of breast cancer had those studies accounted for the above-mentioned variables. In addition, the three studies that had the longest latent periods (ie, Daling [9], Lipworth [11] and Rookus [16]) all showed higher risk than the earlier studies [8, 12, 10] which had shorter latent periods. This would again imply that the risks of breast cancer due to an abortion at a young age are actually higher than the conservative 50% increased risk estimate.

Addendum 6C:
Critique of the Danish Study (researcher: Mads Melbye et al) [22]:

The Danish study was published in the January 9, 1997, edition of *The New England Journal of Medicine*. This prospective study relied on Denmark's National Cancer Registry as well as its National Board of Health to obtain information on the patient's cancer and abortion history, both of which are reported to government agencies in that country. The study's main assets include its size and its freedom from "reporting bias." The study claimed to show a number of findings: 1) the risk of having an abortion before a woman's first full-term pregnancy (FFTP) was negligible, namely an 8% trend: [RR= 1.08 (0.82-1.44)]; 2) the overall risk of an abortion after a woman's FFTP is 1.0; and 3) the risk of breast cancer was increased if one had a late-term abortion. For example, a woman who had an abortion after the 18th week of pregnancy sustained an 89% increased risk of breast cancer.

The study's size was impressive although the data which it presented — and also failed to present — actually supported the hypothesis that abortion causes breast cancer. Two central criticisms have already been mentioned but shall be repeated in addition to others.

- Failing to report the results accurately:

The study claims that "induced abortions have no overall effect on the risk of breast cancer." [22, p.81]. However, this is not what their data show. The authors reported that 1338 (A) cases of breast cancer developed in the group of women who did have abortions (2,697,000 person-years) (B), and that 8,908 (C) cases of breast cancer developed in the group who did not have abortions (25,850,000 person-years) (D). This simple calculation (ie, A/B divided by C/D) yields a 1.44 relative risk or a 44% increased risk for those women who had an abortion.

- *A shorter follow-up time* between the "cohorts" and the "controls":

Brind and Chinchilli noted that Danish women who had abortions were followed up for shorter periods of time than were the "controls." They stated: "Since the [Melbye] study encompasses such a wide range, women who had induced abortion are concentrated in the younger end of the total cohort, resulting in considerably less average follow-up time for them than for women without induced abortions (9.6 versus 20.7 years)" [23]. Melbye et al responded in the same journal to Brind's allegation. Melbye wrote: "They [Brind and Chinchilli] claim that a selection bias is introduced because the average follow-up time for women with induced abortion is shorter than that for women without induced abortions. Such an objection can stem only from lack of insight into the design and analysis of a cohort study. For each woman entering the cohort, we calculated the follow-up time (person-years) and allocated this follow-up time according to the abortion history. The calculation of breast-cancer rates (cases per person-years) thus takes into account differences in follow-up time for women with abortions and women without abortions."

Melbye's response appears to offer a sharp rebuttal to Brind and Chinchilli's remarks. But has Melbye failed to address a basic problem? It would appear that he has. He noted that his study had taken into account the difference in follow-up times by dividing the breast cancer "cases" by "person-years." However, Melbye et al failed to address the larger question; that is: *What about the effect of an inadequate latent period?* Specifically, it may take 15, 20 or even 25 years before the full effect of an abortion at a young age shows up, as concerns breast cancer. *By following the women who had induced abortions for an average of fewer than 10 years, Melbye et al hardly allowed an adequate latent period to pass.* This is crucial if one is to determine the effect of an abortion performed early in a woman's life.

   •   Failure to include basic variables:

Because the study was prospective in nature and obtained its information from government data banks, certain key variables were not adjusted for which include: 1) a family history of breast cancer; 2) a history of oral contraceptive use; 3) a history of alcohol use; 4) age of menarche; and 5) age of menopause. This weakness was even admitted by Patricia Hartge, the woman who wrote an editorial in the *New England Journal of Medicine* that was otherwise "more than complementary" to Melbye et al. An additional problem is that "more than 30,000 women in the study cohort who had abortions were misclassified as having had no abortions." [23, p.1834] Thus, Melbye et al classified 30,000 women who had abortions as women who did not have abortions!

   •   The funding question:

This observation is more of a curiosity than a direct criticism, however this author cannot fail to be puzzled as to *why a Danish medical study which was performed by Danish researchers was partially funded by the U.S. Department of Defense.* The reader will note that Dr. Melbye's research article ends with the disclaimer that: "The views expressed in this paper do not necessarily reflect the position or the policy of the U.S. government." Why a U.S. government agency is funding a Danish study and then feels compelled to publish a disclaimer at the end of the study strikes this author as exceptionally odd. Perhaps the U.S. Department of Defense could offer an explanation to the public as to why U.S. tax dollars that are earmarked for maintaining our defensive forces, have gone to a Scandinavian country to fund a study on breast cancer.

- Failure to stress the risk of abortions after the 12th week of pregnancy:

Melbye et al did note that the risk of breast cancer increased in women who had later term abortions, but this received little attention compared to Dr. Melbye's better known statement, recorded in the *Wall Street Journal*, in which he said, "I think this settles it. Definitely — there is no overall risk of breast cancer for the average woman who has had an abortion." [23]. Most of the public never heard that Melbye found that women who had an abortion after the 12th week of pregnancy sustained a 38% increased risk, and women who had late-term abortions past 18 weeks, sustained an 89% statistically significant risk [1.89 (1.11-3.22)]. Of note, more than 100,000 women in the U.S. had abortions after the 12th week of pregnancy annually in the 1970s and early 1980s [24, p.10].

References:

1. Russo J, Russo IH. Susceptibility of the mammary gland to carcinogenesis. *Am J Pathol.* 1980; 100: 497-512.

2. Russo J, Tay TK, et al. Differentiation of the mammary gland and susceptibility to carcinogenesis. *Breast Cancer Research and Treatment.* 1982; 2: 5-73.

3. Russo J, Russo IH. Toward a physiological approach to breast cancer prevention. *Cancer Epidemiology, Biomarkers and Prevention.* 1994; 3: 353-364.

4. Witt B, Wolf G, et al. Relaxin, CA-125, progesterone, estradiol, Schwangerschaft protein, and human Chorionic Gonadotropin as predictors of outcome in threatened and nonthreatened pregnancies. *Fertility and Sterility.* 1990; 53: 1029-1036.

5. Segi M, et al. An epidemiological study on cancer in Japan. *GANN.* 1957; 48: 1-63.

6. Pike MC, Henderson BE, et al. Oral contraceptive use and early abortion as risk factors for breast cancer in young women. *Br J Cancer.* 1981; 43: 72-76.

7. Rookus MA, Leeuwen FE. Oral contraceptives and risk of breast cancer in women ages 20-54 years. *The Lancet.* 1994; 344: 844-851.

8. Brinton LA, Hoover R, et al. Reproductive factors in the aetiology of breast cancer. *Br J Cancer,* 1983; 47: 757-762.

9. Daling J, Malone K, et al. Risk of breast cancer among young women: relationship to induced abortion. *J Natl Cancer Inst.* 1994; 86: 1584-1592.

10. Lindefors-Harris BM, Edlund G, et al. Risk of cancer of the breast after legal abortion during the first trimester: a Swedish register study. *Br Med J.* 1989; 299: 1430-1432.

11. Lipworth L, Katsouyanni K, et al. Abortion and the risk of breast cancer: a case-control study in Greece. *Int J Cancer.* 1995; 61: 181-184.

12. Rosenberg L, Palmer JR, et al. Breast cancer in relation to the occurrence and time of induced and spontaneous abortion. *Am J Epidemiol.* 1988; 127: 981-989.

13. Parkins T. Does abortion increase breast cancer risk? *J Natl Cancer Inst.* 1993; 85: 1987-1988.

14. Brind J, Chinchilli M, et al. Induced abortion as an independent risk factor for breast cancer: a comprehensive review and meta-analysis. *J Epidemiol Community Health.* 10/ 1996; 50: 481-496.

15. Lagnado L. Study on abortion and cancer spurs fight. *Wall Street Journal.* Oct. 11, 1996.

16. Rookus M, Leeuwen F. Induced abortion and risk for breast cancer: reporting (recall) bias in a Dutch case-control study. *J Natl Cancer Inst.* 1996; 88: 1759-1764.

17. Brind J. U.S. Congress to NCI Chief. *Abortion-Breast Cancer Quarterly Update.* Winter, 1998-1999.

18. Brind J. U.S. Reps call for ABC hearings. *Abortion-Breast Cancer Quarterly Update.* Spring, *1998.*

19. Rohan, et al. *Am J Epidemiol.*1988; 128: 478-89.

20. Brind J. ABC down under. *Abortion Breast Cancer Quarterly Update.* Summer, 1997.

21. Brind J, et al. Induced abortion and the risk of breast cancer. *N Engl J Med.* 1997; 336: 1834.

22. Melbye M, Wohlfahrt J, et al. Induced abortion and the risk of breast cancer. *N Engl J Med.* 1997; 336: 81-85.

23. Lagnado L. Abortion study fuels debate on cancer link. *The Wall Street Journal.* Jan. 9, 1997: B1, B5.

24. Henshaw SK, O'Reilly K. Characteristics of abortion patients in the United States, 1979 and 1980. *Family Planning Perspectives.* 1983; 15: 5-16.

25. Daling J, Brinton L, et al. Risk of breast cancer among white women following induced abortion. *Am J Epidemiol.* 1996; 144: 373-380.

26. Rosenberg L. Induced abortion and breast cancer: more scientific data are needed. *J Natl Cancer Inst.* 1994; 86: 1569-1570.

27. Weed D, Kramer BS. Breast cancer studies aren't "political." The *Wall Street Journal.* March 26, 1997.

28. McGinnis J. The politics of cancer research. *The Wall Street Journal.* Feb. 28, 1997.

Chapter 7:
Breast Cancer and Abortion: Other Questions

Q-7A: What is the link between abortion and breast cancer if the abortion takes place after a woman's *first full-term pregnancy* (FFTP)?

Janet Daling noted a trend of increased risk of 50% [RR=1.5 (1.0-2.2)] in her 1994 study. Melbye et al [1] found a 44% increased risk (ie, risk calculated from their raw data) for abortion in general, but did not specify how many of these abortions were after a woman's FFTP. Nevertheless, most of the abortions presented in his paper are abortions after a woman's FFTP. The most conservative and accurate figure comes from Dr. Brind et al's 1996 meta-analysis, which found that women who had an abortion after their FFTP experienced a 30% increased risk for developing breast cancer [RR=1.3 (1.1-1.5)].

Q-7B: What is the risk of abortion in women who remain nulliparous (ie, women who have not given birth to a child)?

Daling et al [2] found a 70% increased risk of developing breast cancer in nulliparous women who had an induced abortion. Brind et al [3] calculated a 30% overall increased risk in their meta-analysis. One must keep in mind that the 30% risk is the increased risk that nulliparous women who have had an induced abortion ("case group") have *in comparison to other nulliparous women*. Because nulliparity is itself a risk factor that confers an estimated 2-fold risk of developing breast cancer [4], had the "cases" been compared to the general population, the risks would likely have been significantly higher.

Q-7C: Does a late-term abortion result in an even greater risk in breast cancer?

Some studies, but not all, have shown a greater risk of developing breast cancer with late-term abortions. Part of the problem in finding the answer to this question is that one study may be comparing women who have had a late-term abortion before their first full-term pregnancy (FFTP) to other women who have had their abortion after their FFTP, which obviously could affect the result. Melbye et al [1] noted that having an abortion after the 18th week of gestation resulted in an 89% increased risk, but they did not distinguish abortion prior to a FFTP from abortion after a FFTP. Rookus and Leeuwen et al [5] actually obtained a lower risk for later-term abortion as compared to early abortion, but again failed to separate abortion prior to versus after a woman's FFTP (ie, he found a 110% increased risk in abortions of pregnancies of fewer than 8 weeks duration and a 60% increased risk in those abortions occurring after 8 weeks).

Fortunately some authors have examined the "before and after FFTP effect." Daling [2] noted that women who had aborted their first pregnancy between the 1st and 8th week of pregnancy sustained a 40% increased risk of breast cancer, whereas those who had aborted their first pregnancy between the 9th and 12th week had a 90% increased risk [2, p.1588]. This is especially important when one notes that in the late 1970s and 1980s more than 45% of abortions occurred after the 8th week of pregnancy [6]. *She also noted that women younger than the age of 18 had an 800% increased risk if they had their abortions between the 9th and 24th week.* Although the data are limited, it would appear that a trend exists for a higher risk of developing breast cancer with late-term abortion, provided it is before a woman's FFTP.

Q-7D: Do women who have an induced abortion at a later age have an increased risk of breast cancer?

It would appear so. Daling et al [2] noted that women who underwent their first induced abortion at or after the age of 30 had a 110% increased risk of developing breast cancer [RR=2.1 (1.2-3.5)]. Rookus et al [5, p.1762] also found this trend in women who had an induced abortion at an older age [RR= 2.0 (0.9-4.5)].

Q-7E: Can one estimate how many more women will get breast cancer because of induced abortion performed early in a woman's reproductive life?

Daling et al noted that of the "control" women who had abortions, only 28% had them after their first child was born [7, p.377]. Thus 72% of abortions were performed before a woman's first baby was born: 45% of them in women who went on to have a baby and 27% of them in women who were still nulliparous at the time of the study. One will note that about 1.6 million women had abortions each year in the 1980s but because about one third of these were repeat abortions, an estimated 1 million women were having their first abortion each year. If one uses Daling's statistics (ie, 45% of women had their abortion prior to their FFTP), and notes that an abortion performed before a woman's FFTP yields at least a 50% increased risk, it would mean that an extra 27,000 women will be getting breast cancer due to abortions prior to their FFTP, based on a national rate of breast cancer of 12% (ie, 1.0 million x 45% x 12% x 50%). This does not include the extra 9,720 nulliparous women (who had abortions prior to their FFTP) and 10,080 of parous women (who had abortions after their FFTP) who would be expected to get breast cancer from their abortions. *Including these women, one can project that in the U.S. alone, 46,800 additional women would be expected to develop breast cancer each year due to abortion.* Although this effect has already started, it will probably reach its peak after the year 2,000. (For the reader who wishes to see the specific details behind these calculations, see the end of this chapter).

Q-7F: *The AMA (American Medical Association) noted in its 1992 JAMA [8] that the risk of dying from maternal childbirth is nearly 12 times as great as the risk of dying from abortion. Is this a fair statement?*

No, this is an inaccurate statement because it focuses on the short-term mortality statistics surrounding pregnancy and ignores the long-term mortality statistics. When a woman has an abortion the risks of death are far more subtle than were she to deliver her baby. It was noted that because of induced abortion more than 46,000 women are expected to get breast cancer annually in the U.S. If one-quarter of these women die from this cancer, it would mean 10,000 deaths occurring annually due to induced abortion. This is literally dozens of times more deaths than the number of women dying from natural child birth each year. In addition, the woman who carries her pregnancy to term will decrease her risk of developing ovarian cancer.

Another often unaccounted factor regarding mortality from abortion is the subsequent deaths from suicides in women who have had an abortion. "A teenage girl is 10 times more likely to attempt suicide if she has had an abortion in the last six months than is a comparable girl who has not had an abortion." [9] In 1987, Reardon noted that 60% of the group of women who suffered from post-abortion trauma experienced suicidal ideation; 28% of this group had attempted suicide; and 18% had tried it more than once [10]. Finally, in their Finnish study Gissler et al [11] noted that women who had an induced abortion had more than 6 times the suicide rate than women who delivered their baby. If the AMA (American Medical Association) had accounted for these factors, they would have said that an abortion is far more dangerous than childbirth in the long run.

Q-7G: Does having an abortion at an early age lead to an increased risk of a more aggressive type of breast cancer?

It has already been noted that women who have an induced abortion at an early age, especially before a FFTP, have at least a 50% increased risk of developing breast cancer, with one major study showing a 150% increase in women who had their first induced abortion prior to the age of 18 [2]. But what about the level of aggressiveness of the breast cancer which these women get? That is, when a woman gets breast cancer it may spread rapidly (ie, metastasize quickly) or it may spread slowly, or perhaps be cured (ie, the less aggressive type of cancers).

Ownby et al, although they failed to distinguish between induced and spontaneous abortion (ie, miscarriage), noted that women who underwent one or more interrupted pregnancies had shorter time periods for recurrence of their disease. Women who had no abortions had a 10.5% recurrence rate; women who had one abortion had a 20.5% recurrence rate; and women who had 2 or more abortions had a 32.3% recurrence rate [12, p.341]. Meanwhile, Olsson et al noted that women who had an abortion at a young age developed cancers which grew faster (ie, had a higher mitotic rate) and had a higher percentage of aneuploid cells (ie, cells which have an abnormal number of chromosomes and thus are more likely to be tumor cells). He wrote: "These results indicate that the rate of tumor cell proliferation is higher in patients with breast cancer who have used oral contraceptives at an early age or who at a young age have had an early abortion. . ." [13, p.1288]. In general, the scientific evidence supports the finding that women who have had an abortion performed early in a woman's reproductive life develop a more aggressive type of breast cancer.

Q-7H: Do women who have multiple induced abortions have a higher risk of breast cancer?

In the U.S. in 1987, 42% of women having abortions had more than one induced abortion, with 15.5% having more than three and 5.5% having four or more abortions [14]. It was noted that Dr. Ownby found that women with breast cancer who had more than one abortion have a shorter time to recurrence of their disease after initial treatment (although she failed to separate induced from spontaneous abortion) [12]. Dr. Brind et al noted in 1996 that "seven out of the 10 studies reporting the multiple abortion OR (ie, "odds ratio" report slightly (though not significantly) higher ORs for two or more, as opposed to one abortion" [3, p.13]. He also noted that: "the extant data are therefore insufficient to draw any firm conclusions about any overall dose effect of induced abortion at the present time." [3]. Few of the studies, however, measured the effect of consecutive induced abortions, especially before a FFTP. Howe et al did find that "ten cases and no controls had a history of repeated interrupted pregnancies with no intervening live births," which would yield an infinitely increased risk, in this small sample. The data then point to a trend for even more risk with multiple abortions, albeit no one has been able to quantify exactly how much more risk. A meta-analysis is needed.

Q-7I: Do women who had an abortion performed early in their reproductive life sustain an increased risk of developing breast cancer before the age of 35?

It has been noted that women who are less than 45 years old generally have an increased risk in developing breast cancer from having an abortion performed early in their reproductive life. What about women who are even younger? Most major studies show that women who had an abortion at a young age have a higher risk of developing breast cancer before the age of 35. Pike et al [15] showed a 140% increased risk of developing breast cancer in women under the age of 32 if they had an abortion prior to their FFTP. Rosenberg et al [16] showed no overall risk in women under the age of 40, but the age mismatching in that study was so markedly different (ie, a 12-year difference between the median age of the "cases" and "controls") that any result is suspect. Howe et al [4] noted a 90% increased risk in women under the age of 40 for women who had any abortion, and Daling et al [2] noted an 80% increased risk in women under the age of 35 if they had an abortion. There appears to be little doubt that abortion — especially abortion prior to a FFTP — increases the risk of developing breast cancer in women at the age of 35 or younger.

Q-7J: Do chemical abortions result in an increased risk of breast cancer?

A number of chemical abortion methods have been developed including RU-486 (mifepristone) and the Methotrexate/Cytotec methods. (Cytotec [misoprostol] is a drug that is routinely used to prevent ulcers, but is being used by certain people to induce chemical abortions). When RU-486 (which acts as an anti-progesterone) is given to a pregnant woman, it breaks the placental bond between a mother and her unborn child. A prostaglandin (ie, another drug category) is then given which initiates contractions of the mother's uterus, thereby expelling the baby. In the latter type of chemical abortion, methotrexate (a chemotherapy agent) is injected into a woman's muscle. Methotrexate also ruptures the placental bond and after a few days the woman is given Cytotec, another prostaglandin, which serves to start uterine contractions.

Because both combinations cause early abortions, there is every reason to anticipate that they will also cause an increased risk in breast cancer. As Dr. Brind stated: "Thus, there is no reason to suspect that new technologies, (such as mifepristone/misoprostol) that would result in generally earlier terminations, would not also be associated with increased breast cancer risk" [3, p.493]. In addition, no one knows what kind of "hormonal blow" either RU-486 or methotrexate themselves might have on the breast of a pregnant woman (ie, the reader will note the consequences of a drug named DES, discussed in Chapter 10). If RU-486 or methotrexate have an additional deleterious effect such as DES did, women who participate in chemical abortions may be at even higher risk of developing breast cancer than women who had surgical abortions.

Q-7K: Will the new "birth control vaccine," which works by causing an early abortion, elevate the risk of breast cancer?

A birth control "vaccine" has been developed with the help of the World Health Organization and has already been used by Talwar et al upon women in India [17]. It is called the hCG vaccine. When a woman becomes pregnant, the young human embryo forms the early placental bond — consisting of "syncytiotrophoblast cells." These cells secrete the pheromone hCG (Human Chorionic Gonadotropin) which serves to keep the corpus luteum intact (ie, a structure which remains in a woman's ovary after ovulation has occurred). Without hCG, the unborn child cannot survive, because the corpus luteum secretes progesterone which functions to keep the placental bond intact. The "vaccine"* attacks the hCG pheromone, which serves to cause an early abortion. *It is possible that these early abortions could increase the risk of breast cancer, especially when one considers that a woman who is "immunized" with the "vaccine" would experience multiple early abortions each year.* In addition, Russo and Russo have implicated hCG as one of the key pheromones in breast development. *Thus, creating an "antibody" or "vaccine" to hCG would in effect be attacking the key hormone that aids in the protection of the breast from carcinogenesis* [18]. "The vaccines are primarily targeted for women in Latin America, the Caribbean, Africa and the Pacific. Major funders of the research, including the World Bank and the World Health Organization, want to increase the effectiveness of population programs through the use of the vaccine" [19]

*The "vaccine" contains an "antibody-like" protein attached to a "carrier" such as the tetanus toxoid which was used in the experiments in India [17].

Q-7L: Could use of the intrauterine device (IUD) increase the risk of breast cancer?

The IUD does not stop ovulation [20]. It theoretically causes many abortions of unknown gestational (pre-birth) age. IUD use may thus increase a woman's risk of developing breast cancer because early abortions have the potential to elevate a woman's risk of breast cancer. This author is unaware of any long-term studies on the IUD's carcinogenic potential regarding breast cancer.

Q-7M: What other risks interact with an abortion performed early in a woman's reproductive life to increase the risk of breast cancer and how is the combined risk calculated?

In order to calculate the risk of two or more risk factors for a particular cancer one must *multiply their independent risks*. This is termed the "multiplier effect."

Let us take the example of a 21-year-old woman who had an abortion at age 17 and has been taking OCPs for at least 4 years and to date, has no live children. Daling noted that women who have an induced abortion prior to the age of 18 have a 150% increased risk of developing breast cancer, whereas Romieu et al noted that women who use OCPs for 4 or more years prior to a FFTP have a 72% increased risk [RR=1.72 (1.36-2.19)]. According to the multiplier effect, this young woman would now have a relative risk of: 2.5 x 1.72 = 4.3, which is a 330% increased risk! It is common knowledge that young women routinely use OCPs after their abortion. The trend towards an increased use was noted by Campbell et al who wrote: "Our findings on adolescents support those of several authors who stated that adolescent women were more likely to use contraceptives after abortion." [21, p.819] The implications of this are very serious.

Another example of the multiplier effect in regard to a positive family history of breast cancer is noted by a number of authors. Andrieu et al [22] found that women who have a family history of breast cancer and who had two or more induced abortions have a 7-fold risk of breast cancer as compared to the rest of the population. *Daling et al. [2] noted that women who had an abortion prior to the age of 18 and had a positive family history of breast cancer, had an infinitely increased risk* (confidence interval: 1.8 to infinity) *of obtaining breast cancer compared to women who had a family history and had not had an abortion performed early in their reproductive life.* She also noted that women who were 30 years old or older at the time of their abortion and had a positive family history had a 270% increased risk compared to women who had a positive family history and no abortion.

Q-7N: Could oral contraceptives and other hormonal contraceptives such as Depo-Provera and Norplant be causing breast cancer due to their abortifacient properties?

It was already noted in the answer to question 3D that oral contraceptives cause early abortions (as do Depo-Provera and Norplant). Because these early abortions result in rapidly declining hormone levels which may affect a woman's breast cells, it is possible that these contraceptives may be causing breast cancer because they cause early abortions.

Q-7O: Do women who have abortions drink more heavily, and does this lead to an increased risk of breast cancer?

A number of studies have noted that women who drink heavily are at increased risk for breast cancer. The reason for this is not known for sure, although it has been noted by some researchers that women who drink heavily experience an increased estrogen level in their blood and that this may increase a woman's risk of developing breast cancer [23, 24]. Longnecker et al in their large study in 1995, found that women who had about one drink a day experienced a 39% increased risk, whereas women who had two drinks a day had a 69% increased risk of developing breast cancer.

This phenomenon is especially important because women who have had abortions tend to have a higher rate of alcohol consumption after their abortion. Speckhard [25] found that 60% of women admitted to increased alcohol use following their abortion. In their survey published in 1986, Klassen and Wilsnack noted that: "Moderate and heavier drinkers combined, exceeded lighter drinkers on rates of. . . abortion (p< 0.001)." [26, p.376]. Finally, the Elliot Institute noted that: "women who abort are nearly four times more likely to start abusing drugs or alcohol" [27, p.1]. Because women who had an abortion tend to have a higher rate of alcohol use, they would theoretically also experience the "multiplier effect" and may well have a substantially higher risk of breast cancer.

Q-7P: Because many women who have an abortion performed early in their reproductive life also take oral contraceptives, how can one tell which factor is increasing the risk of breast cancer?

Because both an abortion performed early in the woman's reproductive life and OCP use are considered risk factors, a number of researchers have tested for them independently of each other. That is, when they perform their retrospective studies, they "separate out" the effects of an abortion performed early in a woman's reproductive life and/or OCP use in their statistical analysis, so that they can calculate the risk for either risk factor independently.

Q-7Q: Can you give an example of some studies that have done this?

Brinton et al [28], Daling et al [2], and Rosenberg [16], in their studies regarding abortion as a risk factor, all adjusted for OCP use. In a similar way, Brinton et al's study [29, p.834], the CASH study [30, p.1507], and White's study [31, p.1507] all examined the risk of early OCP use and all adjusted for abortion.*

Q-7R: Is there any other way in which one can separate the effects of an abortion performed early in a woman's reproductive life and early OCP use?

Yes. Remennick [32] made two important observations about the Russian people. First, she noted a statistically significant correlation between the percent of abortions in primagravidas (ie, abortions in women who are pregnant with their first child) and the crude breast cancer rate ($r=0.62$, $p<0.05$). (The higher the r value, the higher the correlation, with 1.00 representing a perfect correlation). Second, she stated: "Another relevant peculiarity is the almost complete absence of oral contraceptives among Soviet women, making all the other relationships unconfounded by this potential risk factor." That is, because so few women had used OCPs, one can feel more confident that an abortion performed early in a woman's reproductive life really is a risk factor for breast cancer in Russian women.

Q-7S: If a woman who is pregnant develops breast cancer, will an induced abortion improve or worsen her prognosis?

.Clarck and Chua, in their large classic study noted that: "Those undergoing a therapeutic abortion had a poorer prognosis compared to a live birth. . ." [33, p.13]. In their series, none of the women who had breast cancer while pregnant and chose to have an abortion were alive after 11 years, whereas about 25% of the women who had breast cancer and chose to deliver their baby were alive after 12 years and 20% survived more than 20 years [33, p.14]. One might ask, "Did the women who had induced abortions have more advanced disease than those who had

---

* Because it is abortion performed *early in a woman's reproductive life* and *early* OCP use that appear to be the greatest risk factors, it would appear that adjusting for them might be better than adjusting for abortion or OCP use in general. Future studies which adjust for *early* OCP use and/ or *early* abortion (ie, before a FFTP) might define more clearly if one of these two risk factors is more dominant because there may be some "degree of overlap" (ie, confounding variables) between them.

live births, thus skewing the study results?" Dr. Clarck assured us that this is not the case: "The principal issue was whether therapeutic abortion was only carried out in those patients with more advanced disease. This was not the case." [34] King et al obtained a similar result. ". . .patients who had termination of the pregnancy had a five year survival rate of 43 percent, whereas patients who underwent mastectomy and who went to term had a five year survival of 59 percent." [35, p.231]. Last, Isaacs commented that: "Contrary to common belief, pregnancy does not stimulate the growth of breast cancer. Thus, no justification exists for therapeutic abortion." He also noted that, "there is good evidence to show that patients who go on to become pregnant after treatment for breast cancer have a better survival." [36, p.50]

Q-7T: Do women who have additional children after developing breast cancer have a better prognosis?

In a large Danish study, Kroman et al [37] noted that women who had children after being treated for breast cancer showed a trend toward having a lower mortality rate than women who had no children after treatment [RR: 0.55 (0.28-1.06)]. Clarck and Chua [33, p.15] had noted that in a group of 30 women who became pregnant after being treated for breast cancer, women who had multiple pregnancies had a 96% 5-year survival rate, and women who had a single pregnancy had a 73% 5-year survival rate. [It is not known whether the stage of breast cancer was identical for both groups at the onset of the trial.]

Q-7U: Is the increasing rate of breast cancer, which is most prominent in Western countries, due to the abortion/oral contraception risk or is it simply due to an increase in mammography usage?

There are probably several reasons for the increase in breast cancer rates in most Western countries including lower parity rates, shorter breastfeeding time, and higher rates of abortion and early OCP use. Researcher White noted: "Recently, two other factors have emerged as possible risk factors for breast cancer: oral contraceptive use before first pregnancy and abortion before first term pregnancy" [38, p.242].

Some researchers have pointed to mammography as the culprit, claiming that with increased use of mammography, the rate of breast cancer might increase initially because more cancers would be detected. Mammography can only explain part of the increase in breast cancer, for the following reasons: First, in their study of women aged 25 to 44 years old, White et al found that although their model predicted that the increase in breast cancer incidence due to greater mammography should be 12%, in actuality the incidence of breast cancer grew by 29% between the early 1970s and late 1980s. Thus, mammography accounted for less than half the reason for rising breast cancer rates. White also noted that the increase in breast cancer "occurred proportionately between local and regional/distant stage at diagnosis" [39, p.1551]. Thus, although one might expect that an increase in mammography would result in a rise in the detection of early small tumors, one would not expect the incidence of larger tumors to be affected, which is precisely what White did find. In addition, Newcomb et al [40] noted that mammography failed to account for 40% of the increased incidence of breast cancer in younger women (ie, aged 40-49 years old).

Q-7V: Is there any other reason why mammography alone does not explain the rising incidence of breast cancer in young women?

Yes. Most studies in young women note that few of their cancers are detected by mammography, thus limiting the effect of this variable. For example, Brinton et al [29] noted that most breast tumors in women under 45 were found by themselves or their partners (66.3%), whereas only 19.1% were found by mammography. "There was no evidence that tumors were more often detected by medical methods in oral contraceptive users compared to nonusers, with the respective percentages in users and nonusers being 7.9% and 8.7% respectively, for routine medical examination, and 18.4% and 21.2%, respectively, for routine mammography." [29, p.833]. In a large English study, the authors noted that "less than 3% of breast lumps were found by a doctor." [United Kingdom study, 41, p.981]. As Colditz et al stated: "Because screening causes, at most, a transient rise in incidence and was not widespread at least through the early 1980s, its effect can explain little of the long-term increase in breast cancer incidence." [42, p.1481].

Q-7W: Does the mammography controversy in any way diminish the fact that the major meta-analyses show that both an abortion performed early in a woman's reproductive life and/or early OCP use increase a woman's risk of breast cancer?

No. Even though the rise in breast cancer may, in small part, be due to the increased use of mammography, it gives no reason for the discrepancy in breast cancer rates between women who did or did not have an abortion performed early in their reproductive life and/or who had early OCP use.

Q-7X: Do women who had "(non-specific) miscarriages" (ie, this category would include miscarriages that occur either before or after a woman's first full-term pregnancy (FFTP) have an increased risk of breast cancer?

Table 7A:
RISKS OF BREAST CANCER TO WOMEN
WHO HAD A MISCARRIAGE

AUTHOR	PERCENT CHANGE	YEAR OF PUBLICATION	CONFIDENCE INTERVAL
Daling [2]	10% decrease*	1994	0.9 (0.7-1.2)
Hadjimichael [43]**	no change	1986	unknown
La Vecchia [44]	10% decrease*	1987	0.9 (0.69-1.15)
Lipworth [45]	10% increase*	1995	1.1 (0.82-1.40)
Newcomb [46]	11% increase	1996	1.11 (1.02-1.20)
Parrazini [47]	no change	1992	1.0 (0.9-1.1)
Rohan [48]	20% increase*	1997	1.2 CI unknown
Rookus [5]	10% increase*	1996	1.1 (0.9-1.5)
Rosenberg [16]	30% increase*	1988	1.3 (0.8-2.2)

* This result reflects a trend toward an increased or decreased risk but does not attain statistical significance.
**Women who had their miscarriage after their first full-term pregnancy (FFTP).

Table 7A is a review of the major studies which gave data on the risk of breast cancer and miscarriages. It would appear that women who had "a non-specific miscarriage" would not have an elevated risk of breast cancer.

Q-7Y: Do the studies published after 1980 show that women who have had a miscarriage before their FFTP have an increased risk for breast cancer?

Table 7B:

RISKS OF BREAST CANCER IN WOMEN WHO HAD A MISCARRIAGE BEFORE THEIR FFTP

AUTHOR	YEAR OF PUBLICATION	PERCENT CHANGE	CONFIDENCE INTERVAL
Adami [49]	1990	20% increase*	0.7-2.0
Brinton [28]	1983	9% increase*	0.8-1.5
Daling [2]	1994	10% decrease*	0.6-1.3
Ewertz/Duffy [50]	1988	163% increase*	0.83-8.32***
Hadjimichael [43]	1986	250% increase	1.7-7.4
Pike et al [15]	1981	151% increase	unknown
Rookus [5]	1996	40% increase*	1.0-1.9
Rosenberg [16]	1988	10% decrease*	0.7-1.4**

* This result reflects a trend toward an increased or decreased risk but does not attain statistical significance.

** Inappropriate age matching in this study: median age of "cases" was 52; median age of "controls" was 40.

*** first trimester miscarriage in nulliparous women.

After reviewing the literature, Table 7B exhibits that 6 out of 8 studies show a trend and/or statistically significant increased risk of breast cancer with miscarriage before a first full-term pregnancy (FFTP). The studies noted here appear to show that a miscarriage before a FFTP does elevate the risk of breast cancer but further research is urgently needed to verify this. Hopefully researchers will perform a meta-analysis in this important area in the near future. This may have special implications for work-

**** Calle et al [52] noted that miscarriage before a woman's first term pregnancy did not result in an increased risk of fatal breast cancer ($RR=0.76$), but this prospective study may be particularly weak in measuring this variable for a number of reasons (see end of chapter for explanation).

ing mothers, who have been noted to have an increased risk of miscarriage. "After being adjusted for confounding factors, weekly job hours during the first trimester of pregnancy showed a strong independent association with spontaneous abortion risk; odds ratio 3.0 (1.4-.5.6)" [51].

Q-7Z1: Do multiple miscarriages before a woman's FFTP increase the risk?

Brinton et al [28] found that women who had two or more miscarriages before their FFTP had a relative risk of 2.16 (0.9-5.1), that is, a 116% increased trend toward developing breast cancer.* This is the result of only one study albeit, it does show a tendency toward increased risk.

*For the researchers in the audience: Lehrer et al [65] noted that women who have breast cancer and had multiple miscarriages also have cancers which have a higher incidence of having less estrogen and progesterone receptors, thus carrying a worse prognosis. Whether the miscarriages had an effect on the breast or whether both the miscarriages and the low amount of receptors are a result of the "[genetic] condition" of that person is not known.

Q-7Z2: Does abortion increase the risk of cervical cancer?

Remennick [32] noted a strong statistically significant partial correlation coefficient between abortion rate and cervical cancer: ($r = 0.63$, $p<0.05$). A partial correlation coefficient gives an index of how related a risk is to an effect (breast cancer). No correlation would register as 0.0 whereas a perfect correlation would register as 1.0. Although Zondervan et al [53] and Daling [2] found no increased risk [$RR= 0.66$ (0.04-3.53)], several other studies have suggested a positive association between abortion and cervical cancer [54, 55-61]. Thomas, in his analysis of a WHO study, reported that women who had an induced abortion had at least a 160% increased risk of developing invasive cervical carcinoma [62]. Molina et al [55] noted a 1.38-fold risk and Parrazini et al [60] noted a 2.5-fold risk for cervical carcinoma with induced abortion. Lé et al [63] found nearly a 5-fold risk for cervical cancer in women reporting two or more abortions. Further study of this area is needed.

Addendum 7A:
Calculations of estimated breast cancer mortality due to abortion.

In the early 1980s it was estimated that more than 1.6 million women had abortions each year [64] and that about one-third were repeat abortions. If one counts only those women who are having their first abortion (so that one does not double count women), one estimates that about 1 million women were having their first abortions each year. In Daling's paper [2], of all the "controls" who had abortions, 45% had an abortion prior to their FFTP, 28% had an abortion after their FFTP, and 27% had an abortion and were nulliparous. If 1 million women had abortions for the first time each year this would mean that the respective groups would have 450,000, 280,000, and 270,000, women in them. The conservative rates of breast cancer increase in each of the respective groups based on Brind et al's paper is a 50% increase, a 30% increase, and a 30% increase. If we now use a 12% overall lifetime risk of breast cancer, and if the findings in Dr. Brind's meta-analysis prove true in the long run, we can expect the following increases in breast cancer rates:

For women who had an abortion prior to their FFTP: 450,000 x 12% x 50% = 27,000;

For women who had an abortion after their FFTP: 280,000 x 12% x 30% = 10,080; and

For nulliparous women who had an abortion: 270,000 x 12% x 30% = 9,720.

Adding these together yields an estimate of 46,800 extra women who will be developing breast cancer each year because of abortion. Certainly, this is a low estimate because of the conservative manner in which the calculations were made. For example, estimates for high risk groups were not used: it was noted earlier that young women under the age of 18 who have an abortion performed early in their reproductive life have a 150% increased risk in breast cancer according to Daling [2]. Also, the fact that about 500,000 women were having repeat abortions annually in the early 1980s could put these women at even greater risk. In addition, the national rate of breast cancer is even higher than 12% over the course of a woman's lifetime, and using the higher statistic would have increased the estimate even more than the 46,800 figure.

Addendum 7B:
Why is the study by Calle a weak one?

Calle et al [52] enrolled 579,274 women who did not have breast cancer in a prospective study and recorded the information from those patients who both *developed* and *died* from breast cancer within 7 years of enrollment. There is a problem with this. A study such as this will only measure women who will both develop and die from breast cancer within a 7-year time frame. *This implies that it will be studying those women who are developing particularly aggressive breast cancers.* It is known that women who develop breast cancer at a young age tend to develop more aggressive cancers than those women who develop them at an older age [66]. Thus, in a large cohort of evenly distributed women from the age of 29 years old to over 70 years old, the study may well be focusing on younger women, which in itself narrows the focus of the study. It is also known that women who have early abortions or use OCPs at an early age have more aggressive cancer. Here again the study would be disproportionately focusing on this category of younger women.

A second point is that, if women who have early miscarriages are at increased risk of developing breast cancer, the study could have failed to identify them because it looked at only women who had both *developed and died* of their breast cancer within a 7-year period. Thus, even if miscarriages had resulted in a significantly increased risk of breast cancer, one may never have known this unless the subjects died from that breast cancer within the 7-year study period.

References:

1. Melbye M, Wohlfahrt J, et al. Induced abortion and the risk of breast cancer. *N Engl J Med.* 1997; 336: 81-85.

2. Daling J, Malone K, et al. Risk of breast cancer among young women: relationship to induced abortion. *J Natl Cancer Inst.* 1994; 86: 1584-1592.

3. Brind J, Chinchilli M, et al. Induced abortion as an independent risk factor for breast cancer: a comprehensive review and meta-analysis. *J Epidemiol Community Health.* 10/ 1996; 50: 481-496.

4. Howe H, et al. Early abortion and breast cancer risk among women under age 40. *Int J Epidemiol.* 1989; 18: 300-304.

5. Rookus M, Leeuwen F. Induced abortion and risk for breast cancer: reporting (recall) bias in a Dutch case-control study. *J Natl Cancer Inst.* 1996; 88: 1759-1764.

6. Henshaw SK, O'Reilly K. Characteristics of abortion patients in the United States, 1979 and 1980. *Family Planning Perspectives.* 1983; 15: 5-16.

7. Daling J, Brinton L, et al. Risk of breast cancer among white women following induced abortion. *Am J Epidemiol.* 1996; 144: 373-380.

8. Gans, et al. American Medical Association report: Induced termination of pregnancy before and after Rode versus Wade. *JAMA.* 1992; 268: 3231-3239.

9. Garfinkel, et al. *Stress, Depression and Suicide: A Study of Adolescence in Minnesota,* (Minneapolis: University of Minnesota Extension Service, 1986).

10. Reardon D. *A survey of psychological reactions.* Elliot Institute. 1987.

11. Gissler M, et al. Suicides after pregnancy in Finland, 1987-1994: register linkage study. *Br Med J.* 1996; 313: 1431-1434.

12. Ownby HE, et al. Interrupted pregnancy as an indicator of poor prognosis in T1,2, N0, M0 primary breast cancer. *Breast Cancer Research and Treatment.* 1983; 3: 339-344.

13. Olsson H, Ranstam J, et al. Proliferation and DNA ploidy in malignant breast tumors in relation to early contraceptive use and early abortions. *Cancer.* 1991; 67: 1285-1290.

14. Henshaw S, Koonin L, et al. Characteristics of U.S. women having abortions, 1987. *Family Planning Perspectives.* 1991; 21: 75-81.

15. Pike MC, Henderson BE, et al. Oral contraceptive use and early abortion as risk factors for breast cancer in young women. *Br J Cancer.* 1981; 43: 72-76.

16. Rosenberg L, Palmer JR, et al. Breast cancer in relation to the occurrence and time of induced and spontaneous abortion. *Am J Epidemiol.* 1988; 127: 981-989.

17. Talwar, et al. Phase I clinical trials with three formulations of anti-human Chorionic Gonadotropin vaccine. *Contraception.* 41: 301-316.

18. Russo J, Russo IH. Toward a physiological approach to breast cancer prevention. *Cancer Epidemiology, Biomarkers and Prevention.* 1994; 3: 353-364.

19.   Anonymous. Indian women condemn contraceptive vaccine. *Pittsburgh Catholic*. December 3, 1993: 3.

20.   Cunningham, et al. *William's Obstetrics*. 20th ed. Stanford, CT: Appleton & Lange; 1997: 580 – 581.

21.   Campbell NB, et al. Abortion in Adolescence. *Adolescence*. 1988; 23: 813-823.

22.   Andrieu N, et al. Familial risk of breast cancer and abortion. *Cancer Detection and Prevention*. 1994; 18: 51-55.

23.   Ginsburg ES. Mello NK, et al. Effects of alcohol ingestion on estrogens in postmenopausal women. *JAMA*. Dec. 4, 1996; 276: 1747-1751.

24.   Mendelson, J. Lukas S, et al. Acute alcohol effects on plasma estradiol levels in women. *Psychopharmocology*. 1988; 94: 464-467.

25.   Speckhard A. *Psycho-Social Stress Following Abortion* (PhD Thesis). University of Minnesota, 1985.

26.   Klassen A, Wilsnack S. Sexual experience and drinking among women in a U.S. national survey. *Archives of Sexual Behavior*. 1986; 15: 363-391.

27.   Elliot Institute. New study confirms link between abortion and substance abuse. *The Post-Abortion Review*. Fall, 1993; 1: 1,6.

28.   Brinton LA, Hoover R, et al. Reproductive factors in the aetiology of breast cancer. *Br J Cancer*. 47: 757-762.

29.   Brinton LA, Daling JR, et al. Oral contraceptives and breast cancer risk among younger women. *J Natl Cancer Inst*. 6/7/1995; 87: 827-835.

30.   Wingo PA, Lee NC, et al. Age-specific differences in the relationship between oral contraceptives use and breast cancer. *Cancer* (supplement). 1993; 71: 1506-1517.

31.   White E, Malone K, Weiss N, Daling J. Breast cancer among young U.S. women in relation to oral contraceptive use. *J Natl Cancer Inst*. 1994; 86: 505-514.

32.   Remennick L. Reproductive patterns and cancer incidence in women: a population-based correlation study in the USSR. *Int J Epidemiol*. 1989; 18: 498-510.

33.   Clarck RM, Chua T. Breast cancer and pregnancy: the ultimate challenge. *Clinical Oncology*. 1989; 1: 11-18.

34.   Clarck RM. (personal letter regarding "Breast cancer and pregnancy: the ultimate challenge.") February 10, 1995.

35.   King RM, Welch JS, et al. Carcinoma of the breast associated with pregnancy. *Surgery, Gynecology and Obstetrics*. 1985; 160: 228-232.

36.   Isaacs JH. Cancer of the breast in pregnancy. *Surgical Clinics of North America*. 1995; 75 (1): 47-51.

37.   Kroman N, et al. Should women be advised against pregnancy after breast-cancer treatment? *The Lancet*. 1997; 350: 319-322.

38.   White E, Daling J, et al. Rising incidence of breast cancer among young women in Washington State. *J Natl Cancer Inst*. 1987; 79: 239-243.

39.   White E, Lee C, et al. Evaluation of the increase in breast cancer incidence in relation to mammography use. *J Natl Cancer Inst*. 1990; 82: 1546-1552.

40. Newcomb PA, Lantz PM. Recent trends in breast cancer incidence, mortality, and mammography. *Breast Cancer Research and Treatment.* 1993; 28: 97-106.

41. Chilvers C, McPherson K, et al. Oral contraceptive use and breast cancer risk in young women (UK National Case-Control Study Group). *The Lancet.* May 6, 1989: 973-982.

42. Colditz G. Epidemiology of breast cancer. *Cancer.* 1993; 71: 1480-1489.

43. Hadjimichael OC, et al. Abortion before first live birth and risk of breast cancer. *Br J Cancer.* 1986; 53: 281-284.

44. La Vecchia C, et al. General epidemiology of breast cancer in northern Italy. *Int J Epidemiol.* 1987; 16: 347-355.

45. Lipworth L, Katsouyanni K, et al. Abortion and the risk of breast cancer: a case-control study in Greece. *Int J Cancer.* 1995; 61: 181-184.

46. Newcomb PA, Storer BE, et al. Pregnancy termination in relation to risk of breast cancer. *JAMA.* 1996; 275: 283-322.

47. Parrazini F, La Vecchia, et al. Menstrual and reproductive factors and breast cancer in women with family history of the disease. *Int J Cancer.* 1992; 51: 677-681.

48. Brind J. ABC down under. *Abortion Breast Cancer Quarterly Update.* Summer, 1997.

49. Adami HO, Bergstrom R, Lund E, Meirik O. Absence of association between reproductive variables and the risk of breast cancer in young women in Sweden and Norway. *Br J Cancer.* 1990; 62: 122-126.

50. Ewertz M, Duffy SW. Risk of breast cancer in relation to reproductive factors in Denmark. *Br J Cancer.* 1988; 58: 99-104.

51. Schenker MB, et al. Self-reported stress and reproductive health of female lawyers. *Journal of Occupational and Environmental Medicine.* 1997; 39: 556-568.

52. Calle EE, Mervis CA, Wingo PA, et al. Spontaneous abortion and risk of fatal breast cancer in a prospective cohort of United States women. *Cancer Causes and Control.* 1995; 6: 460-468.

53. Zondervan KT, Carpenter LM, et al. Oral contraceptives and cervical cancer-further findings from the Oxford family planning association contraceptive study. *Br J Cancer.* 1996; 73: 1291-1297.

54. Lé MG, Cabanes PA, et al. Oral contraceptive use and risk of cutaneous malignant melanoma in a case-control study of French women. *Cancer Causes and Control.* 1992; 3: 199-205.

55. Molina R, et al. Oral contraceptives and cervical carcinoma in Chile. *Cancer Research.* 1988; 48: 1011-1015.

56. Harris RW, et al. Characteristics of women with dysplasia or carcinoma in situ of the cervix uteri. *Br J Cancer.* 1980; 42: 359-369.

57. Hulka BS. Risk factors for cervical cancer. *J Chron Dis.* 1982; 35: 3-11.

58. Zanmetti P, et al. Characteristics of women under 20 with cervical intraepithelial neoplasia. *Int J Epidemiol.* 1986; 15: 477-482.

59. Fujimoto I, et al. Epidemiological study of the preinvasive cervical cancer. *Japanese J of Cancer Research*. 1987; 33: 651-660.

60. Parrazini F, et al. Risk Factors for adenocarcinoma of the cervix; A case-control study. *Br J Cancer*. 1988; 57: 200-204.

61. Groenroos M. Etiology of premalignant cervical lesion in teenagers. *Acta Obstet Gynecol Scand*. 1980; 59: 79.

62. Thomas DB, et al. Oral contraceptives and invasive adenocarcinomas and adenosquamos carcinomas of the uterine cervix. *Am J Epidemiol*. 1996; 144: 281-289.

63. Lé MG, Bachelot A, et al. Oral contraceptive use and breast or cervical cancer: preliminary results from a French case-control study. In: Wolff JP, Scott JS. *Hormones and sexual factors in human cancer aetiology*. Excerpta Medica. New York: Elsevier Science Publishers; 1984: 139-147.

64. Henshaw S, Binkin N, et al. A portrait of American women who obtain abortions. *Family Planning Perspectives*. 1985; 17: 90-96.

65. Lehrer S., Levine E, et al. Diminished ration of estrogen receptors to progesterone receptors in breast carcinomas of women who have had multiple miscarriages. *Mount Sinai Journal of Medicine*. 1992: 28-31.

66. Nixon A, Neuberg D, et al. Relationship of patient age to pathologic features of the tumor and prognosis for patients with stage I or II breast cancer. *J Clin Oncol*. 1994; 12: 888-894.

Chapter 8:
Breast Cancer and
Early Oral Contraceptive Use

"Perhaps the greatest interest and controversy in breast cancer epidemiology has surrounded the questions of whether use of oral contraceptives and estrogen replacement therapy affect the risk for breast cancer." [1, p.298]

More than 10 million women in the U.S. currently use oral contraceptive pills (OCPs) [2] and they are used by more than 50 million women worldwide annually. In addition, women are using OCPs earlier in their reproductive lives and for longer periods of time. Obviously, if women who take OCPs — especially those who take them before their first full-term pregnancy (FFTP) — are at risk, it has personal as well as worldwide repercussions. The focus of this chapter will be to answer one specific question, namely:

Is the woman who takes oral contraceptive pills at an early age at increased risk for developing breast cancer?

First, we explore some of the background of the oral contraceptive pill and the history of the OCP/breast cancer debate.

Q-8A: What is an OCP and how does it work?

[A more detailed discussion of what an OCP is and how it works can be found in Appendix 5].

A woman's menstrual cycle is regulated by a small gland in the brain called the pituitary gland. It secretes a number of hormones which include FSH (Follicle Stimulating Hormone) and LH (Luteinizing Hormone), both of which are necessary for ovulation to occur and both stimulate a woman's ovaries to produce two important sexual hormones called progesterone and estradiol-17B.

In the 1920s and 1930s, scientists found methods of obtaining both progesterone and estradiol from animals and discovered their chemical composition. It was soon noted that if either of these compounds were given in high doses, they could inhibit ovulation. Basically, these hormones, when given in high doses, had the effect of "shutting down the pituitary gland" so that the levels of FSH and LH would decrease, thereby inhibiting ovulation.

Researchers soon discovered how to make artificial progestins and estrogens in the laboratory. In the 1950s, it was discovered that the combination of an artificial estrogen and progestin would inhibit ovulation. These were the first OCPs.

Today's OCPs are still made with a combination of an artificial estrogen and progestin. The estrogen is either ethinyl estradiol or mestranol. The body breaks down mestranol into ethinyl estradiol so that the two have very similar effects. The other part of today's OCPs is composed of an artificial progestin. Today's progestins are far more powerful than the body's natural hormone, progesterone. Estranes are the first type of artificial progestin and are about 5 to 10 times more potent than progesterone. They include norethindrone and norethynodrel. A second even more powerful type of progestin are the gonanes, which include norgestrel, gestodene and norgestimate.

Over the years, OCPs have changed. In the 1960s, OCPs were available in sequential or combination form. Sequential OCPs contained an estrogen for 4 weeks of the cycle and added a progestin in the 4th week. They were removed from the market in the 1970s because they increased the incidence of uterine cancer. Combination OCPs contain a fixed amount of an estrogen and progestin, whereas triphasic OCPs, the third type of OCP (also called phasic pills), alternate the ratio of the estrogen and progestin throughout the cycle. Both of these types of OCPs are commonly used today although the use of triphasics has increased over the last 15 years.

How do OCPs work? The combination of these artificial estrogens and progestins function to prevent or stop pregnancy in three ways. First, they inhibit ovulation by inhibiting the pituitary gland and thus FSH and LH. Today's OCPs, which have lower amounts of hormones than the original OCPs, do not totally shut down ovulation. It is estimated that breakthrough ovulation occurs at least 5 to 10% of the time and this is probably a low estimate because some of today's OCPs have estrogen contents as low as 20 micrograms. Second, they may thicken the cervical mucus, making it somewhat more difficult for sperm to travel through. Third, they change the lining of the uterus and often cause an early abortion in those instances when ovulation and conception have occurred. Both pro-life and pro-abortion groups admit to this effect, with the latter doing so publicly in testimony before the Supreme Court in 1989 [3].

(For a detailed discussion of this as well as an examination of the OCPs mechanism of action, see Appendix 5).

Q-8B: Did scientists study the OCP's effect on animals?

Yes, concerns were raised in 1972 when it was noted that an OCP containing mestranol and norethynodrel appeared to cause a case of metastatic breast cancer in *a female rhesus monkey* [4]. This was especially worrisome because rhesus monkeys rarely develop breast cancer. Until that time only three cases of breast cancer in rhesus monkeys were known. Although it was argued that this was simply a "chance finding," concern grew when it was noted that both beagles [5, 6] and rodents [7, 8, 9] developed breast cancer when exposed to the hormones contained in today's OCPs.

Q-8C: What effect does OCP use have on human breast cells?

In 1989, Anderson et al [10] published a classic paper regarding the influence of OCP use on the rate of breast cell division. They found that nulliparous women who took OCPs had a significantly higher rate of breast cell division (measured via thymidine labeling index) than nulliparous women who did not take them. The difference in <u>parous</u> women (ie, women who have had at least one child) who either did or did not take OCPs was not as significant. This is illustrated in Figure 8A where nulliparous women who were either taking or not taking OCPs (ie, labeled "on," or "off") were compared to parous women who were "on" or "off" the Pill.

Figure 8A:

RATE OF BREAST CELL DIVISION
IN WOMEN WHO TAKE THE PILL

(adapted from data from Anderson et al) [10]

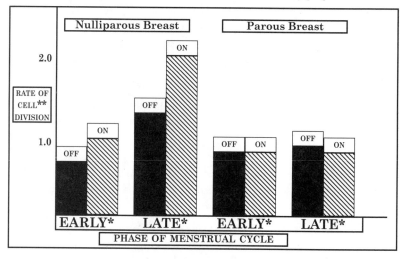

*Early or late phase of the secretory portion of a woman's menstrual cycle.

**Rate of cell division was measured by TLI — (thymidine labeling index).

This was especially significant because it is known that, in general, cells which have an increased rate of cell division are more likely to become cancerous. Another study by Williams et al [11] found that women who took OCPs had a marked reduction of estrogen receptor positive breast cancer cells when their cells were examined (ie, estrogen receptor positive breast cells respond much better to treatment than estrogen receptor negative breast cancer cells). Additional information as to specifically how either estrogen or progestin could cause breast cancer is given in the addendum at the end of this chapter.

Q-8D: Does the fact that OCP use causes early abortions explain why it increases the risk of breast cancer in young women?

Daling [12] and Rookus [13] have noted that abortions prior to 8 weeks of pregnancy result in an increased risk of breast cancer, but do the very early abortions from use of hormonal contraceptives such as the OCP and Depo-Provera also elevate the risk? Stewart et al have shown that estradiol and progesterone levels already start to rise above baseline levels within 4 days of conception, thus prior to implantation and before hCG levels begin to rise [14, p.1472]. An early abortion would cause a sudden fall in the levels of these hormones. Could these early hormonal fluctuations be playing a role? To this author's knowledge, no one has asked or studied this question. Many hormone levels change in pregnancy and perhaps with advances in technology we may be able to measure the hormone levels in early pregnancy more accurately, such as Stewart et al have. Perhaps in time, a variant of Stewart et al's methods may be able to quantify more precisely how often OCP use causes early pregnancy and abortion, in addition to enabling researchers such as Anderson et al to be able to perform studies on breast cells during the very early stages of pregnancy.

Q-8E: What is the historical evidence from studies of humans that oral contraceptives cause breast cancer when taken by women early in their lives?

In 1981, Pike et al [15] noted that women who took OCPs for 4 or more years prior to their first full-term pregnancy (FFTP) experienced a 125% increased risk in breast cancer, whereas women who took them for 8 or more years prior to their FFTP had a 250% increased risk. This startled the research world and led to additional studies, including a very large American study called the CASH trial in the early 1980s (ie, Center for Disease Control's Cancer And Steroid Hormone study). The researchers originally reported in 1983 that: "Oral contraceptive use before a woman's first pregnancy did not increase her risk of breast cancer significantly more than other methods of delaying first pregnancy." [16] As time progressed, however, and further "cases" were included in the study group, the CASH study showed some very disturbing results. By 1993 it showed that women under the age of 44 had a 40% increased risk in breast cancer, which was statistically significant in the 35 to 44 year-old age group [17].

Later in England, Chilvers et al [18] published the results of another large study called the United Kingdom National Study. They showed that young women under the age of 36 who had used oral contraceptives for at least 4 years before their FFTP had at least a 44% increased risk in breast cancer. The last large study was performed in 1995 by Brinton et al [19]. It showed a 42% increased risk for women who used OCPs for more than 6 months prior to their FFTP.

Q-8F: If the major studies showed the risks that you have just mentioned, then why do doctors fail to inform their patients of those risks?

That is a good question. Part of the problem is that because the OCP/breast cancer debate is complicated, most people have to rely on what "the experts" tell them. Unfortunately, it does not help when major medical journals and medical associations fail to stress the dangers of early oral contraceptive use.

A good example of this occurred recently in the study printed in a condensed version in *The Lancet* [20] and in complete form in *Contraception* [21]. This was and remains the largest meta-analysis regarding the studies of OCPs and breast cancer. Researchers from around the world studied and combined data from 54 studies, involving 25 countries and 53,297 women who had breast cancer. It concluded: "Women who are currently using combined oral contraceptives or have used them in the past 10 years are at a slightly increased risk of having breast cancer diagnosed, although the additional cancers tend to be localized to the breast. There is no evidence of an increase in the risk of having breast cancer diagnosed 10 or more years after cessation of use. . ." Unfortunately, this study is known more for what it did say, than what it did not say. There were several major problems with the study, which is analyzed in depth in Appendix 5. The largest weakness was the failure to report any evidence of what the pooled risk of oral contraceptive *use before a FFTP* was in women less than 45 years old. The researchers of the study did examine the risks of women who had used OCPs before age 20, but this certainly is not the equivalent of studying premenopausal women who used OCPs prior to their FFTP. An additional problem is that the Oxford study pooled data from studies which examined women with breast cancer from as far back as the early and mid-1970s [21, p.5S].

Q-8G: Why does the fact that the Oxford study pooled data from early studies affect its results?

The Oxford study pooled the results of studies which interviewed women with breast cancer in the early and mid-1970s [21, p.5S]. *Taking data from studies which interviewed women before 1980 will tend to underestimate the risk of developing breast cancer from early OCP use.* Why? Data from studies before 1980 would be unlikely to show much risk *because the latent period was too short* and few women used OCPs for significant periods of time prior to their FFTP in the late 1960s and early 1970s as compared to women of the late 1970s and 1980s [21, p.9S]. Thomas warned of this problem years before the Oxford study was published: "The major limitation of this effort (ie, the Oxford study), of course, is that all existing data sets have limited information on use of oral contraceptives by young women for a prolonged period." [22, p.362]

Q-8H: What about the question of "length of use" before a FFTP; did the Oxford study address that?

No. One of the biggest problems with the Oxford study is that it failed to ask the question of what the risk of OCP use was prior to a FFTP in premenopausal women. Another major weakness is that the study failed to ask the question of what the risk of long-term OCP use (eg, greater than 4 years) before a FFTP was. This is especially important because women in Western countries today are using OCPs for far longer periods of time than women did in the 1960s and early 1970s. We hope that some researchers will perform a re-analysis of the Oxford meta-analysis and will have the courage to ask the question: What is the risk of breast cancer to women who were under the age of 45 as of 1990 and who used OCPs for 4 or more years prior to a FFTP, when confined to the studies done after 1980, or better yet, after 1985?

Q-8I: Has anyone done a meta-analysis that examined the question of risk to women under the age of 45 who had taken OCPs prior to their FFTP?

Yes. Two different researchers have addressed this question. Thomas et al, in 1991, found that women who took OCPs for extended periods of time prior to their FFTP had a 44% increased risk [$RR=1.44$ (1.23-1.69)] of developing breast cancer [23]. In 1990, Romieu pooled studies of women under the age of 45 who had taken OCPs for 4 or more years prior to their FFTP and found that they had a 72% increased risk [$RR=1.72$ (1.36-2.19)] of developing breast cancer when she restricted her analysis to those studies done after 1980 [24].

Q-8J: What are the largest retrospective studies to date and how does one find them?

This author used *Med-Line*, which is the name of a computer program that allows the researcher to find major journal articles on virtually any medical subject (it can be accessed through the Internet). In addition, the extensive bibliography found in the Oxford study in *The Lancet* [20] was used to obtain virtually every major retrospective study that gathered the bulk of its data after 1980 and examined women under the age of 45, in regard to their history of oral contraceptive use.

After gathering all of the retrospective studies, the largest were selected, specifically, those studies that had about 750 or more women under the age of 45. Some studies made no comment on OCP use prior to a FFTP. When this occurred, this author looked for the next closest approximation to the parameter of "early OCP use." A parameter of OCP use within 5 years of menarche was chosen as a close approximation of OCP use prior to a FFTP, if no data on the latter were available. What, then are the largest studies and what do they show?

Table 8A:
THE FOUR LARGE STUDIES THAT MEASURED
EARLY OCP USE AND THE RISK OF BREAST CANCER
TO WOMEN UNDER THE AGE OF 45

AUTHOR	YEAR	SIZE OF STUDY	FINDINGS
Wingo [17] CASH Study	12/80-82	2089 less than age 45	40% increased risk ages 20-44
Rosenberg [25]*	1977-1992	1427 less than age 45	88% increased risk**
White [26]	1983-1990	747 less than age 45	50% increased risk: for use within 5 years of menarche (parous women)
Brinton [19]	5/90-12/92	1648 less than age 45	42% increased risk (parous women)**

* This study did not control for abortion.

** Calculated from raw data found in their paper — see end of chapter for details.

Q-8K: *What do these results mean?*

In summary, the four largest retrospective studies of parous women under the age of 45 all show at least a 40% increased risk to women who took OCPs prior to their FFTP or within 5 years of menarche.

Q-8L: *Could you explain a little bit about each study?*

(This answer is somewhat technical and may be skipped without a loss of continuity).

Certainly. The CASH study was mentioned earlier. It has the largest group of women under the age of 45, specifically, 2089. Because the CASH data were taken from interviews with women during the years of 1980 through 1982, it means that it detected the risk of early contraceptive use and breast cancer despite the fact that the study had a short latent period. The authors admit this themselves: "However, because oral contraceptives have only been marketed in the U.S. since the 1960s, we were unable to study any possible very late effects of their use" [27, p.409]. As this author noted earlier, because women started taking OCPs more frequently before their FFTP in the 1970s, the effect of earlier OCP use and breast cancer would be picked up more strongly in studies which took their data *after* 1985. In 1993, a *Cancer* supplement issue [17] reported the following results from the CASH study for women who took OCPs prior to their FFTP:

Women aged 20 to 34 years old had a 1.4 (0.9-2.4) risk and women aged 35 to 44 years old had a 1.4 (1.1-1.8) risk (in other words a 40% increased risk). Unfortunately, the authors did not combine the data for the 20 to 44 year-old age group. Because the 35 to 44 year-old age group had about 10 times as many women in it as the 20 to 34 year-old age group, combining the data would have likely yielded a statistically significant risk of 40% for the combined age group of women aged 20 to 44 years old.

Two other researchers have provided helpful insights into the CASH study. Peto's re-analysis of women aged 20 to 44 years old in the CASH study [28] showed a RR of 1.29 (1.03-1.61) in women with 0-3 years of OCP use prior to their FFTP and a RR of 1.48 (1.15-1.91) in women with 4 or more years of OCP use prior to their FFTP. He noted that "whether the results of this and other studies prove a causal relation between OCP use and breast cancer in young women will continue to be debated — but the CASH results, at least for use before first full-term pregnancy, appear to support rather than weigh against the hypothesis." Pike and Bernstein also supported Peto's findings: "The CASH study as reported in women aged 20-44 is thus positive." [29]

Despite these findings, the lead author of the CASH paper, Phyllis Wingo, wrote in her abstract: "Available data provide no reasons to change prescribing practices or the use of OCP that are related to the breast cancer risk." *Why an author would downplay an increased breast cancer risk of 40% to women less than 44 years old is inexplicable.* In addition to this, it must be noted that the CASH study also suffered from a significant stack effect, the "death factor," and a fairly short latent period [30]. Each of these effects would serve to give an even higher risk had they been adjusted for. Therefore, a CASH finding of 40% risk for early OCP use in women less than age 44 is a very conservative estimate.

Rosenberg performed another large study which was published in The *American Journal of Epidemiology* in 1996. She, like the researchers in the CASH study, failed to combine the data for the 25 to 34 and 35 to 44 year-old age groups [25, p.33]. Combining the data leads one to an 88% increased risk for OCP use prior to a FFTP in women aged 24 to 44 years old (for the calculation of this see the end of this chapter). Rosenberg's increased risk is especially significant in that she had a huge stack effect (20% of "controls" were aged 25 to 34 years old, vs. only 9% of "cases") and a short latent period (ie, some of her data came from the late 1970s) Last, the study was supported indirectly through a grant from Merrell Dow Inc. (which has now merged with Hoechst Inc.) and Hoffman-La Roche Inc., both of whom support the Slone Epidemiology Unit, where Dr. Rosenberg works. All three of these weaknesses would tend to diminish the risk (ie, 88%), making it a very conservative estimate.

White and Daling published the third study in the *Journal of the National Cancer Institute* in 1994 [26]. They noted a 50% increased RR of 1.50 (1.1-2.2) in parous women who took the OCP within 5 years of menarche and had taken it for at least 1 year. White's study suffered from the stack effect (9% "cases" and 17% of "controls" in the youngest age group, 21 to 30 year olds) as well as a significant death factor. Over 10% of "cases" died or were too ill to be interviewed. In addition, the study limited its focus to only white women, thereby eliminating young black women who are at particular risk from early OCP use (see Chapter 11). All of these factors would have tended to increase the relative risk had the study been adjusted for them.

Brinton's study [19] from the National Cancer Institute (NCI) is the last of the four research projects which studied a large group of women prior to the age of 45. It has the advantage of a long latent period, which makes it especially significant. In Table 5 of her study, Brinton noted the relative risks for women who took OCPs for different lengths of time prior to their FFTP. All of the four subgroups shown had an increased risk of breast cancer, with two of the subgroups showing a statistically significant result. Women who took OCPs between 6 months and 2 years prior to their FFTP had a 40% increased risk [RR= 1.40 (1.1-1.8)], whereas women who took OCPs between 4 and 5 years prior to their FFTP had a 67% increased risk [RR=1.67 (1.2-2.3)]. However, Brinton et al failed to combine the overall data for all of the women who took OCPs for more than 6 months prior to their FFTP in spite of the fact that this is a simple calculation. Combining the data leads to a calculated odds ratio (OR) of 1.42 (ie, a 42% increased risk) for women who took the OCP prior to a FFTP — a result which would have almost certainly been statistically significant had the authors presented it (see end of this chapter for calculations). Perhaps Dr. Brinton could explain why this pivotal calculation was omitted.

Q-8M: Can you comment on why a recent large study published by researchers at Harvard claimed to show no increased risk of developing breast cancer for women who had taken OCPs for 5 years or more prior to their FFTP?

In 1997, a group of researchers at Harvard Medical School led by Dr. Hankinson published a study in *Cancer Causes and Control* [31]. It based its conclusions on data taken from the Nurses' Health Study and *claimed to show* that women who took OCPs for 5 years or more prior to their FFTP had no increased risk of breast cancer compared to women who never took OCPs [*RR*=0.7 (0.24-1.31)]. Unfortunately, the study's design appears to have been badly flawed.

Q-8N: Can you identify the flaws?

The researchers compared women with breast cancer who took OCPs for 5 years or more prior to their FFTP (eg, let's refer to these women as Group A] *to* women with breast cancer who never took OCPs [eg, Group B).

It is known that women took OCPs *for longer periods of time earlier in their reproductive lives* in the 1980s and 1990s than in the 1960s and 1970s as *was clearly noted* in the Oxford study [21, p.9S; Tables 14 and 15]. So any group of women who had taken OCPs for 5 years or more prior to their FFTP (ie, Group A) would have been more likely to have done so while in their late teens and 20s in the 1980s or 1990s, whereas women in Group B (who never took OCPs) would be more likely to contain a distribution of women who would have been in their late teens and 20s in either the 1960s, 1970s, 1980s or 1990s. *But this strongly supports the contention that women in Group A would have a lower average age and a shorter follow-up time than the women in Group B, which would of course invalidate the study's conclusions.*

It is frightening to note that the Harvard team presented NO DATA *on either the average age of women in the noted groups or their respective lengths of follow-up time. The research team instead chose to follow the noted groups in "person-years"* as their measure of follow-up time. This is the length of a follow-up period derived from the number of women followed, multiplied by the average number of years they were followed. For example, if group A had 100 women who were followed for 10 years, the total amount of follow-up time would be 100 x 10 = 1,000 person-years. But if group A had 250 women who were followed for 4 years it would also have 1,000 person-years of follow-up time. This is totally inadequate because the measure of "person-years" gives no data on the length of follow-up time *in actual years,* and without this information the study must remain suspect *because it was noted that women in group A most likely had both a younger average age and were followed for a shorter period of time than the women in group B.*

Q-8O: Is there any way that the public will ever have access to the necessary data that was not presented in the Harvard study?

I am not sure. This author tried in vain to obtain the answers to three basic questions over a 6 month period of time from three different researchers involved in the Harvard study. Attempts were made via e-mail, phone calls and certified mail. It is ironic that one cannot obtain access to data from these researchers especially because their study obtained its data from the Nurses' Health Study, *a study which is funded by citizen tax dollars through a grant via the National Cancer Institute* (NCI). The simple and necessary questions that need to be answered are presented at the end of this chapter. Until the noted researchers at Harvard make their data available for all to see, the study's conclusions must remain suspect.

Q-8P: What should women who take OCPs prior to their FFTP be told?

They should be told that all of the collective data we have point to an estimated increased risk of breast cancer of 40% to women who have used OCPs before their FFTP.

Addendum 8A:

The following simple questions that were asked of the researchers at Harvard have never been answered:

1) How many women were there in the group who were under the age of 45 and who used oral contraceptives for 5 years or more prior to their FFTP (see page 69, Table 3 of your paper [ie, the women who were followed for 9,741 person-years]). What was the mean age for the women in this group?

2) How many women were there in the group who were under the age of 45 and never used the OCP? (see Table 2 page 68, these women were followed for 176,306 person-years). What was their mean age?

3) How many women were in the group who were under the age of 45 and had used the OCP for 10 years or more of total duration? (Correlating to Table 2 on page 68, the group that had 21,760 person-years of follow-up)

Addendum 8B:

How might the estrogen or the progestin either individually or jointly cause breast cancer?

(The following is a fairly technical answer and may be skipped without loss of continuity).

This is a very difficult question. Researchers know that the cancer cell is first formed by the influence of a <u>carcinogen</u> in a process called <u>initiation</u> and then continues to grow and be influenced by <u>promoters</u> (ie, those risk factors that promote the growth of cancerous breast cells). Many authors claimed that estrogen and progestins simply promote the growth of an already existing breast cancer cell. Others have theorized that they might also play a role as an initiator or as an "aid" to an initiator. *The truth is, no one really knows.* What we do know is that OCPs speed up the rate of breast cell division in nulliparous women, which would theoretically leave breast cells susceptible to the initiation process. We also know that hormone levels at the cellular level may have little to do with the levels measured in the bloodstream. Hulka et al have noted that: "Aspirates from women with normal breasts or benign breast disease have estradiol and estrone levels 10-40 times higher than plasma levels." [32, p.1116]. In addition, "Synthetic estrogens and progestins may possess higher binding affinities for estrogen receptors and progesterone receptors than natural 17B-estradiol and progesterone" [33, p.286]. *This means that the artificial hormones may be more concentrated than thought to be at the level of the breast cell and that we really do not know how potent they are on the cellular level.* What happens when these artificial hormones interact with the hormone receptors on the individual breast cells? As one leading researcher told me confidentially: "(There is) no way to adequately assess the potency of the birth control pill on the in vivo breast."

In summary, "Three types of carcinogenic effects are theoretically possible. The oral contraceptives might act as an initiator and transform a normal cell into a cancer cell through mutation of the genome or alteration of its expression. The oral contraceptives might act as a co-initiator by increasing the division rate of breast cells rendering them more susceptible to chemical, viral or radiation carcinogenesis, all of which require DNA synthesis to establish genetic alteration. Oral contraceptives might act as a tumor promoter and promote the growth of already transformed but latent breast cancer cells." [34, p.765]

In addition to the evidence discussed, researchers in the 1980s began to note that the progestins used in OCPs stimulated the growth of human breast cells. Specifically, norethindrone stimulated the growth of MRC-7 cells (ie, the name of a type of human breast cancer cell which has been grown in a culture dish by researchers) [35]. This is another point of concern because norethindrone was the most common progestin used in OCPs from 1964 to 1988 and is still used in some of today's OCPs such as Ortho-Novum, Brevicon, Loestrin, Norinyl and Ovcon [36]. Jordan et al also noted that other progestins in addition to norethindrone (ie, norethynodrel, norgestrel and gestodene) all stimulated growth of the MRC-7 cells [37, p.1503], and Jeng et al [35] reported similar results. Another researcher named Longman [33] noted that the combination of ethinyl estradiol and norgestrel (eg, found in Ovral and Lo/Ovral) caused the greatest growth response in malignant breast cancer cells [33, p.284].

Addendum 8C: Calculation of Risks
Calculation of Risks for the Brinton et al study [19]:

Table 5 in Brinton's paper [19, p.832] gives the raw data for women under the age of 45 who used OCPs for more than 6 months prior to their FFTP:

The number of "cases" that fit this category was: 243+186+ 141+155=725:

The number of "controls" was: 201+177+92+132=602.

The number of "cases" and "controls" that did not use OCPs or used them less than 6 months was 274 and 322 respectively.

The relative risk estimate or odds ratio is: 725/274 divided by 602/322= 1.4153 or about a 42% increased risk.

Calculation of Risks for the Rosenberg study [25]:

Page 33 of Rosenberg et al's study noted that of the women who were aged 25 to 44, a total of 52+23+136+34=245 "cases" used OCPs for more than 1 year prior to their FFTP whereas 86+30+86+39=241 "controls" did. In addition, 547 "cases" and 1014 "controls" had less than 1 year of OCP use before their FFTP. The odds ratio or estimated relative risk is thus: 245/547 divided by 241/1014 which comes to 1.884 or about an 88% increased raw risk for women aged 25 to 44 years old who used OCPs for more than 1 year prior to their FFTP.

References:

1. Gomes L, Guimaraes M, et al. A case-control study of risk factors for breast cancer in Brazil, 1978-1987. *Int J Epidemiol.* 1995; 24: 292-299.

2. Faust JM. Image change for condoms. ABC News Report. [Internet E-mail]. 6/8/97.

3. Alderson Reporting Company. Transcripts of oral arguments before court on abortion case. *New York Times.* April 27, 1989; B12.

4. Kirschstein RL, et al. Infiltrating duct carcinoma of the mammary gland of a Rhesus monkey after administration of an oral contraceptive: a preliminary report. *J Natl Cancer Inst.* 1972; 48: 551-553.

5. Geil, et al. FDA studies of estrogen, progestogens, and estrogen/progesterone combinations in the dog and monkey. *J Toxicol Environ Health.* 1979; 3.

6. Shubik P. Oral contraceptives and breast cancer: laboratory evidence. In: Interpretation of Negative Epidemiological Evidence for Carcinogenicity. *IARC Sci Pub.* 1985: 65; 33.

7. Lanari C, Molinolo AA, et al. Induction of mammary adenocarcinomas by medroxyprogesterone acetate in balb/c female mice. *Cancer Letters.* 1986; 33: 215-223.

8. Welsch CW, et al. 17B-Oestradiol and enovid mammary tumorigenesis in C3H/HeJ female mice. *Br J Cancer.* 1977; 35: 322.

9. Kahn RH, et al. Effect of long-term treatment with Norethynodrel on A/J and C3H/HeJ mice. *Endocrinology.* 1969; 84: 661.

10. Anderson TJ, Battersby S, et al. Oral contraceptive use influences resting breast proliferation. *Hum Pathol.* 1989; 20: 1139-1144.

11. Williams G, Anderson E, et al. Oral contraceptive (OCP) use increases proliferation and decreases oestrogen receptor content of epithelial cells in the normal human breast. *Int J Cancer.* 1991; 48: 206-210.

12. Daling J, Malone K, et al. Risk of breast cancer among young women: relationship to induced abortion. *J Natl Cancer Inst.* 1994; 86: 1584-1592.

13. Rookus M, Leeuwen F. Induced abortion and risk for breast cancer: reporting (recall) bias in a Dutch case-control study. *J Natl Cancer Inst.* 1996; 88: 1759-1764.

14. Stewart DR, Overstreet JW, et al. Enhanced ovarian steroid secretion before implantation in early human pregnancy. *J Clin Endocrinol Metab.* 1993; 76: 1470-1476.

15. Pike MC, Henderson BE, et al. Oral contraceptive use and early abortion as risk factors for breast cancer in young women. *Br J Cancer.* 1981; 43: 72-76.

16. Ory HW, et al. Long-term oral contraceptive use and the risk of breast cancer (CASH Study). *JAMA.* 1983; 249: 1591-1595.

17. Wingo PA, Lee NC, et al. Age-specific differences in the relationship between oral contraceptives use and breast cancer. *Cancer* (supplement). 1993; 71: 1506-1517.

18. Chilvers C, McPherson K, et al. Oral contraceptive use and breast cancer risk in young women (UK National Case-Control Study Group). *The Lancet.* May 6, 1989: 973-982.

19. Brinton LA, Daling JR, et al. Oral contraceptives and breast cancer risk among younger women. *J Natl Cancer Inst.* 6/7/1995; 87: 827-35.

20. Collaborative Group on Hormonal Factors in Breast Cancer. Breast cancer and hormonal contraceptives: collaborative reanalysis of individual data on 53,297 women with breast cancer and 100,239 women without breast cancer from 54 epidemiological studies. *The Lancet.* 1996; 347: 1713-1727.

21. Collaborative Group on Hormonal Factors in Breast Cancer. Breast cancer and hormonal contraceptives: further results. *Contraception.* 1996; 34: S1-S106.

22. Thomas DB. Oral contraceptives and breast cancer. *J Natl Cancer Inst.* 1993; 85: 359-364.

23. Thomas DB. Oral contraceptives and breast cancer: review of the epidemiologic literature. *Contraception.* 1991; 43: 597-643.

24. Romieu I, Berlin J, et al. Oral contraceptives and breast cancer. Review and meta-Analysis. *Cancer.* 1990; 66: 2253-2263.

25. Rosenberg L, Palmer JR, et al. Case-control study of oral contraceptive use and risk of breast cancer. *Am J Epidemiol.* 1996; 143: 25-37.

26. White E, Malone K, Weiss N, Daling J. Breast cancer among young U.S. women in relation to oral contraceptive use. *J Natl Cancer Inst.* 1994; 86: 505-514.

27. Ory HW, et al. Oral-contraceptive use and the risk of breast cancer (CASH Study). *N Engl J Med*. 1986; 315: 405-411.

28. Peto J. Oral contraceptives and breast cancer: Is the CASH study really negative? *The Lancet*. March 11, 1989: 552.

29. Pike MC, Bernstein L. Oral contraceptives and breast cancer. *The Lancet*. July 15, 1989: 158.

30. Stadel BV, Lai S, et al. Oral contraceptives and premenopausal breast cancer in nulliparous women. *Contraception*. 1988; 38: 287-299.

31. Hankinson SE, et al. A prospective study of oral contraceptive use and risk of breast cancer (Nurses Health Study, United States). *Cancer Causes and Control*. 1997; 8: 65-72.

32. Hulka B, Liu E, et al. Steroid hormones and risk of breast cancer. *Cancer Supplement*. 1994; 74: 1111-1124.

33. Longman SM, et al. Oral contraceptives and breast cancer. *Cancer*. 1987; 59: 281-286.

34. Gay JW, et al. Oral contraceptives and breast cancer. *Missouri Medicine*. 1990; 87: 763-766.

35. Jeng MH, Parker CJ, et al. Estrogenic potential of progestins in oral contraceptives to stimulate human breast cancer cell proliferation. *Cancer Research*. Dec. 1, 1992: 6539-6546.

36. Gerstman BB, Gross TP, et al. Trends in the content and use of oral contraceptives in the United States, 1964-1988. *Am J Public Health*. 1991; 81: 90-96.

37. Jordan C, Jeng MH, et al. The estrogenic activity of synthetic progestins used in oral contraceptives. *Cancer Supplement*. 1993; 71: 1501-5.

Chapter 9:
Breast Cancer and the Pill:
Other Questions

Q-9A: Have there been any other large studies such as those described previously concerning OCP use prior to a first full-term pregnancy (FFTP)?

Yes, another large study of 755 women was done by Chilvers [1], but it confined itself to studying women under the age of 36. It found that women who took OCPs for 4 or more years prior to their FFTP had at least a 44% increased risk of breast cancer.

Table 9A: THE CHILVERS STUDY
OF WOMEN UNDER THE AGE OF 36

AUTHOR	FINDINGS	SIZE OF STUDY	YEAR STUDIED
Chilvers [1] United Kingdom Study	44% increase in women > 4 years use prior to their FFTP	755 less than age 36	1/82-12/85

Q-9B: Have any other studies shown an increased risk in young women less than the age of 36?

Yes, Pike et al showed that women age 32 or less had a 2.25-fold breast cancer risk if they took OCPs for 4 or more years prior to their FFTP [2].

Q-9C: Does OCP use exhibit the multiplier effect when other risk factors are involved?

When two factors affect the risk of obtaining breast cancer, and a woman has both of these risk factors, she can calculate her estimated risk by multiplying the independent risk of both of these factors. Several examples demonstrate that oral contraceptives increase the risk of breast cancer when combined with another risk factor. Brinton et al noted: "Among women with an affected relative, use of oral contraceptives for 5 or more years was associated with a RR of 3.1 (0.7-13.6) compared to a RR of 1.9 (1.2-3.1) among those without such a family history" [3, p.832]. Ravnihar [4] noted that women who have a family history of breast cancer and used OCPs had a 5.2-fold risk over women who had a positive family history and had no use of OCPs. Last, Pike et al [2] noted that women without benign breast disease who used OCPs for at least 49 months prior to their FFTP had a 1.69-fold increased risk of breast cancer, but women who took OCPs and did have a history of benign breast disease had an infinitely increased risk as compared to the "control" population.

Q-9D: What do the other studies (whose data come predominantly after 1980) that have limited themselves to evaluating women under the age of 45 show for women who took OCPs prior to their FFTP?

Chapter 8 addressed the data and results of the four largest retrospective studies known to date. Table 9B shows the results of all of the "case/control" retrospective studies, *the bulk of whose data come primarily after 1980. Eighteen out of 20 studies show an increased trend or significant risk in the development of breast cancer from oral contraceptive use before a woman's FFTP.* In fact, most of the studies show an increased risk of greater than 40%. This means that the breast cancer risk of OCP use prior to a FFTP is almost certainly higher than the conservative estimate of 40% given in Chapter 8.

Table 9B: BREAST CANCER RISK FROM STARTING OCPS BEFORE A FFTP IN WOMEN UNDER THE AGE OF 45

AUTHOR CHANGE	PERCENT CHANGE	YEAR	STUDY SIZE (RR) or Odds Ratio (OR)	FINDINGS
Brinton et al [3]	42% increase*	1990-1992	1648< 45 years old	1.42 OR (calculated)
Chie et al [5]	10% increase*	1993-1994	97 premenopausal	OR= 1.1 (0.2-5.5)
Chilvers [1]	2-51% increase	1982-1985	755 less than 36	1.02 RR for 0-4 yrs; 1.51 for 4-8 yrs; 1.44 > 8 yrs pFFTP
Clavel [6]	50% increase**	1983-1987	358 premenopausal	OR=1.5 (1.0-2.2)
Ewertz [7]	50% increase**	1983-1984	203 less than 40	1.50 (0.87-2.58)
Lee [8]	90% increase**	?1988-1990	about 100 premenopausal	1.9 (0.4-7.7)
McCredie et al [9]	20% decrease**	1992-1995	467 under 40	0.8 (0.6-1.0)
McPherson et al [10]	2-97% increase**	1980-1984	351<45	1.02 (0.5-1.9) 1-12 months pFFTP; 1.97 (1.0-3.8) for 1-4 yrs pFFTP; 2.59 (1.3-4.5) > 4 yrs pFFTP
Meirik et al [11]	0-100% increase	1984-1985	422 less than age 45	1.2 (0.8-1.7) 0-3 yrs; 1.0 (0.6-1.7) 4-7 yrs; 2.0 (1.8-4.2) > 8 yrs pFFTP
Miller et al [12]	100% increase	1983-1986	407 less than 45	2.0 (1.2-3.6)
Olsson [13]	80-110% increase	1979-1985	174 premenopausal	1.8 (1.0-3.2) for 0-3 yrs and 2.1 (1.1-3.8) for 4-7 yrs prior to FFTP
Palmer [14]	60-220% increase	1977-1992	219 less than 45 (black women)	3.2 (1.1-9.2) 0-3 yrs; 1.7 (0.5-5.5) 3-4 yrs: 1.6 (0.4-6.1) > 5 yrs pFFTP
Paul et al [15]	20% decrease**	1983-1987	155 less than 45 (severe stack effect)	0.80 (0.59-1.1)
Rohan et al [16]	93% increase**	1982-1984	113 premenopausal	1.93 (0.44-4.42) for > 19 months use prior to FFTP
Rookus et al [17]	250% increase***	1986-1989	132 less than 36	3.5 (p< 0.01) starting at or before age 19
Rosenberg et al [18]	88% increase*	1977-1992	1427 less than 45	OR = 1.88 (calculated)
Ursin et al [19]	36% decrease to 74% increase	1983-1988	742 less than age 40	OR= 0.64 (0.32-1.27) 1-12 months; 1.74 (0.75-4.03) > 13 months use pFFTP
Weinstein et al [20]	59% increase	1984-1986	about 326 less than or equal to 49	OR= 1.59 (1.02-2.47)
White et al [21]	50% increase***	1983-1990	747 < than 45 (suffers from stack effect)	OR= 1.5 (1.1-2.2) for > 1 yr use within 5 yrs of menarche (in parous women)
Wingo [22] CASH Study	40% increase	12/80-82	2089 less than age 45	1.40 (0.9-2.4) ages 20-34; 1.40 (1.1-1.8) ages 35-44

*Calculated from raw data. **This result reflects a trend toward an increased or decreased risk but does not attain statistical significance.

***FFTP in every study except Rookus and White who measure early OCP use in alternative ways.

The only two studies that showed an overall negative relationship were that of Paul et al [15] and McCredie [9]. The former study suffered from a huge stack effect having more than 6 times as many "controls" compared to "cases" in the 20 to 29 year-old age group (0.1035% vs. 0.0168%). The latter study found that women who had one child were at higher risk for breast cancer than nulliparous women, which raises concerns about the entire study. In addition, McCredie et al used the unconventional tactic of employing a p level greater than 0.05 to compute the data for risk of OCP use prior to a FFTP.

Q-9E: What about those women who used OCPs for a greater number of years prior to their FFTP?

We have already noted that Romieu [23] found a 72% increased risk [$RR=1.72$ (1.36-2.19)] in her meta-analysis from 1990 in women who took OCPs for 4 or more years before their FFTP. In addition, the *Brinton study [3] is significant in that she allowed a longer latent period to pass and found a 210% increased risk of developing breast cancer for young women (ie, under the age of 35) who took OCPs for more than 10 years and began before the age of 18.*

Q-9F: Do OCPs taken after a FFTP cause breast cancer in women under the age of 45, if we confine the studies to those that obtained most of their information after 1980?

We note in Table 9C that most studies whose data comes predominantly after 1980 still show some risk of developing breast cancer from OCP use after a FFTP but in general this does not appear to be as great as the risk of OCP use before a FFTP.

Table 9C:
BREAST CANCER RISK FROM USING OCPS AFTER A FIRST FULL-TERM PREGNANCY (FFTP)

AUTHOR	PERCENT CHANGE	YEAR	STUDY SIZE	FINDINGS (RR) or Odds Ratio (OR)
Brinton et al [3]	15% increase**	1990-1992	1648< 45 years old	OR = 1.15
Chie et al [5]	80% increase*	1993-1994	about 80 less than 45	OR=1.8 (0.7-5.5)
Chilvers et al [1]	23-97% increase	1984-1988	755 less than 36	1.23 for 0-4 yrs; 1.40 for 4-8 yrs; 1.97 for > 8 yrs
Ewertz [7]	no change	1983-1984	203 less than 40	1.00 (0.58-1.72)
McPherson et al [10]	29% decrease**	1980-1984	351 less than 45	OR = 0.71
Miller et al [12]	160% increase	1983-1986	407 less than 45	2.6 (1.5-4.5)
Palmer[14]	20-150% increase*	1977-1992	524 less than 45 (black women)	1.2 (0.6-2.1) < 3 yrs; 2.5 (1.2-5.3) 3-4 yrs; 1.7 (1.0-2.9) > 5 yrs
Rosenberg et al [18]	6% increase**	1977-1992	1427 less than 45	OR=1.06
Ursin et al [19]	30% decrease to 23% increase*	1983-1988	742 less than 40	OR= 0.70 (0.47-1.03) 1-48 months; 0.89 (0.54-1.47) 4-8 yrs; 1.23 (0.63-2.40) > 8 yrs
Weinstein et al [20]	29% increase*	1984-1986	about 326 less than or equal to 49	1.29 (0.89-1.88)
White et al [21]	0-17% increase*	1983-1990	747 less than 45	OR = 1.00 (0.73-1.37) to 1.17 (0.85-1.61)
Wingo [22] CASH Study	0-40% increase*	12/80-82	2089 less than 45	1.40 (0.8-2.4) in age 20-34; 1.0 (0.8-1.3) in age 35-44

* This result reflects a trend toward an increased or decreased risk but does not attain statistical significance.
** OR calculated from raw data; see end of this chapter for details.

Q-9G: How does the risk of taking OCPs before a FFTP compare to taking them after a FFTP?

Table 9D compares the risks of OCP use before a FFTP to after a FFTP. One will note that in general, taking OCPs prior to a FFTP carries a higher risk than taking them after a FFTP.

Table 9D:

COMPARISON OF RISKS OF DEVELOPING BREAST CANCER IN WOMEN WHO TOOK OCPS BEFORE OR AFTER THEIR FFTP

AUTHOR	YEAR	FINDINGS FOR RISK BEFORE FFTP	FINDINGS FOR RISK AFTER FFTP
Brinton et al [3]	1990-1992	42% increase	15% increase
Chie et al [5]	1993-1994	10% increase*	80% increase*
Chilvers [1]	1982-1985	2-51% increase	23-97% increase
Ewertz [7]	1983-1984	50% increase*	no change
McPherson et al [10]	1980-1984	2-97% increase*	29% decrease*
Miller et al [12]	1983-1986	100% increase	160% increase
Palmer[14]	1977-1992	60-220% increase*	20-150% increase*
Rosenberg et al [18]	1977-1992	88% increase	6% increase
Ursin et al [19]	1983-1988	36% decrease to 74% increase*	30% decrease to 23% increase*
Weinstein et al [20]	1984-1986	59% increase	29% increase*
White et al [21]	1983-1990	50% increase	0-17% increase*
Wingo [22] CASH Study	12/80-82	40% increase	0-40% increase

*This result reflects a trend toward an increased or decreased risk but does not attain statistical significance.

Q-9H: Do OCPs "as a whole," that is, when we compare "ever users" to "never users," cause breast cancer in women under the age of 45, when we confine the studies to those which obtained the bulk of their information after 1980?

We can see that the CASH study [22] found a 40% increased risk in women aged 20 to 34. Palmer [14], who studied young black women, found a 120% increased risk. Overall, Table 9E demonstrates clearly that the bulk of the studies since 1980, especially some of the larger ones, point to an increased risk for "ever" versus "never use."

Table 9E: BREAST CANCER RISKS OF EVER VS. NEVER USE OF OCPS IN WOMEN UNDER THE AGE OF 45

AUTHOR	PERCENT CHANGE	YEAR	STUDY SIZE	FINDINGS (RR) or Odds Ratio (OR)
Brinton et al [3]	27% increase*	1990-1992	1648< 45 years old	1.27 (1.1-1.5)
Chie et al [5]	60% increase*	1993-1994	about 80 less than 45	1.6 (0.7-3.8)
Chilvers et al [1]	6% decrease to 57% increase	1984-1988	755 less than 36	0.94 for 0-4 yrs; 1.42 for 4-8 yrs; 1.57 for > 8 yrs
Clavel [6]	50% increase	1983-1987	278 PREMENOPAUSAL	1.5 (1.1-2.1)
Ewertz [7]	18% increase*	1983-1984	203 less than 40	1.18 (0.73-1.91)
Gomes [24]	81% increase	1978-1987	71 < 43	1.81 (1.15-2.1)
La Vecchia [25]	30-90% increase	1991-1993	454 less than 45	OR = 1.3-1.9
Lee [8]	10% decrease	?1988-1990	About 100 PREMENOPAUSAL	0.9 (0.5-1.6)
Lee et al [26]	13% increase	1982-1984	64 less than age 44	OR = 1.13 (Costa Rican women)
Lund et al [27]	29% increase	1984-1985	422 less than 45	OR = 1.29 (calculated)
Mayberry [28]	40-100% increase	1980-1982	177 less than 40 (all black)	1.4 (1.0-1.9) < 5 years: 2.0 (1.1-3.6) > 5 years
McCredie et al [9]	4% increase	1992-1995	467 under 40	OR = 1.04
Miller et al [12]	100% increase	1983-1986	407 less than 45	2.0 (1.4-2.9)
Newcomb [29]	0-40% increase*	1988-1991	1050 < 45	1.4 (0.8-2.3) in women < 35; 1.0 (0.8-1.3) 35-44
Noonan et al [30]	26% increase*	1979-1984	301 less than 35	1.26 (0.95-1.66) severe stack effect
Palmer [14]	120% increase	1977-1992	184 less than 45 (black women)	2.2 (1.5-3.3)
Paul et al [15]	no change	1983-1987	489 PREMENOPAUSAL	1.0 (0.77-1.3) severe stack effect
Primic-Zakelj et al [31]	4% increase*	1988-1990	501 PREMENOPAUSAL	1.04 (0.80-1.37)
Rosenberg [32]	76% increase	1982-1986	79 less than 40 (Canadian women)	OR=1.76

Table 9E is continued on page 156

Table 9E continued

AUTHOR	PERCENT CHANGE	YEAR	STUDY SIZE	FINDINGS (RR) or Odds Ratio (OR)
Rosenberg et al [18]	10% decrease to 70% increase	1977-1992	1427 less than 45	1.7 (1.3-2.3) ages 25-34; 0.9 ((0.7-1.0) ages 35-44
Ursin et al [19]	17% decrease	1983-1988	742 less than age 40	OR= 0.83 (0.62-1.12)
Weinstein et al [20]	68% increase	1984-1986	about 326 less than or equal to 49	OR=1.68 (1.16-2.42)
White et al [21]	2% increase*	1983-1990	747 < than 45	OR=1.02 (0.71-1.48)
Wingo [22] CASH Study	10-40% increase*	12/80-82	2089 less than age 45	1.4 (1.1-2.1) in age 20-34; 1.1 (0.9-1.3) in ages 35-44.

*This result reflects a trend toward an increased or decreased risk but does not attain statistical significance.

Q-9I: Why does Table 9E exhibit that most studies show an increased risk, whereas the recent meta-analysis from Oxford [33] exhibited a far smaller effect?

The complex answer to this can be found in Appendix 4 (Commentary on the Oxford Oral Contraceptive Study). In short, *Table 9E shows the results of the studies which limit their focus to women who were less than 45 years old and obtained the bulk of their data after 1980.* The Oxford study combined the data from *old studies* (ie, before 1980) with data from new ones. The pattern of OCP use was far different in older studies: Women in the 1960s and early 1970s often took OCPs after their FFTP, whereas women in the late 1970s and 1980s started taking them earlier and for longer periods of time [34, p.9S]. In addition, studies before 1980 fail to allow an adequate latent period. Until a meta-analysis is done on the newer studies, the reader might be best served by making his or her own conclusions after reviewing Table 9E.

Table 9F:
BREAST CANCER RISK TO WOMEN WHO TOOK OCPS
FOR AT LEAST 4 YEARS PRIOR TO THE AGE OF 45

AUTHOR	PERCENT CHANGE	YEAR	STUDY SIZE	FINDINGS (RR) or Odds Ratio (OR)
Brinton et al [3]	27% increase*	1990-1992	1648< 45 years old	1.27 (1.0-1.6) > or = 5 yrs. of use
Chie et al [5]	250% increase*	1993-1994	about 80 less than 45	OR=3.5 (0.9-14.3)> or = to 5 yrs. of use
Chilvers [1] United Kingdom Study	43-74% increase	1/82-12/85	755 less than age 36	1.43 (0.97- 2.12) 4-8 yrs; 1.74 (1.15-2.62) for > 8 yrs. of use
La Vecchia [25]	30-60% increase	1991-1993	454 less than 45	OR= 1.3 (0.9-2.0) > 10 yrs use age < 35: OR= 1.6 (0.4-6.0) > 10 yrs. of use ages 35-44
McCredie RE et al [9]	16% increase	1992-1995	467 under 40	OR = 1.16 for > 5 yrs. of use
Mcpherson et al [15]	20-78% increase*	1980-1984	351<45	1.20 (0.78-1.84) 4-12 yrs of use; 1.78 (0.82-3.87) for > 12 yrs. of use
Meirik et al [11]	20-120% increase	1984-1985	422 less than 45	1.2 (0.8-1.0) 4-7 yrs; 1.4 (0.8-2.3) 8-11 yrs; 2.2 (1.2-4.0)> 12 yrs. of use
Miller et al [12]	90-310% increase	1983-1986	407 less than 45	1.9 (1.1-3.3) 5-9 yrs use: 4.1 (1.8-9.3) for more than 10 yrs. of use
Olsson [13]	100-110% increase	1979-1985	174 PREMENOPAUSAL	2.1 (1.1-3.8) 4-7 yrs pFFTP: 2.0 (0.8-4.7) > 8 yrs pFFTP

Table 9F is continued on page 158

Table 9F continued

AUTHOR	PERCENT CHANGE	YEAR	STUDY SIZE	FINDINGS (RR) or Odds Ratio (OR)
Paul et al [15]	0-130% increase*	1983-1987	388 less than 45	1.3 (0.41-4.0) 6-9 yrs in ages 25-34; 2.3 (0.67-7.8) 10-13 yrs ages 25-34; 1.0 (0.62-1.8) 6-9 yrs ages 35-44; 1.0 (0.59-1.8) 10-13 yrs ages 35-44
Rookus et al [17]	110% increase*	1986-1989	132 less than 36	2.1 (1.0-4.5) for 4 or more yrs
Rosenberg [18]	14% increase**	1977-1992	1427 less than 45	OR=1.14** raw for 5 or more years
Ursin et al [19]	29% decrease to 40% increase	1983-1988	742 less than age 40	OR= 0.71 (0.49-1.02) 4-8 yrs; 0.79 (0.52-1.18) 8-12 yrs; 1.40 (0.81-2.40) > 12 yrs.
Weinstein et al [20]	78% increase	1984-1986	about 326 less than or equal to 49	OR=1.78 (1.09-2.93) > 4 yrs
White et al [21]	32% increase*	1983-1990	747 < than 45	1.32 (0.92-1.88) for > 10 yrs use

*This result reflects a trend toward an increased or decreased risk but does not attain statistical significance.

**Calculated risks: see end of this chapter for details.

Q-9J: Do women who were under the age of 45 on or before 1995, and who took OCPs for a longer period of time (eg, 4 years or more), incur an increased risk for breast cancer when one looks at studies since 1980?

Table 9F clearly shows that when one reviews the studies whose data come predominantly after 1980, every one shows an increased trend or an actual statistically significant risk. Many of the studies, including Meirik et al [11], Paul et al [15], Rookus et al [17], and Miller et al [12] point to an increase of over 100% risk when OCPs were taken for a total of 10 to 12 years. The Oxford study did not reflect this risk because of its inclusion of older data that did not allow for a sufficient latent period.

Q-9K: What risks do nulliparous women take when ingesting oral contraceptive pills?

Most studies show a trend toward an increased risk of developing breast cancer. Paul et al's study results must be interpreted in light of both a severe stack effect and the death effect [15, p.367-8] rendering the results of this study extremely questionable.

Table 9G:

BREAST CANCER RISK FROM OCP USE IN NULLIPAROUS WOMEN UNDER THE AGE OF 45

AUTHOR	PERCENT CHANGE	YEAR	STUDY SIZE	FINDINGS (RR)
Chilvers [1]	2% decrease to 130% increase	1982-1985	755 less than 36	0.98 for 0-4 yrs 1.37 for 4-8 yrs 2.30 for > 8 yrs
Ewertz [7]	25% increase*	1983-1984	203 less than 40	1.25 (0.46-3.38)
Lund et al [27]	142% increase	1984-1985	422 less than 45	OR = 2.42 (calculated)
Miller et al [12]	60% increase*	1983-1986	407 less than 45	1.6 (0.8-3.1)
Palmer [14]	150-210% increase*	1977-1992	524 less than 45 (black women)	2.5 (0.5-13) 1-2 yrs: 3.1 (0.5-17) 3-4 yrs; 2.7 (0.8-8.9) > 5 yrs
Paul et al [15]	43% (decrease)*	1983-1987	345 less than 45 (comment: large stack effect)	0.57 (0.25-1.3)
Rosenberg [18]	12% increase*	1977-1992	1427 less than 45	OR=1.12 (calculated)
Ursin et al [19]	43% decrease to 20% increase	1983-1988	742 less than age 40	0.82 (0.5-1.33) 1-4 yrs; 0.57 (0.32-1.02) 4-8 yrs: 0.58 (0.31-1.08) 8-12 yrs; 1.20 (0.58-2.48) > 12 yrs
Wingo [22] CASH Study	0-50% increase*	12/80-82	2089 less than age 45	1.5 (0.8-2.7) ages 20-34; 1.0 (0.7-1.6) ages 35-44

*This result reflects a trend toward an increased or decreased risk but does not attain statistical significance.

The increased overall risk shown by the remaining studies is especially significant for another reason. When a study such as that of Chilvers [1] notes an increased risk of 130% for nulliparous women who have taken OCPs for

more than 8 years, *this represents the increased risk of
these women compared to other nulliparous women* and
not the female population in general. In other words,
women who are nulliparous and have used OCPs for more
than 8 years would experience a 2.3-fold risk compared to
other nulliparous women, *but an even higher risk when
compared to the general population* because nulliparity itself is a risk factor which confers about a 2-fold risk [35].
The combination of nulliparity and an 8-year length of exposure would result in an estimated increase of 4.6 (ie, 2.3
x 2.0) which is a 360% increased risk of developing breast
cancer compared to the general population. This phenomenon was also supported by the finding of another author
of CASH, Bruce Stadel [36, p.288], who pointed out that
nulliparous women aged 20 to 44 who had menarche before age 13 and had used OCPs for 8 to 11 years had a
170% increased risk of developing breast cancer, and if
they used them for 12 or more years they had a 1080% increased risk! In addition, special note should be taken of
Palmer's study [14] which pointed to a very high risk for
black nulliparous women.

Q-9L: Does OCP use after the age of 25 increase the risk of breast cancer in those studies which acquired data since 1980?

Table 9H shows that every study which looked at late
OCP use (ie, after the age of 25) showed an elevated trend
or risk, which increased markedly as the length of time of
total OCP use increased. Although Table 9H lists only a
few studies, the reader will note that in general the degree
of increased risk is not small by any means, with some of
them showing over a 140% increase.

Table 9H:
BREAST CANCER RISK TO WOMEN
WHO TOOK OCPS AFTER THE AGE OF 25

AUTHOR	PERCENT CHANGE	YEAR	STUDY SIZE	FINDINGS
Lund et al [27]	50% increase	1984-1985	422 less than 45	OR = 1.50 (calculated)
Noonan [30]	42% increase	1979-1984	Estimate 600 under age 45	1.42 (1.04-1.58) use after age 35
Olsson [13]	60% increase	1979-1985	174 premenopausal	1.6 (0.9-2.7)
Palmer [14]	0-140% increase	1977-1992	524 less than 45 (black women)	1.0 (0.4-2.5) < 3 yrs; 2.4 (1.3-4.6) > 3 yrs after age 25
Paul et al [37]	170% increase*	1983-1987	891 women aged 25-54*	2.7 (0.97-7.5) for 10 yrs use after age 40
Rosenberg [18]	14% increase*	1977-1992	1427 less than 45	OR=1.14 (calculated)
Rosenberg [32]	no change	1982-1986	79 less than 40 (Canadian women)	OR=1.00 (calculated)
Wang et al [38]	160-300% increase	1985-1986	300 aged 20-55	2.6 (1.2-5.8), < 2 yrs after 35; 4.0 (1.1-15.1) > 2 yrs after 35
Weinstein et al [20]	32% increase	1984-1986	about 326 less than or equal to 49	OR=1.32 (0.87-2.00)
Yuan et al [39]	300% increase	1984-1985	about 200 less than 45	4.0 (1.15-16.59) for use after age 45

*This result reflects a trend toward an increased risk but does not attain statistical significance.

Q-9M: Why do each of the tables show a higher risk of breast cancer than most of the public might be aware of?

Most patients get their information on oral contraceptive pill risks from four main sources: 1) their physician, 2) their pharmacist, 3) the drug insert (ie, from the pharmaceutical company), and 4) from the lay press.

The average physician is often very busy, and he or she often relies on conferences and/or the most popular journal articles to keep him or her updated. Unfortunately, as you may have noticed, information regarding the field of OCP use and its link to breast cancer is found in literally hundreds of medical journal articles and is a complex area. So, although individual physicians should know about this link, most do not. Of course, that does not excuse physicians because any physician ought to be familiar with the dangers of any hormones he/she prescribes. The excuse that "I just followed the practices of my colleagues" will become unacceptable as patients become familiar with the information contained in this book and present it to their physicians and nurses.

Pharmacists have routinely failed to inform patients about the link between OCP use and breast cancer. Part of the reason is that no pharmacist can tell every patient about every side effect. However, this does not mean they should be ignorant of the risks of OCP use, especially in young women. Perhaps this will change as people bring this to their pharmacist's attention.

Pharmaceutical companies do include a drug insert with every drug they manufacture and they do state that: "Some studies have reported an increased relative risk of developing breast cancer particularly at a young age. This increased relative risk appears to be related to duration of use" [40]. *This, however, is hopelessly inadequate because few patients ever read the fine print of their drug inserts and the drug companies know it.* Drug companies have a responsibility to print this birth control risk information in large bold print. Until now, they have been *grossly negligent* in adequately stressing the danger of early OCP use.

The lay press has also paid little attention to this issue but cannot be totally accountable because they literally must rely on the words of "the experts." Unfortunately, many of today's "research experts" are hopelessly dependent on and/or fearful of the biases of their financial supporters (ie, usually the federal government) who cannot be presumed to be unbiased. At the very least, and especially in light of the millions of lives at stake, the scientific community should respond aggressively and candidly to the concerns documented in this book. The evidence can no longer be ignored.

Q-9N: Are there any data from the largest studies that young women who took OCPs more than 10 years ago have an increased risk?

Table 9I:
BREAST CANCER RISKS FROM OCP USE
15-20 YEARS SINCE FIRST USE

STUDY→	BRINTON [3] WOMEN LESS THAN AGE 35	PALMER [14]* BLACK WOMEN LESS THAN 45	MILLER [12]** WOMEN LESS THAN 45	ROSENBERG [18]: WOMEN AGED 25-34
YEAR OF INTERVIEW	1990-1992	1977-1992	1983-1986	1977-1992
INTERVAL SINCE FIRST USE OF OCP				
< 10 YEARS				1.6 (1.1-2.3) = 60%
10-14 YEARS	1.63 (1.1-2.5)=63%			1.8 (1.3-2.6) = 80%
15-19 YEARS	2.02 (1.2-3.4)=102%	2.6 (1.5-4.6) = 160%		1.9 (1.0-3.5) = 90%
>= 20 YEARS	3.01 (0.3-34.9) = 201%***	2.0 (1.0-4.3) = 100%***	6.0 (1.6-22) = 500%	

*In women who used OCPs for more than 3 years.
**In women who used OCPs for more than 5 years.
***This result reflects a trend toward an increased risk but does not attain statistical significance.

Brinton et al [3] noted that young women have a 63-102% statistically significant increased risk of developing breast cancer 14 to 19 years after first OCP use, and a 201% statistically insignificant risk 20 or more years after original OCP use. Rosenberg [18] et al noted similar risks in young women up to 19 years after first OCP use. Miller et al [12] noted an even higher risk 20 years after first use of OCPs and Palmer [14] reported that black women also have elevated risks. *In summary, these results give doctors who gave their patients OCPs reason to be extremely concerned, because every one of the four studies pointed to at least a 90% increased risk of developing breast cancer as one approaches a 20-year latent period.*

Q-9O: If these four studies show an increased risk almost 20 years after women first began their use of OCPs, why do some people continue to claim that OCPs have no long-term risk?

As you will note, the information from the Brinton and Rosenberg studies was confined to women under the age of 35. The trend toward an increased risk 15 years after first use is not as strong in the older age groups in these two studies. There is a good reason for this. Women who were the age of 35 or less in the late 1980s or early 1990s (when the latter two studies obtained their data) would have been far more likely to have used OCPs prior to their FFTP than women in their mid to late forties. The young women under the age of 35 represent a group of women who statistically had far higher and longer OCP use prior to their FFTP than older women. In addition, one must also note that both Miller and Palmer did study women under the age of 45 and found statistically significant elevated risks.

Q-9P: What should doctors be telling their patients regarding the long-term risks of breast cancer from OCP use among young women (under the age of 35)?

At this point doctors need to inform their patients that the studies which looked at the risk of OCP use in young women after almost 20 years since their first use, found statistically significant increases in breast cancer risk of 90% or higher.

Q-9Q: Do women who take OCPs for "irregular cycles" or acne have a higher incidence of breast cancer or other cancers?

This author found no study on this specific group of women although there is every reason to suspect that OCPs would raise the risk of breast and cervical cancer in this group of women as much as it does in other women. However, Dr. Grimes [41] did note that women who took OCPs to regulate their cycles had an increased risk of pituitary adenoma (ie, specifically "prolactinomas" — a type of tumor of the pituitary gland). For example, Shy et al [42] noted that women who took OCPs for irregular cycles had a 670% increased risk of developing prolactinomas: [*RR*= 7.7: (3.7-17.0)]. This should be taken seriously because at least one progestin has been noted to cause growth of the pituitary gland in rats [43]. Young women frequently have irregular cycles and do not necessarily require medical treatment.

Q-9R: *What are the medical alternatives for controlling painful menstrual cramps besides OCPs?*

Menstrual cramps can be controlled by less harmful drugs than OCPs. For example, taking 1,000 mg of Calcium and 399 mg of Magnesium around the time of a woman's onset of menstrual bleeding appears to help with menstrual cramps and migraine headaches. In addition, taking high dose anti-inflammatory agents (eg, ibuprofen) *after* one's menstrual flow has started (and under a doctor's care) will often give relief. Also, the *Journal of Adolescent Medicine* published a case report of a young lady who experienced a 90% reduction in her cramping symptoms when taking Nicardipine *after* her menstrual cramps had begun [37]. Nicardipine is a type of calcium channel blocker that is used for treating hypertension.

Q-9S: *Do women who take OCPs have a higher risk of bilateral breast cancer?*

Ursin et al [45] studied this specific question. They studied 144 "cases" and noted that women who had taken OCPs for more than 1 year had a 70% trend toward an increased risk of developing bilateral breast cancer [1.7 (1.0-2.9)]. When this analysis was restricted to parous women only, the trend toward an increased risk rose to 110% [*RR* = 2.1 (1.0-4.4)].

Q-9T: *Women who take OCPs may have a later age of first birth, thus having two risk factors for breast cancer. Is it possible that researchers have mistakenly attributed the risk of using OCPs to that of an older age at first birth?*

When two factors can both influence the same effect (ie, breast cancer), one must be careful to distinguish between them. Fortunately, almost every major study since the late 1970s has adjusted for age at first birth, thus, clearly separating its effect and the effect of early OCP use.

The converse situation exists with OCP use and the risk factor of family history. Because women with very strong family histories of breast cancer might be less likely to use OCPs — and thus underestimate the relative risk for OCP use — one might think that these risks would be difficult to distinguish. Almost every good study adjusts for the risk factors of family history, except for certain prospective studies [eg, 46, 47].

Q-9U: Does use of the minipill (ie, the OCP that contains only progestin) cause breast cancer?

No one is really sure, although these pills often contain norgestrel (eg, Ovrette) and therefore could carry similar risks. The Oxford study noted an overall increased trend of 19% (ie, 1.19 [0.89-1.49]) in women who had taken progestin-only OCPs for 4 or more years, but this says little about extended use in young women, especially before their FFTP [34, p.98S]. Analysis from the New Zealand study [48] noted that women who had taken progestin only OCPs before age 25 had a 1.5-fold risk (0.73-2.9), although the result did not achieve statistical significance. It must again be noted that the risks for early use prior to a FFTP are most likely quite a bit higher, and as of today, there is no good reason to believe that the oral progestins are any less dangerous than the combination OCPs.

Q-9V: Do women who have used OCPs early in life develop more aggressive breast cancers?

Yes, as noted earlier by Olsson: "these results indicate that the rate of tumor cell proliferation is higher in patients with breast cancer who have used oral contraceptives at an early age or who at a young age have had an abortion performed early in the woman's reproductive life. . ." [49, p.1288-9]. Schonborn et al [50] observed that women who took OCPs had a higher percentage of poorly differentiated tumors. Ranstam et al have also noted that the survival rate of women who have used oral contraceptives — especially at an early age — was less than those who did not use OCPs or used them at later ages [51, p.2044]. It was also noted that women who used OCPs early in their reproductive lives had larger tumors than women who did not use OCPs [52, 267]. The same study found that women who had used OCPs early in life had a significantly lower concentration of estrogen and progesterone receptors on their tumor cells [In general, the lower the concentration of estrogen and progesterone receptors of a breast cancer cell, the worse the prognosis and response to treatment. The converse is also true — the higher the concentration of estrogen or progesterone receptors, the better the prognosis]. "The studies suggest that hormone receptors of the primary tumor are permanently reduced after early OCP use in a dose-dependent manner (the earlier the use, the lower the receptor)." [52, p.1991]. Olsson et al [53] also noted that women who had used OCPs at an early age (ie, on or before the age of 20) had a 5.3-fold risk of having "amplification of Her-2/neu." Her-2/neu is a type of oncogene that is associated with larger tumors, high tumor grade, advanced tumor stage, and an absence of steroid receptors [53, p.1483].

Kooy et al [54] noted that women who used oral contraceptives for more than 9 years had a 2.5-fold (1.4-4.4) increased risk for developing p53+ tumors. Over expression of the p53 gene is commonly regarded as evidence of the presence of a p53 mutation which has been associated with breast cancer. Therefore the question to be answered is: Does long-term use of OCPs act as an oncogene activator by causing over expression of the p53 gene?

Other evidence comes from the Oxford study which found that women who took OCPs before the age of 20 and had used them within the last 5 years had a higher incidence of *local* and *distal* breast cancer. (Local [regional] breast cancer is cancer that is confined to the breast, whereas distal breast cancer means cancer that has spread from its original site. Distal breast cancer is also called <u>metastatic</u> breast cancer). They also noted that women who took OCPs after the age of 20 had a slightly higher risk of regional breast cancer and a slightly lower risk of distal breast cancer [34, p.83S]. Of course this is a critical difference, especially when one notes that most of today's young women are taking OCPs before their FFTP, which is precisely the time interval that correlates with an increased risk of both local and distal breast cancer.

Q-9W: Do women with breast cancer who took OCPs at an early age have a worse prognosis than those who never took them or who took them at a late age?

It would appear that they do. Ranstam et al [51] noted that "cases" who used OCPs before the age of 20 had a 62% 5-year survival rate, whereas "cases" who had never used them or took them after the age of 25 had an 86% 5-year survival rate [51, p.2043].

Q-9X: Do women who have the BRCA1 or BRCA2 oncogene and have taken OCPs have a greater risk of getting breast cancer than women who have the oncogene but have never taken OCPs?

Ursin et al [55] have noted that "Long-term OC use (>48 months) before a FFTP was associated with an elevated risk of being classified as a mutBRCA carrier," (odds ratio 7.8, p=0.004). In other words, if two groups of women both had a mutation of the BRCA gene, then if one group used OCPs for 4 years or more before their FFTP, that group would have a 680% increased risk of getting breast cancer. This is important for Jewish women who have a far higher frequency of carrying a defective BRCA1 gene.

Q-9Y: In light of all the evidence presented, why has the Food and Drug Administration (FDA) continued to allow OCPs to be sold with very little warning, and why do most physicians and pharmacists rarely stress the risk of the OCP causing breast cancer?

The FDA is usually extremely conservative as concerns the approval of new drugs and warnings of their dangers, yet it has failed to pull OCPs off the market despite the evidence. Perhaps the FDA will reconsider this in light of testimony this author recently presented* and the fact that this book has been submitted to the FDA as part of the public record.

*Proceedings of the FDA: *Over-The-Counter Products*. Gaithersburg, Maryland; June 28, 2000. Presenter: Chris Kahlenborn, M.D.: *The Pill and Breast Cancer.*

Physicians and pharmacists should certainly warn their patients about the increased risk of breast cancer. Both financial incentives and an attitude of "medical correctness" may contribute to the failure of physicians, pharmacists, and drug companies to adequately warn their patients. This is unfortunate in light of the proven effectiveness of natural methods of child spacing. (See question 9Z). Until these groups are effectively confronted by the laity or start to lose law suits, little will change. The only way to promote positive change is to present them with the evidence.

Q-9Z: Why have so few couples used Natural Family Planning?

Natural Family Planning (NFP) — methods of family planning based on measurements of cervical mucus viscosity (and basal body temperature for some methods) — has been criticized widely, probably more out of bias and ignorance than an informed opinion. Several good trials have shown that NFP has an effectiveness rate that is on par with OCPs — that is, less than a 3% rate of pregnancies per year. These trials have been done in both industrialized and less advanced countries and have shown low annual pregnancy rates: the United Kingdom — 2.7% [56]; Germany — 2.3% [57]; Belgium — 1.7% [58]; India — 2.0% [59]; Liberia — 4.3% [60]; and China — 4.4% [61]. In addition, "the largest natural family planning study combined effective teaching with high motivation and showed that natural family planning can be extremely effective in the Third World. The study was of 19,843 predominantly poor women in Calcutta, 52% Hindu, 27% Muslim, and 21% Christian. Because of poverty, motivation was high both among the users and among the well trained teachers of natural family planning. The failure rate was similar to that with the combined oral contraceptive pill — 0.2 pregnancy per 100 woman yearly." [62]. (Note: The recent review study by Potter noted a typical failure rate of 7% for women who take OCPs [63]). *Perhaps the greatest reason that so few know of or have used NFP is that there is no economic force behind it.* If couples were to use NFP, drug companies, physicians, pharmacists, and family planning agents such as Planned Parenthood would all suffer financially. Why NFP use in countries such as China, Brazil and other developing countries is not more common, especially given its lack of side effects and monetary advantages over conventional contraception, remains a mystery.

Addendum 9A:

[The following questions have answers that *contain more complex material* and may be omitted without a loss of continuity]

Q-9A1: Does use of oral contraceptives which contain a higher amount of the estrogen hormone have a higher propensity to cause breast cancer?

No one is sure, but so far only a few studies point to an increased risk with higher estrogen or progestin doses, and a number of studies actually show the reverse trend. Most oral contraceptives contained 50 micrograms of ethinyl estradiol in the 1970s, but in the 1980s the "low dose" brands that contained 35 micrograms were increasingly used. Today both types are used, in addition to the more recent "super-low" OCPs which contain 20 micrograms of synthetic estrogen. Although researchers originally claimed that use of the higher dose OCPs caused more breast cancer, several studies since then have contradicted this. Rookus and Leeuwen [17] noted that women who took OCPs for more than 12 years had a 1.2 RR if their brand of OCP contained more than 50 micrograms of estrogen and a 2.9 RR if the OCP had less than 50 micrograms. Thomas et al [64] noted that women who took low dose OCPs for more than 5 years had a 1.69 RR (1.20-2.38) compared to a 1.32 RR (0.96-1.84) for those women who had taken high dose OCPs. Ursin et al [45] noted that women who used OCPs with a low mestranol content (ie, a type of estrogen) had more than twice the risk of those who used OCPs with the medium-dose mestranol content. The strongest evidence, however, comes from the Oxford study, the largest meta-analysis to date concerning OCPs. Surprisingly, it showed a small, non-statistically significant *increase* in risk as the estrogen content of an OCP was *decreased* in women who had taken OCPs more than 10 years ago [34, p.94S]. It also showed an *increased* risk (non-significant) for women who took the *lower* dose triphasic pills compared to those who took the conventional higher dose monophasic pills in the group of women who had taken them more than 10 years ago [34, p.87S]. Women who had taken high dose OCPs more than 10 years ago had less metastatic breast cancer than women who had used low-dose OCPs more than 10 years ago [34, p.96S].

Q-9A2: Will the dose of estrogen in the OCP affect the results of future studies?

No one knows if the lower dose OCPs will be more or less dangerous than higher dose OCPs in the long run. It was noted that some authors have actually found an increased risk for breast cancer in women who used the lower dose estrogen pill and that the Oxford meta-analysis supported this finding in certain subgroups. Brinton's findings also lend support to the finding that low dose OCPs appear to carry a significant risk. In her study, which showed a calculated odds ratio of 42% for women who had used OCPs prior to their FFTP, she noted: "It is doubtful, however, that the relationship will be explained by use of higher dose preparations, since the majority of these younger women would have initiated pill use during an era when both estrogen and progestin doses would have been reduced."[3, p.834]. As the low dose OCPs' estrogen content drops even lower (ie, some now contain 20 micrograms of estrogen), OCPs will cause an even higher number of early abortions because the rate of breakthrough ovulation will increase. Whether a very early abortion could affect the risk of breast cancer will not be known until the physiology of very early pregnancy is understood better, as was noted in the answer to question 8D.

Q-9A3: Are OCPs which contain a potent progestin more dangerous than those with a low potency progestin?

Many studies are finding that the progestin component may actually be the main factor in breast cancer formation, either through a compound effect with estrogen or by an independent process. OCPs contain more modern and potent progestins today and no one really knows if they will be more dangerous, although two studies raise exactly that suspicion. White et al noted that women who took OCPs with a high potency progestin had a 50% increased risk of breast cancer compared to women who took OCPs that contained a low potency progestin. [21, p.509]. Pike et al [65] noted that women who took high potency progestin OCPs before the age of 25 had a far greater risk (ie, infinite risk [2.0 - infinity]) of developing breast cancer than those who took the low potency progestin OCPs [RR=4.9 (1.9-13.4)]. This is especially significant in that the most common types of OCPs used to date, according to information from the Oxford meta-analysis [34, p.88S], use the combination of estradiol and a very high potency progestin (according to Pike [65] named norgestrel (eg, Ovral).

Q-9A4: What about the risks for developing breast cancer in women who took higher vs. lower dose progestins 10 years ago?

The Oxford study showed no difference in women who had taken a high versus a low dose progestin called norethisterone when they had used it more than 10 years ago [34, p.92S].

Q-9A5: In addition to possibly causing a higher rate of breast cancer, does use of OCPs which contain high dose progestins cause a more aggressive type of breast cancer?

Several studies support this statement. "Recent or current use (at time of diagnosis), use of progestin-predominant oral contraceptives, or use before age 20 may increase risk of estrogen receptor negative tumors." [66, p.1118]. (Estrogen receptor negative tumors generally have a worse prognosis than estrogen positive tumors). In addition, Olsson has noted that these same type of progestin OCPs lead to tumors which have much higher INT2 levels than tumors in women who did not take these OCPs [53, p.1486]. A breast cell's INT2 level is felt to be of prognostic importance; in general, the higher it is, the poorer the patient's prognosis.

Q-9A6: Until this point, retrospective studies have been analyzed. Why did this author separate the prospective studies from the retrospective?

The Oxford study gives a complete list of the ten prospective studies which had been done before 1996. In general, these studies cannot be easily analyzed in regard to the OCP/breast cancer link for several reasons: 1) *they examine older patients* — that is, they rarely subdivide their data into age groups that look specifically at those women who are less than the age of 45 on or before 1995. Including older women means that they would have had little access to early OCP use, which makes it almost impossible to measure this variable; 2) *a high drop-out rate*. It is not unusual for a prospective study to lose thousands of participants along the way, due either to apathy or patients moving away, or due to the death of the patients from disease including breast cancer; 3) *a short follow-up period*. Often a prospective study will allow 10 years or less of follow-up time, such as Calle's study [67]. This is hardly enough of a latent period to show much effect. 4) In addition, prospective studies may suffer from "follow-up differentiation," in which the *"cohort" (ie, the women who have either had an abortion or have taken the OCP) are followed up for far shorter periods of time than the "controls"* as is noted in Appendix 1: Q-A1B. A prospective study starts out with thousands of women but only a small percent ever develop breast cancer. Vessey et al studied 17,032 women, 72 of whom developed breast cancer in the 35 to 47 year-old age group [68]. It is obviously difficult to make conclusions based on such a small study size; 5) *a post-menopausal population.* Several of the prospective studies looked at hormone use in post-menopausal women. Because this population involves older women, most of whom are far older than the age of 45, it has little relevance to the question of OCP risk in women under the age of 45; and 6) *a failure to adjust for other variables.* Many prospective studies do not ask their participants about their history of abortion, alcohol use, or even family history. This certainly reduces the accuracy of a study, especially when one notes that all three of the former variables are important risk factors.

Q-9A7: What did the prospective studies show?

Several of the studies confined themselves to the population of post-menopausal women (Hiatt [69], Mills [70], and Schuurman [71]). Two of the studies made no mention of OCP risk at all (Miller [12], Hiatt [69]). The remaining six studies usually showed non-specific risks due to limitations of the study. Some of the relevant findings include: 1) Calle et al [67]: In their cohort of 676,530 several hundred developed breast cancer. It was noted that women who had a family history of breast cancer and used OCP's had a relative risk of 2.82 — this was statistically significant although no age group was given; 2) Vessey et al [68] found no specific relationship between OCP use and breast cancer but only studied 72 women between the ages of 25 and 44 years old;   3) Alexander [72] noted a 4.83 relative risk (1.97-11.87) to women aged 45 to 54 years old who took OCPs for more than 1 year versus women who took it for less than 1 year; 4) In a study of Seventh Day Adventists, Mills [70] found that women who used OCPs post-menopausally had a relative risk of 1.54 (0.94-2.53) compared to nonusers; 5) Kay et al [73] found a 3.33 RR in "ever" versus "never" use in women aged 30 to 34 years old who had breast cancer; and 6) Romieu [74] found a RR of 1.06 (0.96-1.18) for all users of OCPs, noting that the average age of the patients was well over 45. She also noted that patients who were taking OCPs "currently" had a 1.53 (1.06-2.19) increased risk. The Oxford meta-analysis found a 1.15 relative risk in its summary of all the prospective studies for women who used OCPs within 5 years of having their breast cancer diagnosed [34, p.44S].

Q-9A8: Can you summarize the results of the prospective studies?

Yes. In general, the information that can be gathered from prospective studies in regard to early OCP use and the risk of breast cancer before the age of 45 is very limited due to the reasons given. Several of the studies do show increased risks in specific categories, but this is usually in slightly older women. One study [ie, Kay et al, 73] did show a specific statistically significant risk in a specific age group — women aged 30 to 34 with breast cancer.

Addendum:

Rosenberg calculated risks for women who took OCPs for at least 4 years:

"Cases" and "controls" aged 25-44 who had more than 5 years of OCP use were 23+21+34+85= 163, and 30+47+39+149=265 respectively, versus 547 "cases" and 1014 "controls" who had less than 1 year's use of OCPs. The OR (odds ratio) is therefore: 163/547 divided by 265/1014, yielding a 1.14 or 14% increased risk for women who took OCPs for 5 or more years despite a severe stack effect.

Calculation of OR for OCP use after a FFTP for the Brinton [3] and Rosenberg studies [18]:

Brinton noted that 82+45+38+75= 240 "cases" and 69+50+35+92= 246 "controls" used OCPs for at least 6 months or more after a FFTP, whereas 389 "cases" and 431 "controls" had less than 6 months of OCP use prior to the age of 25. The OR would be:

240/389 divided by 246/431=1.08 or an 8% increased risk.

In the Rosenberg study, the number of women aged 25 to 44 years old with and without breast cancer who used OCPs for more than 1 year after a FFTP was 36+21+134+85=276 (ie, "cases") and 102+47+186+149 =484 (ie, "controls"), whereas 547 "cases" and 1014 "controls" used OCPs for less than 1 year. The estimated relative risk is therefore: 276/547 divided by 484/1014 which yield an OR of 1.06 (ie, a 6% increased risk).

References:

1. Chilvers C, McPherson K, et al. Oral contraceptive use and breast cancer risk in young women (UK National Case-Control Study Group). *The Lancet.* May 6, 1989: 973-982.

2. Pike MC, Henderson BE, et al. Oral contraceptive use and early abortion as risk factors for breast cancer in young women. *Br J Cancer.* 1981; 43: 72-76.

3. Brinton LA, Daling JR, et al. Oral contraceptives and breast cancer risk among younger women. *J Natl Cancer Inst.* 6/7/1995; 87: 827-35.

4. Ravnihar B, et al. A case-control study of breast cancer in relation to oral contraceptive use in Slovenia. *Neoplasma.* 1988; 35: 109-121.

5. Chie, et al. Oral contraceptive and breast cancer risk in Taiwan, a country of low incidence of breast cancer and low use of oral contraceptives. *Int J Cancer.* 1998; 77: 219-223.

6. Clavel F, Andrieu N, et al. Oral contraceptives and breast cancer: A French case-control study. *Int J Epidemiol.* 1991; 20: 32-38.

7. Ewertz M. Oral contraceptives and breast cancer risk in Denmark. *Eur J Cancer.* 1992; 28A: 1176-1181.

8. Lee HP, Gourley L, et al. Risk factors for breast cancer by age and menopausal status: a case-control study in Singapore. *Cancer Causes and Control.* 1992; 3: 313-322.

9. McCredie MER, et al. Breast cancer in Australian women under age of 40. *Cancer Causes and Control.* 1998; 9: 189-198.

10. McPherson K, Vessey MP, et al. Early oral contraceptive use and breast cancer: Results of another case-control study. *Br J Cancer.* 1987; 56: 653-660.

11. Meirik O, Lund E, Adami HO, et al. Oral contraceptive use and breast cancer in young women. *The Lancet.* Sept. 20, 1986: 650-653.

12. Miller D, Rosenberg L, et al. Breast cancer before age 45 and oral contraceptive use: new findings. *Am J Epidemiol.* 1989; 129: 269-279.

13. Olsson H, Moller TR, Ranstam J. Early contraceptive use and breast cancer among premenopausal women: Final report from a study in southern Sweden. *J Natl Cancer Inst.* 1989; 81: 1000-1004.

14. Palmer J, Rosenberg L, et al. Oral contraceptives use and breast cancer risk among African-American women. *Cancer Causes and Control.* 1995; 6: 321-331.

15. Paul C, Skegg DC, et al. Oral contraceptives and risk of breast cancer. *Int J Cancer.* 1990; 46: 366-373.

16. Rohan T, McMichael A. Oral contraceptive agents and breast cancer: a population-based case-control study. *The Medical Journal of Australia.* 1988; 149: 520-526.

17. Rookus MA, Leeuwen FE. Oral contraceptives and risk of breast cancer in women ages 20-54 years. *The Lancet.* 1994; 344: 844-851.

18. Rosenberg L, Palmer JR, et al. Case-control study of oral contraceptive use and risk of breast cancer. *Am J Epidemiol.* 1996; 143: 25-37.

19. Ursin RK, et al. Use of oral contraceptives and risk of breast cancer in young women. *Breast Cancer Research and Treatment.* 1998; 50: 175-184.

20. Weinstein A, Mahoney M, et al. Breast cancer risk and oral contraceptive use: results from a large case-control study. *Epidemiology.* 1991; 2: 353-358.

21. White E, Malone K, Weiss N, Daling J. Breast cancer among young U.S. women in relation to oral contraceptive use. *J Natl Cancer Inst.* 1994; 86: 505-514.

22. Wingo PA, Lee NC, et al. Age-specific differences in the relationship between oral contraceptives use and breast cancer. *Cancer* (supplement). 1993; 71: 1506-17

23. Romieu I, Berlin J, et al. Oral contraceptives and breast cancer. Review and meta-Analysis. *Cancer.* 1990; 66: 2253-2263.

24. Gomes L, Guimaraes M, et al. A case-control study of risk factors for breast cancer in Brazil, 1978-1987. *Int J Epidemiol.* 1995; 24: 292-299.

25. La Vecchia C, Negri E, et al. Oral contraceptives and breast cancer: A cooperative Italian study. *Int J Cancer.* 1995; 60: 163-167.

26. Lee NC, Rosero-Bixby L, et al. A case-control study of breast cancer and hormonal Contraception in Costa Rica. *J Natl Cancer Inst.* 1987; 6: 1247-1254.

27. Lund E, et al. Oral contraceptive use and premenopausal breast cancer in Sweden and Norway: Possible effects of different pattern of use. *Int J Epidemiol.* 1989; 18: 527-532.

28. Maybery RM. Age-specific patterns of association between breast cancer and risk factors in black women, ages 20 to 39 and 40 to 54. *Ann Epidemiol.* 1994; 4: 205-213.

29. Newcomb PA, Longnecker MP, et al. Recent oral contraceptive use and risk of breast cancer (United States). *Cancer Causes and Control.* 1996; 7: 525-532.

30. Thomas DB, Noonan EA. Breast cancer and combined oral contraceptives: results from a multinational study (The WHO collaborative study of Neoplasia and steroid contraceptives). *Br J Cancer.* 1990; 61: 110-119.

31. Primic-Zakelj, et al. Breast-Cancer risk and oral contraceptive use in Slovenian Women aged 25-54. *Int J Cancer.* 1995; 62: 414-420.

32. Rosenberg L, Palmer JR, et al. A case-control study of the risk of breast cancer in relation to oral contraceptive use. *Am J Epidemiol.* 1992; 136: 1437-1444.

33. Collaborative Group on Hormonal Factors in Breast Cancer. Breast cancer and hormonal contraceptives: collaborative reanalysis of individual data on 53,297 women with breast cancer and 100,239 women without breast cancer from 54 epidemiological studies. *The Lancet.* 1996; 347: 1713-1727.

34. Collaborative Group on Hormonal Factors in Breast Cancer. Breast cancer and hormonal contraceptives: further results. *Contraception.* 1996; 34: S1-S106.
35. Kelsey J. A review of the epidemiology of human breast cancer. *Epidemiologic Reviews.* 1979; 1: 74-109.
36. Stadel BV, Lai S, et al. Oral contraceptives and premenopausal breast cancer in nulliparous women. *Contraception.* 1988; 38: 287-299.
37. Paul C, Skegg C, et al. Oral contraceptive use and risk of breast cancer in older women (New Zealand). *Cancer Causes and Control.* 1995; 6: 485-491.
38. Wang Q, Ross R, et al. A case-control study of breast cancer in Tianjin, China. *Cancer Epidemiology.* 1992; 1: 435-439.
39. Yuan J, Yu M, et al. Risk factors for breast cancer in Chinese women in Shanghai. *Cancer Research.* 1988; 48: 1949-1953.
40. Schlesselman J, Stadel B, et al. Breast cancer detection in relation to oral contraception. *J Clin Epidemiol.* 1992; 45: 449-459.
41. Grimes DA. Neoplastic effects of oral contraceptives. *Int J Fertility.* 36; 1991: 19-24.
42. Shy KK, et al. Oral contraceptive use and the occurrence of pituitary prolactinoma. *JAMA.* 1983; 249: 2204-2207.
43. Benagiano G. Long-acting systemic contraceptives. In: Diczfalusy E. ed. *Regulation of Human Fertility.* Copenhagen: Scriptor; 1977: 323-360.
44. Earl DT, et al. Calcium channel blockers and dysmenorrhea. *Journal of Adolescent Medicine.* 1992; 13: 107-108.
45. Ursin G, Aragaki C, et al. Oral contraceptives and premenopausal bilateral breast cancer: a case-control study. *Epidemiology.* 1992; 3: 414-419.
46. Lindefors-Harris BM, Edlund G, et al. Risk of cancer of the breast after legal abortion during the first trimester: a Swedish register study. *Br Med J.* 1989; 299: 1430-1432.
47. Melbye M, Wohlfahrt J, et al. Induced abortion and the risk of breast cancer. *N Engl J Med.* 1997; 336: 81-85.
48. Skegg D, et al. Progestogen-only contraceptives and risk of breast cancer in New Zealand. *Cancer Causes and Control.* 1996; 7: 513-519.
49. Olsson H, Ranstam J, et al. Proliferation and DNA ploidy in malignant breast tumors in relation to early contraceptive use and early abortions. *Cancer.* 1991; 67: 1285-1290.
50. Schonborn I, Nischan P, et al. Oral contraceptives use and the prognosis of breast cancer. *Breast Cancer Research and Treatment.* 1994; 30: 283-292.
51. Ranstam J, Olsson H, et al. Survival in breast cancer and age at start of oral contraceptive usage. *AntiCancer Research.* 1991; 11: 2043-2046.
52. Olsson H, Borg A, et al. Early oral contraceptive use and premenopausal breast cancer-A review of studies performed in southern Sweden. *Cancer Detection and Prevention.* 1991; 15: 265-271.

53. Olsson H, et al. Her-2/neu and INT2 prot-oncogene amplification in malignant breast tumors in relation to reproductive factors and exposure to exogenous hormones. *J Natl Cancer Inst.* 1991; 83: 1483-1487.

54. Van der Kooy K, Rookus MA, et al. P53 protein overexpression in relation to risk factors for breast cancer. *Am J Epidemiol.* 1996; 144: 924-933.

55. Ursin G, et al. Does oral contraceptive use increase the risk of breast cancer in women with BRCA1/BRCA2 mutations more than in other women? *Cancer Research.* 1997; 57: 3678-3681.

56. Clubb EM, et al. *A pilot study on teaching NFP in general practice: current knowledge and new strategies for the 1990s.* Washington, D.C.: Georgetown University; 1990: 130-132.

57. Frank-Hermann P, et al. Effectiveness and acceptability of the symptothermal method of NFP in Germany. *Am J Obstet Gynecol.* 1991; 165: 2045-2052.

58. De Leizaola MA. De premiere d'une etude prospecive d'efficacite du planning famillial naturel realisee en Belgique francophone. *J Gyncol Obstet.* Biol. Rev. 1994, 23: 359-364.

59. Dorairaj K. The modification mucus method in India. *Am J Obstet Gynecol.* 1991; 165: 2066-2067.

60. Gray RH, et al. Evaluation of NFP program in Liberia and Zambia. *J Biosoc Sci.* 1993; 25: 249-258.

61. Zhang DW, et al. The effectiveness of the ovulation method used by 688 couples in Shanghai. Reprod. *Contraception.* 1993; 13: 194-200.

62. Ryder RE. Natural Family Planning: effective birth control supported by the Catholic Church. *Br Med J.* 1993; 307: 723-726.

63. Potter LA. How effective are contraceptives? The determination and measurement of pregnancy rates. *Obstet Gynecol.* 1996; 88: 13S-23S.

64. Thomas DB, Noonan EA, et al. Breast cancer and specific types of combined oral contraceptives. *Br J Cancer.* 1992; 65: 108-113.

65. Pike MC, Henderson BE, et al. Breast cancer in young women and use of oral contraceptives: possible modifying effect of formulation and age at use. *The Lancet.* October 22, 1983: 926-929.

66. Hulka B, Liu E, et al. Steroid hormones and risk of breast cancer. *Cancer Supplement.* 1994; 74: 1111-1124.

67. Calle EE, Mervis CA, Wingo PA, et al. Spontaneous abortion and risk of fatal breast cancer in a prospective cohort of United States women. *Cancer Causes and Control.* 1995; 6: 460-468.

68. Vessey MP, McPherson K, et al. Breast cancer and oral contraceptives: findings in Oxford-Family planning Association contraceptive study. *Br Med J.* 1981; 282: 2093-2094.

69. Hiatt RA, et al. Exogenous estrogen and breast cancer after bilateral oophorectomy. *Cancer.* 1984; 54: 139-144.

70. Mills PK, et al. Prospective study of exogenous hormone use and breast cancer in seventh day Adventist. *Cancer.* 1989; 64: 591-597.

71. Schuurman A, et al. Exogenous hormone use and the risk of postmenopausal breast cancer: results from the Netherlands Cohort Study. *Cancer Causes and Control.* 1995; 6: 416-424.

72. Alexander FE, et al. Risk factors for breast cancer with applications to selection for the prevalence screen. *J Epidemiol Community Health.* 1987; 41: 101-106.

73. Kay CR, Hannaford PC. Breast cancer and the pill-A further report from the Royal College of General Practitioners' oral contraception study. *Br J Cancer.* 58: 675-680.

74. Romieu I, Willett W, et al. Prospective study of oral contraceptive use and risk of breast cancer in women. *J Natl Cancer Inst.* 1989; 81: 1313-1321.

Chapter 10:
Learning from a Mistake?
The History of
DES (Diethylstilbestrol)

DES is the abbreviation for a synthetic estrogen called diethylstilbestrol, which was given to pregnant diabetic mothers because certain researchers (ie, White and Hunt in 1943) reported that it would decrease a pregnant diabetic woman's risk of having a miscarriage. It was later used for other indications such as pre-eclampsia, premature labor, etc. It was usually given between the 8th and the 15th week of pregnancy and continued until well into the third trimester. The initial trials started in the late 1940s but women took it regularly from the 1950s until the 1960s. In the mid 1950s, it was noted that DES did not decrease a woman's rate of miscarriage and over time it was discovered that *the daughters* of the women who had taken *DES experienced a higher incidence of both vaginal and cervical cancer* [1]. But what about the *mothers* who took DES? Did they need to worry about getting any particular cancer? After all, DES is an artificial estrogen and it was given during the first trimester of pregnancy. Either of these two facts should give a woman cause to worry.

Researchers continued to monitor women for any observation of cancer, especially breast cancer. For almost 25 years, researchers claimed that there was no link between DES and breast cancer risk in the women who had used it. Finally, in 1978, Bibbo et al published a study which showed a 47% increased risk of developing breast cancer, but the authors under-emphasized the findings because they were not statistically significant: "We detected no statistically significant differences between the two groups in the frequency and types of uterine, ovarian, breast and other reproductive-tract abnormalities." [2, p.766] Studies in the 1980s confirmed what many had feared: DES causes a statistically significant increase in breast cancer.

How much does DES elevate the risk of breast cancer? Colton et al published a classic article [3] which provided a detailed account of this. Two tables which contain information from that article serve to illustrate:

Table 10A:
RISKS OF DES FOUND IN VARIOUS STUDIES

AUTHOR	PERCENT INCREASE	YEAR OF STUDY	NUMBER OF SUBJECTS	RESULTS: RELATIVE RISK
Bibbo et al [2]	46% increase*	1978	693	1.46 (not significant)
Beral & Colwell [1]	infinite risk	1980	79	infinite risk CI's not given
Vessey et al [see 3]	not reported	1983	319	not reported
Hadjimichael et al [see 3]	37% increase*	1984	1531	1.37 (0.83-2.28)
Colton et al [3]	35% increase	1993	2864	1.35 (1.05-1.74)

*This result reflects a trend toward an increased risk but does not attain statistical significance.

Table 10A shows the progression of data from the various studies since 1978. Every study points to an increased risk of breast cancer from DES, except the Vessey study, which did not report any results. Perhaps the most significant result is found in the study by Colton et al, especially given the size of the study and the fact that it had the longest latent period. Note that it calculated a *statistically significant 35% risk overall.* Data and results from the Colton study [3] give us more important information as noted in Table 10B, which follows:

Table 10B:
BREAST CANCER RISK TO WOMEN WHO TOOK DES

TIME SINCE EXPOSURE (years)	PERCENT INCREASE	RELATIVE RISK
0-9	13% increase*	1.13 (0.38-3.37)
10-19	13% increase*	1.13 (0.70-1.81)
20-29	36% increase*	1.36 (0.93-1.99)
30 or more	33% increase*	1.33 (0.95-1.87)
AGE AT DIAGNOSIS		
less than 40	22% increase*	1.22 (0.48-3.09)
40-49	18% increase*	1.18 (0.74-1.87)
50-59	18% increase*	1.18 (0.82-1.71)
60 or over	47% increase	1.47 (1.02-2.13)

*This reflects a trend toward an increased or decreased risk but does not attain statistical significance.

What lesson should we learn from Table 10B? First, it should be noted from the upper half of the table, that it took more than 20 years before the risk of DES and breast cancer began to show a trend toward an increased risk. Second, we see that even after 30 years, the trend toward an increased risk of DES remained high — over 30%. Third, the bottom half of the table shows us an extremely important finding: *The risk of DES appears to be greatest in women older than 60.*

Q-10A: Why does the present author bring up the example of DES?

DES is extremely important because it provides us with a historical lesson of how a synthetic estrogen, when given during pregnancy, caused a significant increase in breast cancer 20-30 years after its first use. DES provides us with a possible medical corollary to both the oral contraceptive pill (OCP) and/or abortion. What is that correlation? DES contained a synthetic estrogen; today's OCPs contain synthetic estrogens. Although the estrogens are certainly different (ie, DES was a non-steroidal whereas today's OCPs contain steroidal estrogens) and are given at different times and doses, one fact stands out: *DES, a synthetic estrogen, causes breast cancer despite studies which found no risk for almost 25 years.* Just as important, *DES was noted to have its greatest effect in women after the age of 60.* This same phenomenon may be happening in regard to early OCP use. It was already noted in Chapters 8 and 9 that virtually every study since 1980 to date, which looked at women who took oral contraceptives before their first full-term pregnancy (FFTP) and were under the age of 45 on or before 1995, showed an increased risk in breast cancer. *In the past, some researchers have imprudently reassured women "not to worry"* because they predict that this increased risk will not be sustained as women approach their 50s and 60s. *This sort of statement must be evaluated in light of the historical example of DES and its increasing risk in women 60 years of age and older.* Better for the laity to make this decision than the "experts."

Q-10B: Does the historical example of DES shed any light on the question of the link between an abortion performed early in a woman's reproductive life and breast cancer?

It may. As was noted, DES was given to pregnant mothers in an attempt to prevent miscarriages. Thus, DES and induced abortion have one thing in common: *they both are a "hormonal blow" to the body at a very sensitive time in the development of the breast.* When DES was given, especially between the 8th and 15th weeks of pregnancy, it introduced a foreign synthetic estrogen into a woman's body at a critical stage — when she was pregnant and her breast cells were dividing rapidly. In an analogous way, an early induced abortion results in an *abrupt decrease* in a woman's hormone levels during this very same critical stage. Thus, although different, *each one is a "hormonal blow" to the body at a time when the breast may be especially sensitive — during early pregnancy. If we recall that it took about 25 years to note the true dangers of DES and the increased risk of breast cancer in mothers who took it, similarly, we may just be beginning to see the real increase in breast cancer in women who had abortions performed early in their reproductive lives as data from the late 1990s and early 21st century come in. In addition, if induced abortion follows a similar pattern as DES, we may notice the biggest increases in breast cancer in women after the age of 60.*

Q-10C: Is there any similarity between the fertility drug Clomid and DES?

There may be. Clomid®* (clomiphene), made by Hoechst Marion Rousel, is a fertility drug which acts upon the pituitary gland, so that it increases the hormones involved in ovulation (called LH and FSH), which results in a tremendous increase in ovarian activity. Clomid® "is capable of interacting with estrogen receptors." [4] It is therefore possible that it may affect a woman's risk of developing breast cancer years after it is first used.

Clomid and the other commonly used fertility drugs have been noted to markedly increase the risk of ovarian cancer. In a large collaborative study which pooled the results of several studies, Whittemore et al [5] found that women who used fertility drugs and who did not get pregnant had a 2600% increased risk in obtaining ovarian cancer compared to women who never took fertility drugs. Spiritas recalculated the data and noted that Whittemore's data actually resulted in an 1100% increased risk [6].

Q-10D: It was noted that daughters of women who took DES experienced a higher incidence of both vaginal and cervical cancer [1]. Could the daughters of women who took Clomid® or OCPs also experience such effects?

The PDR (*Physicians' Desk Reference*) states that "Newborn rats, injected (with Clomid®) during the first few days of life, also developed metaplastic changes in uterine and vaginal mucosa. . ." (PDR, 1997). Thus, theoretically the daughters who are born to women who have recently taken Clomid® could also experience an increased risk of cervical and vaginal cancer.

The same question could be asked of women who become pregnant while taking OCPs. In 1996 Potter [7] found that the pregnancy rate for "typical use" in women using OCPs was 7%. This means that tens of thousands of women have and will continue to become pregnant while taking OCPs. In these incidences DES and the OCP are both artificial hormones that would have been taken at some point in pregnancy, so it is not unreasonable to ask: *Will the daughters of women who take OCPs have higher incidences of breast, cervical, vaginal or other cancers?* What about the effects on the sons of these women? *For example the rate of testicular cancer has risen by 50% over the past 25 years. Is it possible that these men were conceived while their mothers were taking oral contraceptives? The answers to these questions may have catastrophic consequences and yet to the best of this author's knowledge, the questions have never been asked. A formal study of these areas is urgently needed.*

References:

1. Beral V, Colwell L. Randomized trial of high doses of stilboestrol and ethisterone in pregnancy: long-term follow-up of mothers. *Br Med J.* 1980; 281: 1098-1101.

2. Bibbo M, Haenszel W, et al. A twenty-five-year follow-up study of women exposed to diethylstilbestrol during pregnancy. *N Engl J Med.* 1978; 298; 763-767.

3. Colton T, Greenberg ER, et al. Breast cancer in mothers prescribed diethylstilbestrol in pregnancy. *JAMA*, 1993; 269: 2096-3000.

4. *Physicians' Desk Reference* (1997). Description of Clomid (R).

5. Whittemore AS, et al. Characteristics relating to ovarian cancer risk: collaborative analysis of 12 U.S. case-control studies. II. Invasive epithelial ovarian cancers in white women. Collaborative Ovarian Cancer Group. *Am J Epidemiol.* 1992; 136: 1184-1203.

6. Spiritas R, et al. Fertility drugs and ovarian cancer: Red alert or red herring. *Fertility and Sterility.* 1993; 59: 291.

7. Potter LA. How effective are contraceptives? The determination and measurement of pregnancy rates. *Obstet Gynecol.* 1996; 88: 13S-23S.

Chapter 11:
Black Women and Breast Cancer

"Breast cancer is the second leading cause of cancer death among African-American women" [1, p.13]. (Lung cancer is first). "For the period of 1985-1989, the incidence for each 5-year age group younger than 40 years, was higher among black women than among white women" [2]. The incidence of breast cancer is increasing in both the black and white population, but young black women are getting more breast cancer and dying from it more often than young white women. Why? Researchers are well aware that two major risk factors have been more prevalent in young blacks than in whites, namely the incidence of early oral contraceptive use and having an abortion performed early in a woman's reproductive life. White and Daling addressed this issue in 1987. They noted that young black women had almost double the rate of increased breast cancer incidence compared to the rest of the population when comparing incidence rates from the mid 1970s to the late 1980s. In discussing possible reasons for the increase they stated: "Recently, two other factors have emerged as possible risk factors for breast cancer: oral contraceptive use before first pregnancy and abortion before first term pregnancy." [3, p.242]. It would seem to be *very reasonable* to propose that these two risk factors are at least partly responsible for the marked increase in breast cancer incidence and mortality of young black women compared to young white women over the past 15 years.

Q-11A: What has happened to the incidence of breast cancer in young black and white women over the past 25 years?

Figure 11A (constructed from data from the National Cancer Institute [4]) shows the incidence of breast cancer in both young black and white women, ages 20 to 44 years old, from the block of years of 1975 to 1979 as compared to 1988 to 1992. *Young white women experienced a 10.1% increase* (ie, going from 36.6 to 40.3 breast cancer "cases" per 100,000 women in the 20 to 44 year-old age group), *whereas young black women experienced a 12.6% increase,* going from a rate of 40.8 to 45.6 per 100,000 women.

Figure 11A:

RISING RATES OF BREAST CANCER IN WHITE AND BLACK WOMEN

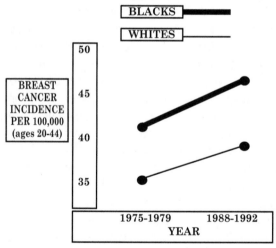

Q-11B: What about the mortality rate in young white and black women?

Figure 11B [5, p.124] shows the relative death rates per 100,000 women for those under the age of 50. The mortality rate of young white females *fell* from 6.7 (in 1975) to 5.9 (in 1990), whereas the rate for young black women actually *rose* from 7.9 in 1975 to 8.9 in 1990. So from 1975 to 1990, although breast cancer mortality *decreased* in white women by about *9%*, it *increased* in young black women by over *12%*.

Figure 11B:
MORTALITY FROM BREAST CANCER IN
WHITE AND BLACK WOMEN

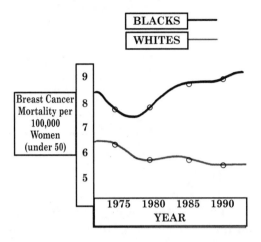

Q-11C: In accordance with these findings, one might expect young black women to have a higher incidence of abortions performed early in their reproductive lives and/or a history of early OCP (oral contraceptive pill) use. Does the historical data support this?

Absolutely. Table 11A shows the abortion rates for both black and white women for different age groups. Data on the abortion rate for young black women became available in 1981, and the rates of abortion for this period as well as for the 1990 to 1991 period are shown.

Table 11A:
ABORTION RATES IN YOUNG
WHITE AND BLACK WOMEN*

AGE	WHITES	BLACKS	WHITES	BLACKS
	1981	1981	1990-1991	1990-1991
UNDER 15	5.1*	27.0*	(0.8)**	(5.4)**
15-17	26.0*	51.5*	21.0*	57.7*
18-19	56.6*	87.9*	46.5*	117.4*

* Sources: [6] and [7] (rates in abortions per 1,000 women).

** The data for women under age 15 in the 1990-1991 years was computed on a different scale than the rates for the under age 15 women in 1981.

The data show that young black women obviously had a higher rate of abortions performed early in their reproductive lives than young white women. Although few statistics are available from the 1970s, it is highly probable that this trend was also true for the 1970s. One can also see that very young blacks (ie, those under 15) have an especially high relative rate of abortion compared to young whites — *specifically they have more than 5 times the abortion rate at this age, for both the 1981 and the 1990 to 1991 time periods.*

Q-11D: *Young black women also have more early live births than young white women. Does this not protect them from breast cancer, because having a child at a younger age decreases a woman's risk of developing breast cancer?*

It is true that young black women have about twice as many live births per 1,000 women as young white women, but those who have a live birth, in any given year, are almost always different women than those who had an induced abortion that year. Young black women have a higher abortion rate as well as a higher birth rate than young white women. It is also likely that many women who had an abortion performed early in their reproductive lives, especially those under the age of 15 and many of those aged 15 to 17 years old, will have chosen to abort their first child. These young women would be at an especially high risk, because the risk of having an abortion before a <u>first full-term pregnancy</u> (FFTP) in young women has been noted to carry a 150% increased risk according to at least one large study [8].

Q-11E: *What do the records show concerning early OCP use among young white and black women?*

It is clear that young black women have had a higher rate of early OCP use than young white women. This trend has continued from the mid-1970s through at least the early 1990s and is even noted in the very young women aged 15 to 17 according to the cited data from 1982. The early use of OCPs by young black women could certainly account for their increasing breast cancer rates. It should also be noted that many young black and white women have used OCPs either before a FFTP or after an induced abortion, making them especially vulnerable because they would now have two risk factors. We must remember that early OCP use, especially when used before a woman has ever had a child, increases the risk of breast cancer. In 1990, Romieu et al's meta-analysis showed women under the age of 45 who had taken OCPs for 4 or more years prior to their FFTP had a 72% increased risk of breast cancer [RR=1.72 (1.36-2.19)] [9].

Table 11B:
PERCENTAGE OF WOMEN AGED 15 TO 19 YEARS OLD USING ORAL CONTRACEPTIVES [10, 11, 12]

YEAR→	1976	1982	1988	1990
WHITES (15-19)	28.4%*	12.6%	18.9%	16.7%
BLACKS (15-19)	47.0%*	20.5%	26.9%	19.0%
WHITES (15-17)		7.6%		
BLACKS (15-17)		11.8%		

* The 1976 data is based upon the category of: "Percentage of women aged 15-19 who ever used a contraceptive method, by first method used" [10].

Q-11F: Do women who have abortions really have a higher rate of OCP use?

It would appear so. Campbell et al noted that: "Our findings on adolescents support those of several authors who cited that adolescent women were more likely to use contraceptives after abortion" [13, p.819].

Q-11G: Have any researchers commented upon the probable connection between early OCP use, abortion, and breast cancer when taken/performed by/on young women?

Yes. It was already noted that White et al commented that oral contraceptive use before a first pregnancy and abortion before a FFTP could be risk factors. [3, p.242]. Kelsey (1993) also noted that "below age 45, the higher rates (of breast cancer) in blacks than in whites in recent years have been hypothesized to reflect more frequent abortion and use of oral contraceptives among young women" [14, p.14]. Last, Mayberry et al noted that ". . .the higher breast cancer incidence rate among young black women may be explained by a higher prevalence and duration of oral contraceptive use" [15, p.1454].

Q-11H: What have the specific studies of oral contraceptive pill use and breast cancer shown in young black women?

Several authors have performed research specifically on black women who have breast cancer, as noted in Table 11C.

Table 11C:
BLACK WOMEN AND RISK OF NON-SPECIFIC OCP USE

AUTHOR OF STUDY	PERCENT CHANGE	FINDINGS
Brinton [16]	110% increase	2.1 RR (1.2-3.5) in women under 35 who had used OCPs for more than 5 years
Laing [17]	450% increase	5.5 RR (1.1-27.1) in women < 47 for ever use
Mayberry [18]	270% increase	3.7 (1.3-10.3) in women age 20-39 who took OCPs for more than 10 years
Palmer [19]	90% increase	1.9 RR (1.3-2.7) in women <44 who used OCPs for more than 1 year

Table 11C presents a number of specific studies regarding OCP use and young black women. These results should certainly be taken seriously, especially because each of them is statistically significant. Although none of the studies specifically examined OCP use prior to a FFTP (first full-term pregnancy), these studies certainly serve as a warning that early OCP use could carry at least as much risk as those presented in Table 11C.

Q 11-I: Could the use of Depo-Provera be another part of the explanation as to why young black women are getting breast cancer more frequently than young white women?

It has already been noted by Skegg et al [20] that women who take Depo-Provera (DMPA) for 2 years or more before the age of 25 have at least a 190% increased risk of developing breast cancer. According to a recent article in the *Wall Street Journal* [21], Depo-Provera accounted for 19% of all contraceptive use in black women aged 15 to 19 years old, but only 8% of all contraceptive use in white women aged 15 to 19 years old. Hence, one might reasonably expect to find more DMPA related breast cancer among black women.

Q-11J: What about the risk of abortion as concerns breast cancer in young black women?

Mayberry [18] noted an odds ratio of 1.1 (0.5-2.3) for developing breast cancer with one induced abortion and 1.4 (0.5-3.8) for two or more abortions in women aged 20 to 39 years old. Laing [17] noted a 50% increased trend [$RR=$ 1.5 (0.7-3.5)] in women under the age of 40, a 180% increase [$RR=2.8$ (1.0-8.1)] in women aged 41 to 49 years old and a 370% increase [$RR=$ 4.7 (2.6-8.4)] in women over the age of 50, who had ever had an abortion. In a later study [22] Laing noted a 144% increase (RR = 2.44) in a comparison of sisters, one of whom had an abortion performed early in her reproductive life. Although this author found no study which specifically examined the effect of abortion prior to a FFTP in young black women, Mayberry and Laing's work certainly serves to warn that abortion performed early in a woman's life is likely to carry significant risk.

Q-11K: Do black women have "worse" breast cancer than white women?

Yes, black women generally have more aggressive breast cancers and poorer survival rates compared to white women. Eley et al [23, p.953] estimated that when comparing white and black women who had breast cancer, black women had between a 70 to 90% increased risk of dying from breast cancer than white women, independent of the stage in which the cancer was diagnosed. He also found that black women had a 2.3-fold risk (ie, a 130% increased risk) of having estrogen negative breast tumors. (In general, estrogen negative tumors respond more poorly to treatment than do estrogen positive tumors.) Some have argued that the difference in breast cancer mortality between black and white women is a reflection of the different standards of care of women who have different incomes. Although this statement could certainly be true, it does not answer the question of why in general, black women have more aggressive breast cancer than white women, *nor does it answer the question as to why breast cancer mortality rates have risen faster in young black women than in young white women.*

Q-11L: Could the fact that Eley et al found that black women had more estrogen negative tumors be a result of their increased early OCP use and history of more frequent abortions?

Yes, it is possible, but not proven. As noted earlier, Olsson et al [24] found that women who took OCPs early in life developed a more aggressive type of breast cancer. The same phenomenon may certainly be occurring in black women who have a higher rate of estrogen negative tumors.

Q-11M: Are black women in any other countries at high risk of developing breast cancer?

Yes, it would appear so. It was noted earlier that women who take Depo-Provera (DMPA) for 2 years or more before the age of 25 have at least a 190% increased risk of developing breast cancer according to Skegg et al [20]. But a study performed on South African women in 1997 found that 72% of black women had used an injectable progestin contraceptive and that 30% of women had used one for 5 years or more [25]. The progestin used most often was either DMPA or norethisterone and these injectable hormones have been used there since the mid 1960s. The study noted that white South African women had a far lower use of these progestin hormones. In general, any race of people — black or white — that has a high rate of OCP or Depo-Provera use, is certainly at increased risk for developing breast cancer.

References:

1. Cancer Facts & Figures for African Americans. American Cancer Society. 1996.
2. Miller BA, et al. Cancer Statistics Review: 1973-1989. Bethesda, MD: National Cancer Institute, 1992. [NIH Publication Number 92-2289]

3. White E, Daling J, et al. Rising incidence of breast cancer among young women in Washington State. *J Natl Cancer Inst.* 1987; 79: 239-243.

4. National Cancer Institute. *SEER Cancer Statistics Review.* 1973-1992: Tables and Graphs. Bethesda, Maryland. Incidence rates of breast cancer in Black and White women age 20-44.

5. National Cancer Institute. *SEER Cancer Statistics Review.* 1973-1992: Tables and Graphs. Bethesda, Maryland.

6. Ventura S, Taffel S, et al. Trends in pregnancies and pregnancy rates, United States, 1980-1992. *Monthly Vital Statistics Report.* 1995; 43: 1-24.

7. Hayes CD. *Risking the Future.* Washington, D.C.: National Academy Press. 1987.

8. Daling J, Malone K, et al. Risk of breast cancer among young women: relationship to induced abortion. *J Natl Cancer Inst.* 1994; 86: 1584-1592.

9. Romieu I, Berlin J, et al. Oral contraceptives and breast cancer. Review and meta-analysis. *Cancer.* 1990; 66: 2253-2263.

10. Zelnik M, Kantner J. Sexual activity, contraceptive use and pregnancy among metropolitan-area teenagers: 1971-1979. *Family Planning Perspectives.* 1980; 12: 230-237.

11. Bachrach C, Mosher W. Use of Contraception in the United States, 1982. Vital and Health Statistics of the National Center for Health Statistics [U.S. Dept. of Health and Human Services]. Dec. 4, 1984; Number 102: 1-8.

12. U.S. Government statistics regarding OCP use in black and white women. Source cannot be specifically cited until government publication is made public (work currently in progress).

13. Campbell NB, et al. Abortion in Adolescence. *Adolescence.* 1988; 23: 813-823.

14. Kelsey J, Horn-Ross P. Breast cancer: magnitude of the problem and descriptive epidemiology. *Epidemiologic Reviews.* 1993; 15: 7-16.

15. Mayberry RM, Stoddard-Wright C. Breast cancer risk factors among black women and white women: similarities and differences. *Am J Epidemiol.* 1992; 136: 1445-1456.

16. Brinton LA, Daling JR, et al. Oral contraceptives and breast cancer risk among younger women. *J Natl Cancer Inst.* 6/7/1995; 87: 827-35.

17. Laing AE, Demenais FM, et al. Breast cancer risk factors in African-American women: The Howard University tumor registry experience. *Journal of National Medical Association.* 1993; 85 (12): 931-939.

18. Maybery RM. Age-specific patterns of association between breast cancer and risk factors in black women, ages 20 to 39 and 40 to 54. *Ann Epidemiol.* 1994; 4: 205-213.

19. Palmer J, Rosenberg L, et al. Oral contraceptives use and breast cancer risk among African-American women. *Cancer Causes and Control.* 1995; 6: 321-331.

20. Skegg DCG, Noonan EA, et al. Depot medroxyprogesterone acetate and breast cancer [A pooled analysis of the World Health Organization and New Zealand studies]. *JAMA*. 1995: 799-804.

21. Freedman AM. Why teenage girls love the shot; Why others aren't too sure. *The Wall Street Journal*. October 14, 1998.

22. Laing AE, Bonney GE, et al. Reproductive and lifestyle factors for breast cancer in African-American women. *Genet Epidemiol*. 1994: A300.

23. Eley JW, Hill HA, et al. Racial differences in survival from breast cancer. *JAMA*. 1994; 272: 947-954.

24. Olsson H, Borg A, et al. Early oral contraceptive use and premenopausal breast cancer-A review of studies performed in southern Sweden. *Cancer Detection and Prevention*. 1991; 15: 265-271.

25. Bailie R, et al. A case-control study of breast cancer risk and exposure to injectable progestin contraceptives. *S Afr Med J*. 1987; 87: 302-305.

Chapter 12:
The Progestins

Progestins are a class of female sexual hormones that have been used by millions of women around the world over the past 25 years. They come in several forms: 1) the all-progestin oral contraceptive pill (ie, the minipill which women may know as Ovrette®, Nor-QD®, or Micronor®); 2) the injectable contraceptives such as Depo-Provera®, which is injected into a woman's muscle; or 3) an implantable contraceptive (ie, Norplant®) which is surgically implanted under a woman's skin. These progestins work by diminishing a woman's frequency of ovulation, by changing the lining of the uterus, and by thickening cervical mucus. The minipill was introduced in 1973 in the U.S., whereas Depo-Provera was approved by the Food and Drug Administration in 1992. Norplant was approved in 1991 and was used by about 1 million Americans in 1995 [1]. The central question of this chapter is: *Do progestins cause breast cancer when used by women at a young age?*

Q-12A: Is there any evidence that progestins cause breast cancer in vitro (ie, in a laboratory setting)?

Yes. Progestins began to receive more attention when it was noted that the rate of breast cell division was highest during the luteal phase of a woman's menstrual cycle at which time progesterone levels are highest. Further studies by researchers Pike [2] and White [3] noted that oral contraceptive pills (OCPs) with potent progestins carried higher risks for causing breast cancer than combination OCPs that contained less potent progestins. But do progestins actually affect breast tumor cells when one studies this in vitro (ie, in a laboratory setting)?

Anderson et al [4] noted that women who were given OCPs that contained only progestin, had the highest rate of breast cell division, even higher than standard combination OCPs. In addition, Schoonen et al [5] noted that pregnanes, which are a specific class of progestin (medroxyprogesterone acetate, found in Depo-Provera, is a type of pregnane), enhanced the growth of human breast cancer cells. Catherino et al [6] also noted that norgestrel — which is the hormonal agent in Norplant and which is also found in Ovral and Ovrette, stimulated MCF-7 cells, another type of human breast cancer cell.

Q-12B: Does use of progestins cause early abortions, and if so could this be playing a role?

Progestin use appears to cause more early abortions than use of combination OCPs (ie, those that contain both an estrogen and a progestin), primarily because they allow such a high rate of breakthrough ovulation. *William's Obstetrics* comments specifically on Norplant: "Up to one third of cycles may be ovulatory based upon serum progesterone determinations." [7] (ie, a woman may be having three or four abortions per year while on Norplant if she conceives during those cycles). (For details concerning how Norplant or OCPs work, see Appendix 5). Although the studies regarding breakthrough ovulation have been done on Norplant, the same phenomenon probably occurs with all of the other progestins in addition to Depo-Provera. It was noted earlier in Chapter 6 that the effect of a very early abortion (ie, within the first week of gestation) regarding breast cancer is difficult to know, but that a very early "hormonal blow" may or may not have an effect on the risk of breast cancer.

Q-12C: Could you explain the history of Depo-Provera and why it has caused so much controversy?

Depo-Provera is a type of progestin (ie, medroxyprogesterone acetate) which is given to women via an intramuscular injection. It has been used by over 30 million women in more than 90 countries [8] and by about 2 million in the U.S. annually [1]. It is manufactured by the drug company Pharmacia-Upjohn.

The original New Drug Application for Depo-Provera was filed in 1967. Controversy arose in the mid 1970s, after it was noted that Depo-Provera led to a notable increase in breast cancer in dogs and uterine cancer in monkeys. In spite of evidence that Depo-Provera caused an increase in the breast cancer rate in mice and dogs, and its rejection by the FDA in 1978, the World Health Organization (WHO) initiated a worldwide trial, experimenting on women in the Third World!

There have been three fairly large "trials" including the WHO study, each of which has showed a marked increase in the rate of breast cancer in younger aged women who have used Depo-Provera for a number of years. In spite of this, on October 29, 1992, in what can only be described as a gravely irresponsible decision, the FDA formally approved Depo-Provera as a contraceptive for use in the U.S.! [8]

Q-12D: What did the animal trials show regarding Depo-Provera?

Lanari et al [9] gave 40 mice an injection of DMPA (depot-medroxyprogesterone acetate: the hormone in Depo-Provera) and 40 mice did not receive it (ie, the controls). Breast cancer developed in 16 out of 40 of the DMPA treated mice and 0 out of 40 in the controls. Another classic study by Larsson [10] showed that 5 out of 20 beagles that received DMPA developed malignant breast cancer (ie, 25%) whereas none of the 40 control dogs did.

Q-12E: When an animal study shows a significant risk, is that not a clear warning that the drug carries a high risk in humans?

Absolutely. It is virtually impossible to conceive of how the WHO went on to test this drug on an experimental basis in women in the Third World after noting that the FDA had rejected its approval in 1978. Researchers began to argue that the beagle was a poor model on which to perform clinical trials with DMPA. In a thorough analysis of the subject, Rutteman, a veterinarian researcher from the Netherlands, disputed the claims that the beagle was a poor model: "It has been claimed that the dog is unique in its sensitivity to the mammary tumor promoting effect of progestins and that this tumorigenic effect results from progestin-induced growth hormone (GH) induction. A thorough review of the literature does not support these claims" [11]. In regard to the FDA's later approval of DMPA in 1992, a high ranking person who had direct access to the FDA proceedings told this author (confidentially) that there was nothing wrong with the trials in the dogs and that it was inappropriate for the FDA to have approved Depo-Provera. In addition to these comments, one must also wonder why so few were alarmed about DMPA's effects in mice.

Q-12F: What did the WHO experiments on Third World women show?

There were two large trials of women who used DMPA and one smaller one:

1) *The WHO trial* [12]: A study of 869 women with breast cancer, 377 of whom were under the age of 45. It acquired data from four different countries from 1979 to 1988. The WHO study found that women who had used DMPA at least 3 years before the age of 25 had a 141% increased risk: [RR = 2.41 (0.59-9.87)] of getting breast cancer. Overall risk for any use was 1.21 (0.96-1.52) and use before a first full-term pregnancy (FFTP) was 1.35 (0.3-6.12).

The WHO study suffered from some obvious problems. First, it had a huge *stack effect* (13.5% of "cases" vs. 27.6% of "controls" were under the age of 35). Second, very few women took DMPA before their FFTP (first full-term pregnancy) so it was difficult to measure its effect on this select population. Third, women who had taken DMPA for a period of time at a young age would barely have experienced a 10-year latent period. The effects of DMPA in young women who took it early in life might not have shown up because too short of a latent period was used.

2) *The New Zealand study* [13]: A study of 891 women, 388 of whom were under 45. Overall risk for all women and any use was 1.0 (0.8-1.3). Women who used DMPA for 2 to 5 years before the age of 25 had a 4.6 (1.4-15.1)-fold risk and women who used DMPA for 2 to 5 years before their FFTP had a 3.2 (0.41-24.3)-fold risk.

The New Zealand study suffered from the same problems as the WHO study, including an egregious stack effect (ie, 7.2% "cases" vs. 21.7% "controls" under the age of 35) as well as the death effect. It too examined few young women who had taken DMPA before their FFTP.

3) *The Costa Rican study* [14]: A study of 171 women, 60 of whom were under the age of 45. Overall DMPA use conferred a 2.6-fold risk (1.4-4.7). The risk of use at a young age was elevated but the authors did not give details regarding specific risks. The risk of using DMPA after 10 years since first use was 4.0 (1.5-10.3)

The Costa Rican trial suffered from a severe stack effect. In addition, it was a rather small trial. Its greatest strength is that because Costa Ricans began using DMPA earlier than other countries, it had a statistic for a longer latent period (ie, a 300% increase in breast cancer after 10 years since first use). The study was funded by USAID and Family Health International — hardly unbiased observers.

Q-12G: Did the stack effect have a bearing on the studies?

Yes. If the stack effect had been properly avoided in the design of the trials, the risks for DMPA use in young women would almost certainly have been significantly higher.

Q-12H: Could you summarize the most worrisome finding of the trials?

The most concerning finding is the fact that each study found an increased risk of at least 2.0 in women who had taken DMPA for more than 3 years before the age of 25 (Costa Rica's results were not printed, but a 2-fold risk deduced from their data is most likely a conservative estimate).

These findings were summarized nicely by Skegg et al [15] who pooled the results of the largest two studies — the WHO and the New Zealand studies. After pooling the data, he found that women who had taken DMPA for between 2 and 3 years before the age of 25 *had a 310% statistically significant risk* of getting breast cancer [*RR*=4.1 (1.6-10.90)] whereas women who had taken DMPA for more than 3 years prior to the age of 25 had a *190% increased risk* that was also significant [*RR*=2.9 (1.2-7.1)]. Because women around the world are now taking contraceptives at an earlier age, these findings should have stunned the WHO into stopping the trials immediately.

Q-12I: What happened instead?

In spite of the findings alluded to above, Thomas and Noonan, in summarizing the WHO findings wrote: "These results provide reassurance that women who have used DMPA for a long time and who initiated use many years previously are not at increased risk of breast cancer." [12, p.833]. In contrast, Paul et al (author of the New Zealand study) at least admitted in the abstract of his 1989 paper that: "Despite the lack of an overall association, these findings suggest that medroxyprogesterone may increase the risk of breast cancer in young women." [13, p.759]. In addition, in a paper written in March 1992 and sponsored by Upjohn (a pharmaceutical company) [16], Staffa et al noted that "There is need for further study, particularly of patients in potentially high-risk groups, including those with (1) extended hormone exposure before age 25 and/or first full-term pregnancy and (2) exposure in the post menopausal period." Even with these warnings, the FDA went on to approve Depo-Provera for women in the U.S. on October 29, 1992!

Q-12J: Which parties bear the largest responsibility for the failure to warn women of Depo-Provera's noted risks in young women who take it for extended periods of time?

The drug manufacturer of Depo-Provera (ie, Pharmacia-Upjohn), the WHO, and the FDA bear direct responsibility. One's physician most certainly also bears a great share of responsibility because there are only three main studies which he or she should be aware of.

Q-12K: Are black women in the U.S. at especially high risk of developing breast cancer from Depo-Provera?

It would appear so. It has already been noted by Skegg et al [15] that women who take Depo-Provera (DMPA) for 2 years or more before the age of 25 have at least a 190% increased risk of developing breast cancer. But according to a recent article in the *Wall Street Journal*, Depo-Provera accounted for 19% of all contraceptive use in black women aged 15 to 19 years old, but for only 8% of all contraceptive use in young white women aged 15 to 19 years old [17].

Q-12L: Are black women in South Africa at especially high risk of developing breast cancer from Depo-Provera?

Yes, it would appear so. A study performed on South African women in 1997 found that 72% of black women had used an injectable progestin contraceptive and that 30% of women had used one for 5 years or more [18]. The progestin used most often was either DMPA or norethisterone and these injectable hormones have been used there since the mid 1960s. The study noted that white South African women had a far lower use of these progestin hormones.

Q-12M: In regard to the risks of breast cancer, why has Depo-Provera received so much attention, whereas Norplant and the other progestins have received so little?

Depo-Provera was developed long before Norplant and thus has received the most study. Whatever results apply to it, may apply to the other progestins.

Q-12N: Would use of Norplant (which is made of levonorgestrel) and other progestins carry a risk as high as DMPA (Depo-Provera)?

White et al [3] noted that use of norgestrel containing oral contraceptives (eg, Ovral, which is made by Wyeth-Ayerst), gave rise to a 50% increased risk of breast cancer. Pike et al [2] lists Ovral among those OCPs containing the "highest potency progestins." In his study, high potency progestins carried an infinitely increased risk in women who took them for more than 6 years when under the age of 25. Thus, there is no reason to believe that Norplant is any less dangerous than Depo-Provera, and when one considers the fact that women keep this hormone in their bodies for 5 years at a time, it could cause a significantly higher risk than Depo-Provera.

Q-12O: How dangerous are the progestin "minipills?"

No one is really sure, although they may contain norgestrel which was noted to stimulate the growth of breast cancer cells by two different researchers [19, 20]. The Oxford study noted an overall increased risk of 19% (ie, 1.19 [0.89-1.49]) in women who had taken progestin only OCPs (ie, minipills) for 4 or more years, but the Oxford study said nothing about extended use in young women, especially before their FFTP [21, p.98S]. The New Zealand study [22] noted that women who had taken progestin only OCPs before age 25 had a 1.5-fold risk (0.73-2.9), although the result did not achieve statistical significance.

Q-12P: Does DMPA use cause any other changes?

Yes. "Prolonged DMPA use may be associated with reversible reduction in bone density, probably related to suppression of endogenous production of estrogen" [8]. In addition, women who used DMPA had a 1.2 non-significant relative risk of developing cervical cancer in two large trials [23, p.673]: (ie, [RR=1.2 (0.3-4.5)] in the Costa Rican trial; [RR= 1.2 (0.84-1.72)] in the WHO trial). Last, "although significant findings differed among centers, overall DMPA users had higher low-density lipoprotein (ie, the 'bad cholesterol') and lower high-density lipoprotein levels (ie, the 'good cholesterol')." [8, p.1546]

Q-12Q: Has anyone studied the effect of the progestins on cervical cancer in humans?

Yes, in a large study Herrero et al [24] found that women who had received injectable progestins (ie, usually DMPA [depot-medroxyprogesterone] or norethisterone enanthate) for at least 5 years and who had used them at least 5 years ago, suffered a 430% increased risk of developing cervical cancer [RR=5.3 (1.1-10.0)].

Q-12R: Has any progestin been withdrawn by its manufacturer?

Yes, Deladroxate was pulled by its original manufacturer because "this drug induced a high number of breast cancers in dogs. . ." [25]. In spite of this, other smaller manufacturers have now started making it, and it is used in Latin American countries.

Q-12S: Are there any countries where women may be at particular risk from the injectable progestin contraceptives?

Yes, China, New Zealand, South Africa, and some Latin American countries such as Costa Rica have extensive use of the injectable progestin contraceptives and their women, especially those who used these hormones for extended periods of time (ie, over 2 years) at a young age, are at increased risk for breast cancer [16, 18].

Q-12T: Why has no one said anything to women who get Norplant or Depo-Provera injections?

Actually, some people have tried, but the monetary, political, and media forces have blocked any headway. Staffa, commenting on the studies on DMPA wrote: ". . .two potential high-risk groups were suggested: women who used Depo-MPA (ie, DMPA) at least 2 years before age 25 and long-term users of Depo-MPA before first full-term pregnancy" [16]. In addition to this, a special panel advised the FDA not to approve Depo-Provera at all: "In the end, Weisz and Stolley concluded that the FDA should not sanction contraceptive uses of the drug at all. Ross, however, advised the agency to approve it for women who are mentally retarded or drug addicts." [26]

Q-12U: Does use of the artificial progestins increase the ease of HIV transmission?

Preston Marx, a virologist, exposed two groups of monkeys to an immune virus called SIV (Simian immunodeficiency virus), which is similar to HIV. He gave 10 of these monkeys a placebo and 18 other monkeys received progesterone. Only one of the placebo group contracted SIV whereas 14 out of the 18 monkeys who had received progesterone contracted the virus [27]. "Three of the progesterone group went on to be rapid progressors, developing AIDS in a few weeks and dying within three to four months. Normal disease course in monkeys is two years," according to Marx [27]. In 1996, researchers found that giving progesterone to female monkeys increased their risk of getting AIDS [27]. This makes sense biologically because progesterone is known to thin the vaginal mucosal lining which may reduce the barriers to viruses or bacteria.

Preston's work is supported by studies of women in Thailand, Rwanda, and Kenya. *Ungchusak et al. have noted that prostitutes who used injectable contraceptives (which consist of progestins) had a 240% increased risk [RR = 3.4 (1.2-13.2)] of contracting HIV when compared to those prostitutes who did not use it [28].* Allen et al [29] noted that women in the general population of Rwanda who used injectable contraceptives, had about a 25% higher HIV infection rate than women who did not use them (ie, 38% vs. 30% repectively). Plourde [30] noted that Kenyan women who were positive for HIV, had used medroxprogesterone (ie, the ingredient in Depo-Provera) over 5 times longer, as a group, than women who did not have HIV.

Another important finding by Mostad et al in the 1997 *Lancet* [31] reported that in a group of 318 Kenyan women who had the human immunodeficiency virus, those who were users of depot medroxyprogesterone were 2.9 times more likely than women who did not use hormonal contraceptives to have HIV-1 cells in their cervical secretions. These women would theoretically be more likely to spread the virus.

These findings should shock Africans and Asians because the injectable progestins are widely used in such countries as Indonesia, Thailand, Kenya, Botswana, and Rwanda, where the current ramifications and future implications are especially *serious because these countries are among the hardest hit by AIDS* [1].

References:

1. Garrett L. Contraceptive linked to AIDS risk. *Pittsburgh Post-Gazette.* May 7, 1996.

2. Pike MC, Henderson BE, et al. Breast cancer in young women and use of oral contraceptives: possible modifying effect of formulation and age at use. *The Lancet.* October 22, 1983: 926-929.

3. White E, Malone K, Weiss N, Daling J. Breast cancer among young U.S. women in relation to oral contraceptive use. *J Natl Cancer Inst.* 1994; 86: 505-514.

4. Anderson TJ, Battersby S, et al. Oral contraceptive use influences resting breast proliferation. *Hum Pathol.* 1989; 20: 1139-1144.

5. Schoonen W, et al. Effects of two classes of progestagens, pregnane and 19-nortestosterone derivatives, on cell growth of human breast tumor cells: II. T47D cell lines. *J Steroid Biochem Mol Biol.* 1995; 55: 439-444.

6. Catherino WH, Jeng MH, et al. Norgestrel and gestodene stimulate breast cancer growth through an oestrogen receptor mediated mechanism. *Br J Cancer.* 1992: 945-952.

7. Cunningham FG, et al. *William's Obstetrics.* Stamford, CT: Appleton & Lange; 1993: 1321-1340.

8. Kaunitz A. Long-acting injectable Contraception with depot medroxyprogesterone acetate. *Am J Obstet Gynecol.* 1994; 170: 1543-1549.

9. Lanari C, Molinolo AA, et al. Induction of mammary adenocarcinomas by medroxyprogesterone acetate in balb/c female mice. *Cancer Letters.* 1986; 33: 215-223.

10. Laarsson KS, et al. Predictability of the Safety of Hormonal Contraceptives from Canine Toxicology Studies. In: Michal, F. ed. *Safety Requirements for Contraceptive Steroids.* Cambridge, Cambridge University Press; 1989: 203-269.

11. Rutteman GR. Contraceptive steroids and the mammary gland: is there a hazard? *Breast Cancer Research and Treatment.* 1992; 23: 29-41.

12. Thomas DB, et al. Breast cancer and depot-medroxyprogesterone acetate: a multinational study. *The Lancet.* 1991; 338: 833-838.

13. Paul C, Skegg DCG, Spears GFS. Depot medroxyprogesterone (Depo Provera) and risk of breast cancer. *Br Med J.* 1989; 299: 759-762.

14. Lee NC, Rosero-Bixby L, et al. A case-control study of breast cancer and hormonal contraception in Costa Rica. *J Natl Cancer Inst.* 1987; 6: 1247-1254.

15. Skegg DCG, Noonan EA, et al. Depot medroxyprogesterone acetate and breast cancer [A pooled analysis of the World Health Organization and New Zealand studies]. *JAMA.* 1995: 799-804.

16. Staffa JA, Newschaffer CJ, et al. Progestins and breast cancer: an epidemiologic review. *Fertility and Sterility.* 1992; 57: 473-491.

17. Freedman AM. Why teenage girls love the shot; Why others aren't too sure. *The Wall Street Journal.* October 14, 1998.

18. Bailie R, et al. A case-control study of breast cancer risk and exposure to injectable progestin contraceptives. *S Afr Med J.* 1987; 87: 302-305.

19. Jordan C, Jeng MH, et al. The estrogenic activity of synthetic progestins used in oral contraceptives. *Cancer Supplement.* 1993; 71: 1501-1505.

20. Jeng MH, Parker CJ, et al. Estrogenic potential of progestins in oral contraceptives to stimulate human breast cancer cell proliferation. *Cancer Research.* Dec. 1, 1992: 6539-6546.

21. Collaborative Group on Hormonal Factors in Breast Cancer. Breast cancer and hormonal contraceptives: further results. *Contraception.* 1996; 34: S1-S106.

22. Skegg D, et al. Progestogen-only contraceptives and risk of breast cancer in New Zealand. *Cancer Causes and Control.* 1996; 7: 513-519.

23. Boyle P, Chilvers C, et al. Depot-medroxyprogesterone acetate (DMPA) and cancer: Memorandum from a WHO meeting. *WHO Bulletin OMS.* 1993; 71: 669-676.

24. Herrero, et al. Injectable contraceptives and risk of invasive cervical cancer: evidence of an association. *Int J Cancer.* 1990; 46: 5-7.

25. Koetsawang S. Once-a-month injectable contraceptives: efficacy and reasons for discontinuation. *Contraception.* 1994; 49: 387-398.

26. Sun M. Panel says Depo-Provera not proved safe. *Science.* 1984; 226: 950-951.

27. Marx PA, et al. Progesterone implants enhance SIV vaginal transmission and early virus load. *Nature Medicine.* 1996; 2: 1084-1089.

28. Ungchusak, et al. Determinants of HIV infection among female commercial sex workers in northeastern Thailand: results from a longitudinal study. *J Ac Immune Defic Syn Hum Retro.* 1996; 12: 500-507.

29. Allen S, et al. Human immunodeficiency virus infection in urban Rwanda. *JAMA.* 1991; 266: 1657-1663.

30. Plourde, et al. Human immunodeficiency virus type 1 infection in women attending a sexually transmitted disease clinic in Kenya. *J Infect Dis.* 1992; 166: 86-92.

31. Mostad SB, et al. Hormonal contraception, vitamin A deficiency and other risk factors for shedding HIV-1 infected cells from the cervix and vagina. *The Lancet.* 1997; 350: 922-927.

Chapter 13:
Oral Contraceptives and Cervical Cancer

In 1999, about 4,800 women died from cervical cancer in the U.S. [1]. In addition cervical cancer is the second most prevalent cancer of women in developing countries [2].

Q-13A: Do any animal studies link the risk of using artificial hormones contained within today's contraceptives to an increased risk of cervical carcinoma?

Yes. Rhesus monkeys that were given high doses of medroxyprogesterone (Depo-Provera®) developed cervical cancer [3]. In addition, animal cells have turned cancerous in the presence of the human papilloma virus (HPV) and norgestrel, a common type of progestin found in many of today's oral contraceptives [4]. Last, norethynodrel, another artificial progestin found in today's OCPs, caused cervical cancer in mice [5].

Q-13B: Are there any specific studies that have noted that OCP use increases the risk of invasive cervical cancer?

Yes, there are many studies that link OCP use to an increased risk of cervical carcinoma but before proceeding further it should be noted that there are three main types of invasive cervical cancer. Squamos cervical cancer comprises about 90% of all types, and adenosquamos and adenocarcinoma make up the remaining 10% [6].

In 1992, Delgado-Rodriguez [7] published a meta-analysis which showed that "ever" versus "never" use of OCPs resulted in a 21% increased risk [RR=1.21 (1.1-1.4)]

211

for invasive cervical cancer and a 1.52-fold risk (1.3-1.8) for carcinoma in situ (ie, the preliminary stage of cervical cancer). *Unfortunately*, much of their data came from studies which took their information *before* the 1980s. Because women were taking OCPs for far shorter periods of time in the 1960s and 1970s than in the 1980s and 1990s, and because these earlier studies *did not have an adequate latent period*, the inclusion of the earlier studies in the meta-analysis results in an underestimate of the relative risk.

In 1993, the most massive worldwide study [8] known to date (conducted by the World Health Organization) was published which examined the risk of OCP use and invasive squamos cervical carcinoma (ie, the most prominent type). *It examined more than 2,300 women who had cervical carcinoma* and noted some critical results: 1) if a woman had ever taken an OCP her risk of invasive cervical carcinoma increased by 31% (statistically significant at the 95% confidence level); 2) women who took OCPs for over 5 years had a 51% increased risk [RR= 1.51 (1.22-1.86)] and those who took them for over 8 years had a 123% increased risk [RR= 2.23 (1.84-2.70)]; 3) *women who had taken OCPs before the age of 25 had a 45% increased risk [RR=1.45 (1.24-1.70)];* and 4) women who first started using OCPs as long as 15 years ago had a 37% increased risk of developing cervical carcinoma [RR=1.37 (1.19-1.57)].

Q-13C: What have the studies which took the bulk of their information after 1980 *shown?*

Tables 13A, 13B, 13C, and 13D give the reader an idea of just how strong the link between OCP use and invasive cervical cancer is. The calculations for the weighted average risks are given at the end of the chapter and allow us to estimate a crude estimate for the relative risk for each of the tables. Table 13A yields an elevated risk of 29.66% for cervical cancer if a woman ever used OCPs. Table 13B yields a risk of 61.97% for long-term use of 5 to 10 years of use or more. In Table 13C one sees that OCP use before the age of 20 increases the risk of developing invasive cervical cancer by 80.01%, whereas Table 13D shows that use before age 25 yields a 64.51% increased risk.

Table13A:
EVER VS. NEVER USE OF ORAL CONTRACEPTIVES
AND RISK FOR INVASIVE CERVICAL CANCER

AUTHOR	PERCENT CHANGE	YEARS STUDIED	PATIENTS IN CATEGORY	RESULTS
Beral et al [9]	80% increase*	1987	49	1.8 (1.0-3.3)
Brinton et al [10]	21% increase*	1986-1987	759 Latin-American women	1.21 (0.9-1.6)
Brinton et al [11]	49% increase	1982-1984	479: stack effect	1.49 (1.1-2.1)
Celentano et al [12]	52% (decrease)	1982-1984	85 less than age 45	0.48 (0.22-0.95)
Daling et al [13]	no change	1986-1992	221	1.0 (0.6-1.6)
Ebeling et al [14]	51% increase*	1983-1985	129	1.51 (0.78-2.92)
Irwin et al [15]	20% (decrease)*	1982-1984	149: stack effect	0.8 (0.5-1.3)
Kjaer et al [16]	30% increase*	1987-1988	58: stack effect	1.3 (0.5-3.3)
Parrazini et al [17]	no change*	1981-1993	257: stack effect	1.0 (0.7-1.6)
Peters et al [18]	no change	1980-1981	198	1.0 (no CI's given)
Thomas et al [19] WHO s	50% increase	1979-1988	376	1.5 (1.1-1.9)
Thomas et al [8]	31% increase	1979-1988	2,361	1.31 (1.19-1.45)
Ursin et al [20]	110% increase	1977-1991	195	2.1 (1.1-3.8)

*This result reflects a trend toward an increased or decreased risk but does not attain statistical significance.

Table 13B:
LONG-TERM USE OF ORAL CONTRACEPTIVES AND
RISK FOR INVASIVE CERVICAL CANCER

AUTHOR	PERCENT CHANGE	YEARS STUDIED	PATIENTS IN CATEGORY	RESULTS
Brinton et al [10]	37% increase*	1986-1987	759 non-U.S. women	1.37 (0.9-2.0) for 5-9 years use
Brinton et al [11]	82% increase	1982-1984	479: stack effect	1.82 (1.1-3.1) for >5 years use
Daling et al [13]	30% increase*	1986-1992	221	1.3 (0.7-2.2) for > 5 years use
Ebeling et al [14]	76% increase*	1983-1985	129	1.76 (0.95-3.82) for > 7 years use
Irwin et al [15]	10% (decrease)*	1982-1984	149: stack effect	0.9 (0.5-1.6) > 5 years use
Kjaer et al [16]	30% increase*	1987-1988	56: stack effect	1.3 (0.5-3.5) for > or = to 6 years use

Table 13B is continued on page 214

Table 13B continued

AUTHOR	PERCENT CHANGE	YEARS STUDIED	PATIENTS IN CATEGORY	RESULTS
Parrazini et al [21]	147% increase	1981-1987	367: stack effect	2.47 (1.19-5.13) for > 2 years use
Thomas et al [19] WHO	120% increase	1979-1988	376	2.2 (1.4-3.5) for > 8 years use
Thomas et al [8]	51% increase	1979-1988	2,361	1.51 (1.22-1.86) for more than 5 years use
Ursin et al [20]	340% increase	1977-1991	195	4.4 (1.8-10.8) for > 12 years use

Table 13C: USE OF OCPs BEFORE THE AGE OF 20 AND RISK FOR INVASIVE CERVICAL CANCER

AUTHOR	PERCENT CHANGE	YEARS STUDIED	PATIENTS IN CATEGORY	RESULTS
Brinton et al [10]	46% increase*	1986-1987	759 Latin-American women	1.46 (0.8-2.6) before age 20
Brinton et al [11]	28% increase*	1982-1984	479: stack effect	1.28 (0.8-2.1) before age 20
Daling et al [13]	130% increase*	1986-1992	221	2.3 (1.4-3.8) before age 18
Kjaer et al [16]	30% increase*	1987-1988	56: stack effect	1.3? (0.5-3.5) before age 20
Thomas et al [19] WHO	230% increase	1979-1988	376	3.3 (1.7-6.6) before age 20
Ursin et al [20]	10% increase*	1977-1991	195	1.1 (0.3-3.3) before age 17

Table 13D: RISKS FOR WOMEN WHO USED OCPS BEFORE THE AGE OF 25

AUTHOR	PERCENT CHANGE	YEARS STUDIED	NUMBER OF PATIENTS	RESULTS
Ebeling et al [14]	204% increase	1983-1985	129	3.04 (1.14-8.13) before age 25
Parrazini et al [21]	141% increase*	1981-1987	367: stack effect	2.41 (0.98-5.93) before age 25
Thomas et al [8]	45% increase	1979-1988	2,361	1.45 (1.24-1.70) before age 25

*This result reflects a trend toward an increased or decreased risk but does not attain statistical significance.

Perhaps the most alarming statistic is the one based on the data from Table 13C. If women who use OCPs before the age of 20 truly end up having a long-term increased risk of cervical cancer of over 80%, then these women ought to be made aware of their increased risk and receive frequent Pap smears. A meta-analysis in this area is desperately needed.

Q-13D: Has anyone studied the effect of progestin use on cervical cancer in humans?

Yes. Herrero et al [22], in a large study, found that women who had received injectable progestins (ie, usually DMPA [depot-medroxyprogesterone] or norethisterone enanthate) for at least 5 years and who had used them at least 5 years ago suffered a 430% increased risk of developing cervical cancer [RR=5.3 (1.1-10.0)].

Q-13E: Human Papilloma virus (HPV) has been identified as a causative factor for developing cervical cancer. How do researchers know whether it is the OCPs or the infection with HPV that is increasing the risk of cervical cancer?

Brinton et al [10] in their fairly large study of 759 women who had cervical cancer noted that OCP use increased the risk for cervical cancer although the study controlled for the variable of HPV status. In addition, the authors of the large WHO study [8] believed that HPV and OCP use were not confounding variables because they found no evidence of confounding in those variables closely related to HPV such as anal or genital warts. It would probably be wise to perform more studies which specifically control for HPV status in the future. Until more studies are performed, it would appear that both HPV status and OCP use are real factors in elevating a woman's risk for invasive cervical carcinoma. One animal study [4] and one human study [23] have suggested that OCPs actually accelerate or enhance the process of cervical carcinogenesis in the woman who is already infected with HPV.

Addendum:

How does one calculate the risk of cervical cancer from different types of OCP use after examining Tables 13A, 13B and 13C?

Let us take the information provided in the first section of Table 13C. We note below that it provides us with the risk of cervical cancer for women who had taken OCPs before age 20. The second column (A) shows how much a particular study increased the risk of cervical cancer, whereas the third column (B) shows how many patients were involved in the study. In order to estimate what the total effect of OCP use before the age of 20 is, as concerns the risk of cervical cancer, one must estimate the risk of each individual study and sum up their risks. To do this, one must factor in two parameters for each study. The first is the percentage change that a study showed (column A) and the second is the size of the study (column B). Multiplying these two parameters (A x B) yields the "weighted contribution" of increase for each study. Totaling each of the weighted contributions yields a total of 1671.68. If one now divides this number by the total number of patients (ie, the sum of column C, or 2086) one obtains an estimate for the effect of OCP use on the risk of cervical cancer. That is: (1671.68/2086) = 80.01%.

In other words, if one takes into account the *relative contribution* of each of the studies that examined the risk of OCP use in women under the age of 20 and the corresponding increased risk of cervical cancer, one would find an 80.01% increased risk.

This same technique was applied to the other categories of OCP use and the risk of cervical cancer to yield the results that OCP use prior to the age of 25 yielded a 64.51% increased risk in cervical cancer whereas long-term OCP use led to a 61.97% increased risk and the risk for "ever" versus "never" use was a 29.66% increased risk.

Table 13E:
EARLY USE OF OCPs AND RISK FOR INVASIVE CERVICAL CANCER

RISKS FOR WOMEN WHO USED OCPS BEFORE THE AGE OF 20			
AUTHOR	PERCENT CHANGE (A)	NUMBER OF PATIENTS (B)	Weighted Contributions (A x B)
Brinton et al [10]	46% increase*	759 non-U.S. women	349.14
Brinton et al [11]	28% increase*	479: stack effect	134.12
Daling et al [13]	130% increase*	221	287.30
Kjaer et al [16]	30% increase*	56: stack effect	16.80
Thomas et al [19] WHOs	230% increase	376	864.80
Ursin et al [20]	10% increase*	195	19.50
Totals →	→ → →	2086	1671.68

* This result reflects a trend toward an increased or decreased risk but does not attain statistical significance.

References:

1. Parkin DM, Pisani P., Ferlay J. Global cancer statistics. *CA Cancer J Clin.* 1999; 49:33-64.

2. Landis SH. Murray T. Bolden S. Wingo PA. Cancer statistics, 1999. *CA Cancer J Clin.* 1999; 49:8-31.

3. Dallenbach-Hellweg. On the origin and histological structure of adenocarcinoma of the endocervix in women under 50 years of age. *Path Res Pract.* 1984; 179: 38-50.

4. Pater A, Bayatpour M, et al. Oncogenic transformation by human papillomavirus type 16 deoxyribonucleic acid in the presence of progesterone or progestins from oral contraceptives. *Am J Obstet Gynecol.* April, 1990; 162: 1099-1103.

5. Kahn RH, et al. Effect of long-term treatment with Norethynodrel on A/J and C3H/HeJ mice. *Endocrinology.* 1969; 84: 661.

6. Brinton LA, et al. Risk factors for cervical cancer by histology. *Gynecologic Oncology.* 1993; 51: 301-306.

7. Delgado-Rodriguez M, Sillero-Arenas, et al. Oral contraceptives and cancer of the cervix uteri. *Acta Obstet Gynecol Scand.* 1992; 71: 368-376.

8. Thomas DB, et al. Invasive squamos-cell cervical carcinoma and combined oral contraceptives: Results from a multinational study. *Int J Cancer.* 1993; 53: 228-236.

9. Beral V, Hannaford P, et al. Oral contraceptive use and malignancies of the genital tract. *The Lancet.* Dec. 10, 1988. 1331-1334.

10. Brinton LA, Reeves WC, et al. Oral contraceptive use and risk of invasive cervical cancer. *Int J Epidemiol.* 1990; 19: 4-11.

11. Brinton LA, et al. Long-term use of oral contraceptives and risk of invasive cervical cancer. *Int J Cancer.* 1986; 38: 339-344.

12. Celentano DD. The role of contraceptive use in cervical cancer: the Maryland cervical cancer case-control study. *Am J Epidemiol.* 1987; 126: 592-604.

13. Daling JR, et al. The relationship of HPV-related cervical tumors to cigarette smoking, oral contraceptive use, and prior herpes virus type 2 infection. *Cancer Epidemiology, Biomarkers & Prevention.* 1996; 5: 541-548.

14. Ebeling K, et al. Use of oral contraceptives and risk of invasive cervical cancer in previously screened women. *Int J Cancer.* 1987; 39: 427-430.

15. Irwin KL, Rosero-Bixby L, et al. Oral contraceptives and cervical cancer risk in Costa Rica. *JAMA.* 1988; 259: 59-64.

16. Kjaer SK. Risk factors for cervical neoplasia in Denmark. *Acta Pathol Microbio, Immunol Scand, Supplement* 80. 1998; 80: 5-42.

17. Parrazini F, et al. Determinants of risk of invasive cervical cancer in young women. *Br J Cancer.* 1998; 77: 838-841.

18. Peters K, et al. Risk factors for invasive cervical cancer among Latinas and non-Latinas in Los Angelos County. *J Natl Cancer Inst.* 1986; 77: 1063-1077.

19. Thomas DB, et al. Oral contraceptives and invasive adenocarcinomas and adenosquamos carcinomas of the uterine cervix. *Am J Epidemiol.* 1996; 144: 281-289.

20. Ursin G, Peters RK, et al. Oral contraceptive use and adenocarcinoma of cervix. *The Lancet.* November 19, 1994; 344: 1390-1393.

21. Parrazini F, et al. Oral contraceptive use and invasive cervical cancer. *Int J Epidemiol.* 1990; 19: 259-263.

22. Herrero, et al. Injectable contraceptives and risk of invasive cervical cancer: evidence of an association. *Int J Cancer.* 1990; 46: 5-7.

23. Gitsch G, Kainz C, et al. Oral contraceptives and human papillomavirus infection in cervical intraepithelial neoplasia. *Arch Gynecol Obstet.* 1992; 252: 25-30.

Chapter 14:
Oral Contraceptives and Other Types of Cancer and Non-cancer Risks

Oral Contraceptives and Hepatoma (Liver Cancer):

In 1996, more than 6,500 women died from liver cancer in the U.S. [1]. Although liver cancer is less frequent than breast or ovarian cancer in the U.S., this is not the case in the rest of the world. *Harrison's Internal Medicine* noted: "(Liver cancer) is especially prevalent in regions of Asia and sub-Saharan Africa where the annual incidence is up to 500 cases per 100,000 population" [2, p.579]. In developing countries it is the 7th most common cancer [3]. It occurs 4 times as often in men as in women and most patients die within 1 year of being diagnosed with this cancer.

Q-14A: What implications do these facts have for women who take OCPs?

The high prevalence of liver cancer in Asia and Africa means that if OCP use increases the risk of this type of cancer, they could be putting millions of women at increased risk of getting liver cancer.

Q-14B: What do the studies of long-term OCP use and risk of liver cancer show?

Stanford and Thomas reported the results of a large WHO sponsored study [4] and found that *short-term use* of oral contraceptives *did not* increase the risk of liver cancer. But what is the risk for women who take oral contraceptives for several years? Kenya et al [5] quoted two studies in their 1990 paper. Kenya noted that two authors found an increased risk of hepatocellular carcinoma with long-term OCP use: Forman (1986) found a 20.1-fold risk whereas Neuberger (1986) found a 340% increased risk [*RR*= 4.4 (1.5-12.8)] in women who took OCPs for more than 8 years. Prentice [6] cited two other studies, one by Henderson et al, and the other by La Vecchia et al that both found increased risk for OCP use greater than 5 years: 13.5 RR (1.2-152.2) and 8.3 RR (1.4-48.1) respectively. Finally, in a large study published in 1993, Tavani et al [7] noted that women who used OCPs for more than 5 years had a 290% increased risk [*RR*=3.9 (0.6- 24.5)].

Q-14C: What implications does this data have for the world?

We do not know if the increased risk of hepatocellular carcinoma for *long-term* OCP users applies to Asian and African countries, because most of the studies were done on patients from Western countries. If the risk of long-term OCP use does result in a 4-fold increased risk of hepatocellular cancer, the implications could already be severe. It was noted earlier that the rate of liver cancer in some Asian and African countries is 500 per 100,000 people. If a country had 200 million adults and therefore approximately 100 million men and 100 million women, it could be expected that 400,000 men and 100,000 women would get liver cancer every year. If even 20% of the female population used OCPs for a long-term basis (ie, greater than 5 years) one could expect an additional 60,000 cases of liver cancer in women annually based on a 4-fold risk (see calculations at the end of this chapter). There are many large Asian and African countries as well as other countries that have high rates of liver cancer, so one would have to multiply this number several fold in order to obtain the cumulative increased risk which could be several hundred thousand women every year — most of whom would die from their liver cancer!

Q-14D: The increased risk of long-term OCP use was addressed, but what about the increased risk for long acting progestins such as Norplant or Depo-Provera?

This author does not know of any recent world trial studying the effects of long-term progestins on the risk of liver cancer, so no one knows if they carry less, equal or more risk than long-term OCP use. An article cited in *The Lancet* in 1994 noted that at least one researcher had found that a specific progestin "induces DNA damage in cultured rat hepatocytes (liver cells)." [8] At this point one must be cautious. It is possible that long-term progestins will cause the same increased risk of developing liver cancer as long-term OCP users have.

Oral Contraceptives and Endometrial (Uterine) Cancer:

In 1999 about 6,400 women died from uterine cancer in the U.S. [1]. It has been observed by several authors that OCP use decreases the risk of uterine cancer. Oral contraceptives thin the lining of the uterus, resulting in a decreased monthly menstrual flow for women, as well as a decreased rate of mitosis (division) for a woman's endometrial cells. This results in an overall decreased risk of uterine cancer.

Table 14A:
THE RISK OF OCPS AND UTERINE CANCER

AUTHOR	PERCENT CHANGE	YEARS STUDIED	NUMBER OF PATIENTS	RESULTS
Ory et al (CASH)[9]	40% (decrease)	1980-1982	433: stack effect	0.6 (0.3-0.9) for "ever" use; 0.4 (0.2-0.8) > 10 years; 0.4 (0.2-0.7) 20 yrs since first use
Levi et al [10]	50% (decrease)	1988-1990	122: stack effect	0.5 (0.3-0.8) for "ever" use; 0.3 (0.1-0.7) for > 5 yrs use; 0.8 (0.3-2.2), 20 yrs since last use
Jick et al [11]	52% (decrease)	1979-1989	142	0.48 (0.26-0.89) for "ever" use; 0.32 (0.11-0.87) for > 5 yrs use; 0.62 (0.19-2.07) 20 yrs since first use
Stanford et al [12]	60% (decrease)	1987-1990	297	0.4 (0.3-0.7) for "ever" use; 0.17 (0.1-0.5) for > 10 yrs use; 0.74 (0.4-1.4) 25 yrs since first use

What does Table 14A tell us? Several trends are noticeable. The largest study — the CASH study — notes a 40% decreased risk in uterine cancer for "ever" versus "never" use of OCPs, although the severe stack effect artificially inflates their degree of decreased risk. Overall however, it appears that OCPs confer a 40 to 50% decreased risk for uterine cancer. They further decrease the risk of uterine cancer if they are taken for longer lengths of time. Taking OCPs for more than 5 years would appear to lower the risk of uterine cancer by up to 60 to 70%.

Q-14E: What about the long-term "protective effect" of OCP use relative to uterine cancer?

Several studies [10, 11 and 12] show that the protection from developing uterine cancer from OCP *use tends to decrease as time goes by.* In each of these studies noted in Table 14B, *there was less protection from uterine cancer from OCP use when one looked at the data for women who had used OCPs more than 20 years ago.*

Table 14B:
WHAT IS THE LONG-TERM RISK OF OCP USE AND UTERINE CANCER?

AUTHOR→	Levi et al [10]	Jick et al [11]	Stanford et al [12]
Time since last use:			
10 years	0.3 (0.1-0.9) 70% decrease	0.35 (0.11-1.09) 65% decrease*	0.19 (0.0-0.3) 81% decrease
11-19 years	0.4 (0.2-1.0) 60% decrease*	0.45 (0.14-1.49)** 55% decrease*	0.38 (0.1-0.8) 62% decrease
> 20 years	0.8 (0.3-2.2) 20% decrease*	0.62 (0.19-2.07) 38% decrease*	0.71 (0.4-1.3) 29% decrease*

*This result reflects a trend toward an increased or decreased risk but does not attain statistical significance.

**Estimated from combining data from the 10 to 14 and 15 to 19 "years after last OCP use" groups.

Q-14F: Does OCP use increase the risk of developing any other type of cancer of the uterus?

Yes, OCP use increases the risk of *choriocarcinoma* and the *invasive hydatidiform mole.* Both of these cancers occur rarely in pregnancy. Palmer [13] noted that 5 years or more of OCP use results in a 6-fold risk (1.3-28) of choriocarcinoma and a 2.8-fold trend toward (0.8-4.8) invasive hydatidiform mole. About 1 in every 6000 pregnancies result in an invasive mole and about 1 out of every 20,000 results in a choriocarcinoma. Of note, choriocarcinoma is more common in Asia, where it may constitute 1 out of every 5000 pregnancies.

Oral Contraceptives and Malignant Melanoma: Table 14C:

RISKS OF MALIGNANT MELANOMA TO WOMEN WHO HAD A HISTORY OF LONG-TERM ORAL CONTRACEPTIVE USE

AUTHOR	PERCENT CHANGE	YEARS STUDIED	NUMBER OF PATIENTS & LENGTH OF USE	RESULTS
Adami et al[15]	57% increase*	1971-1976	6 used OCPs for 5 or more yrs.	1.57 (0.83-3.03)
Bain et al [16]	20% (decrease)*	1979-1981	23 with 5 or more yrs.	0.8 (CI not given)
Beral et al [17]	50% increase	1974-1980	28 with 5 or more yrs.	1.5 (1.03-2.14)**
Hannaford et al [18]	2% (decrease)*	1974-?1989 prospective	#? 10 or more yrs. Oxford data	0.98 (0.24-3.09)
Hannaford et al [18]	77% increase*	1974-?1989 prospective	#? 10 or more yrs. RCGP data	1.77 (0.8-3.9)
Helmrich et al [19]	no change	1976-1982	5 with 10 or more yrs.	1.0 (0.4-2.9)
Holly et al [20]	110% increase	1976-1979	#? 10 or more yrs.	2.1 (CI not given)
Holly et al [21]	17% (decrease)*	1981-1986	#? (not given) for 10 or more yrs.	0.83 (0.54-1.3)
Lé et al [22]	110% increase*	1982-1987	13 with 10 or more yrs.	2.1 (0.7-5.9)
Osterlind et al 23	no change	1982-1985	30 with 10 or more yrs.	1.0 (0.6-1.7)
Palmer et al [24]	45% increase	1979-1991	25 with 10 or more yrs.	1.45 raw risk**
Westerdahl [25]	no change	1988-1990	19 with > 8 yrs.	1.0 (0.5-2.0)

*This result reflects a trend toward an increased or decreased risk but does not attain statistical significance.

Malignant melanoma is one of the most dangerous and rapidly spreading cancers known. There has been a steady increase in melanoma in women in the U.S. In 1962, about 1054 women died from it. By 1996 it was estimated that 2,700 women would die from melanoma. Is there a link between OCP use and malignant melanoma? A review by

Osterlind [14] found that there was not much increase in melanoma for women who took OCPs when comparing "ever" versus "never" use. However, 4 out of 7 studies showed a trend toward increased risk when OCPs were taken for longer than 5 years. Since then, more studies have been done and Table 14C summarizes studies which have examined the risk of taking OCPs for 5 years.

Six out of 12 studies show a trend toward an increased risk for malignant melanoma due to long-term OCP use but only two results are likely statistically significant (ie, the studies with the double asterisk next to them). No study shows a *statistically significant* decrease. *Thus, the evidence would indicate that there is a trend for a possible increased risk for malignant melanoma in a number of studies with long-term OCP use. No formal risk estimate can be made until a researcher or research team performs a complete meta-analysis on all the long-term studies done to date.* This would be important to do, because even a 30% increase in malignant melanoma in women who take OCPs for longer periods of time would be important to know about.

Oral Contraceptives and Ovarian Cancer

Ovarian cancer was estimated to claim the lives of about 14,800 women in the U.S. in 1996 [1]. The medical literature indicates that having children, breastfeeding, and using OCPs all decrease the risk of ovarian cancer.

Q-14G: How much does OCP use decrease the risk of ovarian cancer?

Hankinson, Colditz et al [26,] performed a meta-analysis in 1992 which showed that "ever" versus "never" use of OCPs resulted in a 36% overall decreased risk of ovarian cancer and 5 or more years of use resulted in a 50% overall reduction of ovarian cancer. These results are fairly well accepted, however a number of other questions have received far less attention.

Q-14H: Is the reduced risk of ovarian cancer from OCP use a "long-term" phenomenon?

Hankinson et al [26] reported that the reduced risk of taking OCPs seems to last for up to 10 years after taking them, but two issues are raised. First, most of their data came from studies from the 1960s and 1970s when OCP estrogen and progestin doses were higher than in OCPs of the 1980s and 1990s. *Lowering the hormonal content of OCPs has led to more ovarian activity* (ie, a higher rate of breakthrough ovulation). Thus today's low dose OCPs may offer less protection against ovarian cancer than those of the 1960s and 1970s. A leading oral contraceptive researcher (Goldzieher) has stated as late as 1994: ". . .the protection against these types of reproductive cancers (ie, ovarian and endometrial) have been shown repeatedly with high-dose oral contraceptives but not, to date, with lower dose oral contraceptives." [27].

The second problem is that few studies have commented on the reduced risk of ovarian cancer for longer periods of time after last OCP use. A study published in 1994 of over 1400 patients with ovarian cancer by Rosenberg et al [28] measured the effects of OCP use in women who had taken them for at least 3 years and took them for the last time over 20 years ago. *In Table 14D her results show a reduced long-term effect of OCP protection as the length of time since last use of OCP increases.*

Table 14D:

**WOMEN WHO USED OCPS FOR 3 OR MORE YEARS
AND THE RISK OF OVARIAN CANCER
IN THE ROSENBERG STUDY**

Time since last OCP use in years	PERCENT CHANGE	RELATIVE RISK	CONFIDENCE INTERVAL
No use	no change		
<15	60% decrease	0.4	0.2-0.8
15-19	50% decrease*	0.5	0.3-1.0
20 or more years ago	20% decrease*	0.8	0.4-1.5

*This result reflects a trend toward an increased or decreased risk but does not attain statistical significance.

Q-14I: Do women who have more children have a decreased risk in ovarian cancer?

Results from a pooled analysis of 12 studies in 1993 by Whittemore [29] showed that white women had about a 15% reduction in ovarian cancer for every child they delivered. This result corroborates the findings in the CASH trial reported by Gwinn et al [30] which found that women who had three children had a 40% reduction in ovarian cancer whereas *women who had five or more children, had a 70% reduced risk of ovarian carcinoma. In contrast, Whittemore and Spiritas noted that women who remain infertile after taking fertility drugs have a staggering 1100% increased risk of developing ovarian cancer, according to the large collaborative study which pooled the results of twelve studies* [31, 32].

Q-14J: Does breastfeeding decrease the risk of ovarian cancer?

Yes. Whittemore et al [29] also noted that white women who had "ever breastfed" had about a 19% decreased risk of ovarian cancer which continued to decrease for every month that a woman breastfed. Gwinn et al [30] noted that women who breastfed for more than a cumulative length of 2 years had a 70% decreased risk in ovarian cancer.

Q-14K: Do these same statistics apply when the black population is studied?

They appear to apply. John et al [33] found that black women who had four or more children had a 47% decreased risk of ovarian cancer. Women who breastfed for at least 6 months had a 15% reduction and women who used OCPs for 6 years or longer had a 38% decreased risk.

Q-14L: Are there "any other" ovarian tumors that are affected by OCP use?

Yes. Usually when doctors speak about ovarian cancer they are speaking about a particular type called "epithelial ovarian cancer" which is the most common type. Nonepithelial cancers comprise about 7% of the rest of the malignant ovarian cancers. The two main types of non-epithelial cancers are called germ cell and stromal cell ovarian cancers. They both tend to occur in younger women. Oral contraceptives increase the trend toward developing a germ cell tumor: 2.0 (0.77-5.10) and reduce the risk of stromal cell tumors by 63%: [RR=0.37 (0.16-0.83)] according to one collaborative study [33].

Q-14M: What is the overall risk of early OCP use, when one summarizes the risk for all cancers?

The results presented here indicate that OCP use increases the risk of breast cancer, cervical cancer, and liver cancer, whereas they decrease the risk of uterine and ovarian cancer. In order to estimate the overall risk we must admit that no one really knows what the long-term effect of early OCP use is on any of these cancers. That is, we do not know if the trend for an increased risk in breast cancer or the decreased risk in ovarian cancer from early OCP use will get bigger or smaller as women approach their 60s and 70s. Because women are taking OCPs for longer periods of time and earlier in their lives the appropriate question to ask is:

Do women who use OCPs for 4 or more years before their first full-term pregnancy (FFTP) sustain an overall risk of more or less cancers if we base our answer on studies that predominantly take their information after 1980? (data taken from American Cancer Society: [1])

Table 14E:

CUMULATIVE EFFECT OF LONG-TERM*
EARLY OCP USE ON THE TOTAL NUMBER OF
REPRODUCTIVE CANCERS IN THE USA

TYPE OF CANCER	NUMBER OF CASES FROM 1996 ESTIMATE	NUMBER OF DEATHS FROM 1996 ESTIMATE	ESTIMATED RATE OF INCREASE OR DECREASE	NUMBER OF ADDITIONAL OR REDUCED "CASES"
BREAST CANCER	184,300	44,300	44% to 72% increase	+59,400 to 97,200
CERVICAL CANCER	15,700	4,900	50% increase	+ 5,750
OVARIAN CANCER	26,700	14,800	50% decrease	- 9,779
UTERINE CANCER	34,000	6,000	50% decrease	-12,452
TOTAL				+42,919 to 80,719

*Long-term is defined here as at least 4 years of use before a first full-term pregnancy.

If one takes the statistics from the 1976 to 1980 database regarding early OCP use in women under the age of 24, one can estimate how many women used OCPs prior to their FFTP. (A detailed account of how the estimates were obtained is provided for at the end of this chapter). If the current trends continue, *between 42,919 to 80,719 additional women will be expected to get cancer annually due to early, long-term OCP use as shown in Table 14E.* The cumulative effect of early long-term OCP use is certainly negative.

Q14N: What about the extra cases of liver cancer that would be caused by early OCP use?

Table 14F:
CUMULATIVE EFFECT OF LONG-TERM OCP USE*
ON THE TOTAL NUMBER OF LIVER
AND MELANOMA CANCERS IN THE USA

TYPE OF CANCER	NUMBER OF CASES FROM 1996	NUMBER OF DEATHS FROM 1996	ESTIMATED RATE OF INCREASE	NUMBER OF ADDITIONAL CASES
LIVER CANCER	9,100	6,800	300% increase	+ 19,997
MALIGNANT MELANOMA	16,500	2,700	? increase	?

* Long-term use is defined as at least 5 years of use, not necessarily before a first full-term pregnancy.

Table 14F shows that if long-term OCP use truly increases the risk of liver cancer, then an additional 19,997 women will be expected to develop liver cancer annually in the U.S. in future years. *A worldwide figure would be many times higher if the conservative estimate of a 300% increased risk ends up applying to women in Asia and Africa as well.* It was noted earlier that if the rate of long-term OCP use in an Asian or African country is 20%, and if long-term OCP use truly does result in a 300% increased risk, an extra 60,000 women will get liver cancer each year, based on a sample size of 100 million women. If one includes a larger population by including the other Asian and African countries as well as other countries from around the world, one would note an increase of 300,000 "cases" per year for a population of 500 million women.

The cure rate of liver cancer is very low; thus, many of these women would end up dying from their liver cancer. In addition, it will be extremely helpful if researchers perform a meta-analysis regarding long-term OCP use and the risk of malignant melanoma, because that would allow estimates of how many women would be at risk of developing malignant melanoma.

Oral Contraceptives and Non-cancer Risks:

Q-14O: Does OCP use have any other risks that should be mentioned? (Most of the following information was taken from the 1996 drug insert of the OCP named Orthocept [34]).

In addition to the elevated risks of breast, cervical, and hepatic cancer, OCP use carries an increased risk of other major side effects which include:

-heart attacks primarily in women with other risk factors such as diabetes, smoking, hypertension, or severe obesity.

-blood clots and pulmonary embolism*

-hypertension

-worsening of cholesterol levels

-causing or worsening of depression

-worsening of headaches, especially migraines

-development of melasma (ie, "dark skin spots") especially in the facial area

Q-14P: Does OCP use protect against osteoporosis?

Carson performed an overview of OCP use and osteoporosis, presenting both positive and negative studies [*Journal of Reproductive Medicine*, 1993]. Unfortunately, the two largest studies which were claimed to be positive were either too old (eg, the Goldsmith study in 1975) or had severe design errors. For example, Carson cites the Kleerekoper study [36] which found that women who did not take OCPs had a lower bone mineral density than

---

*It should be noted that today's low-dose OCPs may contain one of the new types of synthetic progestins called gestodene or desogestrel which apparently increase a woman's susceptibility to thrombosis (blood clots) [35].

women who did take OCPs. This study examined women ranging in age from 15 to 91 years old. This basically invalidates the study because most women over 60 years old never had the opportunity to take OCPs, therefore women with the least OCP use (ie, the older women) had the most osteoporosis. This type of error is called a failure to properly age-match. The study should have limited itself to studying women of the same age group (eg, women ages 52-55 years old) who would then theoretically have had similar exposures to OCP availability.

Other studies have suggested that OCP use plays a role in causing osteoporosis. Register et al [37] have noted that oral contraceptive use inhibits the normal acquisition of bone mineral in skeletally immature young adult female monkeys and Cooper et al [38], in a large British study, noted that women who took oral contraceptives actually had a statistically significant 20% *increase* in the occurrence of osteoporotic fractures in later life [$RR = 1.20$ (1.08-1.34)]. Few women have heard this information.

Q-14Q: *Does OCP use increase the likelihood of transmitting the HIV virus?*

It was noted previously that injectable progesterone thins the vaginal mucosal lining and that the use of injectable progestins has been implicated in the transmission of HIV (Human Immunodeficiency Virus) in both monkeys [39] and in women in Thailand, Kenya, and Rwanda [40, 41]. Because OCPs contain artificial progestins, their use also might cause increased risk. Several studies support this. Allen et al [41] found that 38% of Rwandan women with HIV had used OCPs versus only 30% of women who did not use OCPs. *Simonsen et al noted that prostitutes from Nairobi, Kenya, had an 80% increased risk of acquiring the HIV if they had used OCPs [42].* One study, by Mati et al [43] found a 50% (statistically non-significant) increase in the risk of HIV infection for women who took OCPs for more than 2 years. This study did not study prostitutes, but instead examined "women thought not to be of high-risk behavior." Because most of the women in this study were married and the number of sexual partners was low, one must question the validity of the study. Obviously, the latter study could fail to pick up the real risk of OCP use if a significant number of women who were faithfully married to a man who did not carry HIV, were on the Pill. These women would not get HIV, independent of whether or not they were using OCPs.

In addition, Mostad et al in the 1997 *Lancet* [44] reported that in a group of 318 Kenyan women who had the human immunodeficiency virus, those who were users of low-dose OCPs were 3.8 times more likely than women who did not use hormonal contraceptives to have HIV-1 cells in their cervical secretions whereas women who used high-dose OCPs were 12.3 times more likely to shed the virus. These women would theoretically be more likely to spread the virus.

Addendum 14A:
Estimates for Risks of Liver Cancer Due to OCP Use:

For a population containing 200 million adults, it is estimated that 100 million will be female. Because the rate of liver carcinoma is 500 per 100,000 in certain Asian and African countries and because it occurs 4 times as frequently in men as in women, an annual incidence of 400,000 "cases" for men and 100,000 "cases" for women is predicted (ie, the rate in men is 400 per 100,000 and the rate in women is 100 per 100,000). Now if 20% of the women had used OCPs on a long-term basis (ie, 5 years or longer)*, it would mean that 20 million women had used them on a long-term basis whereas 80 million had not. These 20 million women would now sustain a risk of 400 per 100,000 (ie, 4-fold their normal rate), and would be expected to develop 80,000 "cases" every year in addition to the 80,000 "cases" from the 80 million women who did not use OCPs on a long-term basis. Thus, in this sample population in which 20% of the women used OCPs on a long-term basis, one would expect 160,000 women to get liver

*In Brinton's study of OCPs, she noted that 37% of women took them for 5 years or more [45, p.830].

cancer every year, which is 60,000 more than the figure of 100,000 which one would expect if no women took OCPs. This example is based on the predictions made for only one country of 200 million adults; its implications would have to be markedly increased for the cumulative populations of Asia and Africa. Often African or Asian women take injectable progestins instead of OCPs. If progestins end up causing a risk similar to that from OCP use, the above statistics would apply to those populations as well.

Addendum 14B:
Calculating the Cumulative Cancer Risk for Early Long-Term OCP Use:

How were the data in Table 14E calculated? The estimates were made using data from Brinton's large study [45] as well as the cited statistic that currently about 10 million women in the U.S. are using OCPs. How can one estimate how many young women were using OCPs for 4 or more years prior to their first full-term pregnancy (FFTP)?

Brinton et al [45] noted in their study that 28.7% of women who had taken OCPs (520/1813) had taken them for 4 or more years prior to their FFTP. Two factors must be taken into account before estimating how many women took OCPs for 4 years or more prior to their FFTP. First, if there are currently 10 million women each year who took OCPs, it does not mean that over 4 years 40 million women will have used OCPs. Why? Because some women use OCPs for less than a year and some use them for several years. One cannot count the latter group as new women using OCPs each year or one would in effect "over count." Second, one must note that women have been using OCPs earlier in their lives and for longer periods of time today than back in the 1960s and 1970s [46, p.9S]. So instead of simply stating that 28.7% of all of the 10 million women using OCPs today are taking them for 4 years or more prior to their FFTP, it is conservatively estimated that 11.25% of women are. [One lowers the base projection by one-third to conservatively correct for over counting and multiplies by an additional 17.6% to account for the increased use of OCPs for longer periods of time at an early age today: (28.7% x 1/3 x 1.176 = 11.25%)]. In order to calculate how many additional breast cancer cases will be caused by early long-term OCP use in the U.S., one multiplies 1.125 million (11.25% x 10 million) by 12% (ie, today's life-time breast cancer risk is conservatively estimated at 12%), which yields the number 135,000. This is the number of breast cancer cases that would be expected to develop in a group of 1.125 million women over a lifetime. If one multiplies 135,000 by either 44% or 72% (which is the estimated increased risk of breast cancer for 4 years of OCP use prior to a FFTP), one obtains 59,400 to 97,200, which represents the number of additional cases of breast cancer due to early long-term OCP use.

In order to calculate the estimated number of cases for each of the other cancers, one simply multiplies the number of women at risk (ie, 1.125 million) by the expected prevalence of the cancer. The expected prevalence for cervical cancer would be a fraction of the rate of breast cancer. Because there were 15,700 cases of cervical cancer and 184,300 cases of breast cancer, cervical cancer has an incidence of: 15,700/184,300 or 0.0852 times the prevalence of breast cancer. Because about 12% of the female population will obtain breast cancer over a lifetime, it means that roughly 12% x 0.0852 or 1.0222% of the female population will get cervical cancer over a lifetime. Multiplying 1.0222% by the number of women at risk (1.125 million) yields 11,500 which is the expected number of these women who would normally get cervical cancer over a lifetime. Multiplying this by a 50% increased risk yields a number of 5,750 which is the expected number of new "cases" of cervical cancer that one would see using an estimate of 50% increased risk for women who took OCPs for 4 years or more prior to their FFTP.

Four years of OCP use would be expected to prevent ovarian cancer and so in the same way one can calculate that 9,779 "cases" of ovarian cancer would be prevented as well as 12,452 "cases" of uterine cancer. The total number of new "cases" would then be (59,400 to 97,200) + 5,750-

9,779-12,452 = (42,919 to 80,719) new cases of cancer in women due to long-term early OCP use.

The additional cases of liver cancer were not included in this projection, but if one notes that at least 1.125 million women would be at risk for using OCPs for 5 years or longer (despite the longer length of time of 5 years used here, this statistic no longer specifies that the OCP use be before a FFTP so at least this many women would be at risk), one would find that an additional 19,997 cases of liver cancer would be expected to develop annually in future years based on a 300% increased risk (ie, 9100/ 184,300 *135,000*300%=19,997). Unfortunately, the decrease in liver cancer that might be expected due to a decrease in the hepatitis incidences in modern countries, may be offset by the increase due to early long-term OCP use.

References:

1. Parkin DM, Pisani P, Ferlay J. Global cancer statistics. *CA Cancer J Clin.* 1999; 49: 33–64.

2. Fauci AS, et al. *Harrison's: Principle of Internal Medicine.* 14th ed. New York: McGraw Hill; 1998.

3. Parkin, et al. Estimates of the worldwide frequency of sixteen major cancers in1980. *Int J Cancer.* 1988; 41: 184-197.

4. Stanford JL. Combined oral contraceptives and liver cancer. *Int J Cancer.* 1989; 43: 254-259.

5. Kenya PR. Oral contraceptive use and liver tumours: a review. *East African Medical Journal.* 1990; 67:146-153.

6. Prentice RL. Epidemiologic data on exogenous hormones and hepatocellular carcinoma and selected other causes. *Preventive Medicine.* 1991; 20: 38-46.

7. Tavani A, et al. Female hormone utilisation and risk of hepatocellular carcinoma. *Br J Cancer.* 1993; 67: 635-637.

8. Rabe T, et al. Liver tumors in women on oral contraceptives. *The Lancet.* 1994; 344: 1568-1569.

9. Ory HW, et al. Combination oral contraceptive use and the risk of endometrial cancer. *JAMA.* 1987; 257: 796-800.

10. Levi F, et al. Oral contraceptive and the risk of endometrial cancer. *Cancer Causes and Control.* 1991; 2: 99-103.

11. Jick S, et al. Oral contraceptives and endometrial cancer. *Obstet Gynecol.* 1993; 82: 931-935.

12. Stanford JL, et al. Oral contraceptives and endometrial cancer: Do other risk factors modify the association? *Int J Cancer.* 1993; 54: 243-248.

13. Palmer JR. Oral contraceptive use and gestational choriocarcinoma. *Cancer Detection and Prevention*. 1991; 15: 45-48.

14. Osterlind A. Hormonal and reproductive factors in melanoma risk. *Clinics in Dermatology*. 1992; 10: 75-78.

15. Adam SA, Sheaves JK, et al. A case-control study of the possible association between oral contraceptives and malignant melanoma. *Br J Cancer*. 1981; 41: 45-50.

16. Gallagher RP, Elwood JM, et al. Reproductive factors, oral contraceptives and risk of malignant melanoma: Western Canada melanoma study. *Br J Cancer*. 1985; 52: 901-907.

17. Beral V, Evans S, et al. Oral contraceptive use and malignant melanoma in Australia. *Br J Cancer*. 1984; 50: 681-685.

18. Hannaford PC, et al. Oral contraceptives and malignant melanoma. *Br J Cancer*. 1991; 63: 430-433.

19. Helmrich S, Rosenberg L, et al. Lack of elevated risk of malignant melanoma in relation to oral contraceptive use. *J Natl Cancer Inst*. 1984; 72: 617-620.

20. Holly EA, Weiss NS, et al. Cutaneous melanoma in relation to exogenous hormones and reproductive factors. *J Natl Cancer Inst*. 1983; 70: 827-831.

21. Holly E, Cress R, Ahn DK. Cutaneous melanoma in women. *Am J Epidemiol*. 1995; 141: 943-950.

22. Lé MG, Cabanes PA, et al. Oral contraceptive use and risk of cutaneous malignant melanoma in a case-control study of French women. *Cancer Causes and Control*. 1992; 3: 199-205.

23. Osterland A, et al. The Danish case-control study of cutaneous malignant melanoma *Int J Cancer*. 1988; 42: 821-824.

24. Palmer Jr, et al. Oral contraceptive use and risk of cutaneous malignant melanoma. *Cancer Causes and Control*. 1992; 3: 547-554.

25. Westerdahl J, et al. Risk of malignant melanoma in relation to drug intake, alcohol, smoking and hormonal factors. *Br J Cancer*. 1996; 73: 1126-1131.

26. Hankinson SE, et al. A quantitative assessment of oral contraceptive use and risk of ovarian cancer. *Obstet Gynecol*. 1992; 80: 708-714.

27. Goldzieher JW. Are low-dose oral contraceptives safer and better? *Am J Obstet Gynecol*. 1994; 171: 587-590.

28. Rosenberg L, et al. A case-control study of oral contraceptive use and invasive epithelial ovarian carcinoma. *Am J Epidemiol*. 1994; 139: 654-661.

29. Whittemore AS. Personal characteristics relating to risk of invasive epithelial ovarian cancer in older women in the United States. *Cancer Supplement*. 1993; 71: 558-564.

30. Gwinn ML, et al. Pregnancy, breastfeeding and oral contraceptives and the risk of epithelial ovarian cancer. *J Clin Epidemiol*. 1990; 43: 559-568.

31. Whittemore AS et al. Characteristics relating to ovarian cancer risk: collaborative analysis of 12 U.S. case-control studies. II. Invasive epithelial ovarian cancers in white women. Collaborative Ovarian Cancer Group. *Am J Epidemiol.* 1992; 136: 1184-1203.

32. Spiritas R, et al. Fertility drugs and ovarian cancer: Red alert or red herring: *Fertility and Sterility.* 1993; 59: 291.

33. John EM, et al. Characteristics relating to ovarian cancer risk: Collaborative analysis of seven U.S. case-control studies. Epithelial Ovarian Cancer in Black Women. *J Natl Cancer Inst.* 1993; 85: 142-147.

34. Orthocept: Drug Insert. Ortho Pharmaceuticals. 1996.

35. Herman R. New birth control pills increase clotting danger. *Pittsburgh Post-Gazette.* June 3, 1997: F4.

36. Kleerekoper M, et al. Oral contraceptive use may protect against low bone mass. *Arch Intern Med.* 1991; 151: 1971-1976.

37. Register TC, et al. Oral contraceptive treatment inhibits the normal acquisition of bone mineral in skeletally immature young adult female monkeys. *Osteo Int.* 1997; 7: 348-353.

38. Cooper C, et al. Oral contraceptive pill use and fractures in women: a prospective study. *Bone.* 1993; 14: 41-45.

39. Marx PA, et al. Progesterone implants enhance SIV vaginal transmission and early virus load. *Nature Medicine.* 1996; 2: 1084-1089.

40. Ungchusak, et al. Determinants of HIV infection among female commercial sex workers in northeastern Thailand: results from a longitudinal study. *J Ac Immune Defic Syn Hum Retro.* 1996. 12: 500-507.

41. Allen S, et al. Human immunodeficiency virus infection in urban Rwanda. *JAMA.* 1991; 266: 1657-1663.

42. Simonsen, et al. HIV infection among lower socioeconomic strata prostitutes in Nairobi. *AIDS.* 1990: 139-144.

43. Mati, et al. Contraceptive use and the risk of HIV in Nairobi, Kenya. *Int J Gynecol Obstet.* 1995; 48: 61-67.

44. Mostad SB, et al. Hormonal contraception, vitamin A deficiency and other risk factors for shedding HIV-1 infected cells from the cervix and vagina. *The Lancet.* 1997; 350: 922-927.

45. Brinton LA, Daling JR, et al. Oral contraceptives and breast cancer risk among younger women. *J Natl Cancer Inst.* 6/7/1995; 87: 827-835.

46. Collaborative Group on Hormonal Factors in Breast Cancer. Breast cancer and hormonal contraceptives: further results. *Contraception.* 1996; 34: S1-S106.

Chapter 15:

World Ramifications of Oral Contraceptive Pill Use and Abortion Performed Early in a Woman's Reproductive Life

Many of the researchers who studied oral contraceptive use or abortion performed early in a woman's reproductive life are from the U.S. Because this country has a high rate of both early OCP use and abortion, we are certainly one of the countries at highest risk for the development of new cases of breast cancer. What about the rest of the world? A number of the women in other countries are at increased risk for breast cancer, especially if they had, have, or will have a high rate of either early OCP use or induced abortion at a young age. It should be remembered that countries whose women take OCPs are at increased risk for cervical cancer (ie, a conservative estimate for 4 years of use is a 50% increase, see Chapter 13). Finally, *it must again be emphasized that women who live in Asian or African countries, or any other country with high rates of liver cancer, are at extreme risk if they take hormonal contraceptives for more than 5 years, because they have been estimated to increase the risk of liver cancer fourfold* [1].

Risks for Women of Specified Countries:

Africa: Africa will be at especially high risk for accelerating its liver cancer rate as the rate of oral contraceptive use is increased, noting that long-term OCP use increases liver cancer rates by 300%. In addition, if OCP use and/or use of progestins such as Depo-Provera and Norplant increase the transmission of the HIV virus, as is *strongly suggested* by the literature [2], it may be contributing to an even faster growth in the number of AIDS "cases."

Australia: Rohan et al [3] wrote in 1988 that: "Australia was one of the first countries in which oral contraceptive agents became available for use. The uptake of the use of oral contraceptive agents was extensive, and by the late 1960s they were used more commonly in Australia than elsewhere." His study showed a 1.93 RR (0.44-4.4) in a group of 113 premenopausal women who had used OCPs for 19 months or more before their <u>first full-term pregnancy</u> (FFTP). A small study by Ellery et al [4] showed no risk with early OCP use but one cannot put much stock in a study that was so small (ie, it had only about 35 women under the age of 45). Australia's younger women may be at enormous risk because nearly 100% of women born after 1950 have reportedly used OCPs [5, 36S]. In addition, Australia has had selective use of DMPA (depot-medroxyprogesterone), which has been noted to cause a 190% increase (or more) in breast cancer in women who took it before the age of 25 for more than 2 years [6, 7]. As concerns induced abortion, Brind noted that Rohan's work showed a 160% increased risk for Australian women who had had an induced abortion [8, p.7]. Last, Australia has one of the highest rates of childless women, in those women born after 1950, putting its women at even higher risk for breast cancer because women who are nulliparous (ie, have no children) are at increased risk for developing breast cancer [9].

Brazil: According to *Population Reports* [10], Brazil experienced one of the fastest increases in the use of OCPs in young women, from 1968 to 1980, in comparison to all the Latin and South American countries. This would put Brazilian women at especially high risk. A study of "ever" versus "never" oral contraceptive use done by Gomes et al and published in 1995 [11] showed a 1.81 RR (1.15-2.85). Brazil had the third highest cumulative amount of OCP use when measured in total number of prescriptions used in a given country in a comparison of major developed and underdeveloped countries [10].

Canada: Hislop noted that in the early 1980s in British Colombia, over 95% of women born after 1950 had taken OCPs [5, p. 36S]. Another Canadian study — the "Canadian National Breast Screening Study" — noted that over 80% of women born after 1940 had used OCPs [5, p.36S]. These are both very high prevalence rates — women who took them for prolonged periods of time or who began using them before their first child was born ought to be warned of their increased breast and cervical cancer risk especially in the late 1990s and after the year 2000.

China: It is estimated that at least 14 million abortions are performed annually on its people [12, p.250]. According to Henshaw: "Among the developing countries, China appears to have the highest legal abortion rate (62 abortions per 1000 women aged 15 to 44 years old), but this figure may be inflated" [12, p.251]. In addition, in 1993 at least 1 million of China's people were using injectable progestin contraceptives [13]. As contraceptive use and chemical abortion increase in China (the use of chemical abortion such as RU-486 like drugs, is reportedly very high in China [14]), one can expect a further increase in the rates of breast, cervical, and liver cancer. This is critical when one notes that cervical cancer is the 2nd most prevalent cancer in developing countries whereas liver cancer is the 7th most prevalent [15].

Two specific studies concerning OCP use were performed on East Asian women. Lee et al [16] in a small study published in 1992 found that 91 women who took OCPs prior to their FFTP had a 1.9 RR (0.4-7.7) of getting breast cancer compared to "controls." In another small study, Wang et al [17] found that Chinese women who started using OCPs after the age of 35 sustained at least a 2.6-fold statistically significant relative risk. Data for OCP risk for women who took them before the age of 20 or before their FFTP was not presented. Wang also noted that women who breastfed more than 6 years had a 0.3-0.4 relative risk of developing breast cancer. According to both Wang and Yuan, China traditionally has had few young women who have used OCPs [5, p.36S].

As concerns the risk of induced abortion performed early in a woman's reproductive life, Yuan et al [18] noted that women who had an abortion prior to their FFTP, had a 2.4-fold increased risk of developing breast cancer than "controls." They also noted that women who used OCPs after the age of 45 had a 4.00 (1.1.-16.59) relative risk. In addition, China has a high rate of childless women in those women born after 1950 [5, p.46S] and China's women have the latest age at first birth among all nations as per the Oxford study [5, p.48S]. The average age at first birth was over 26 years old, and because young Chinese women have far fewer children than any other country, this again puts them at high risk for increasing breast cancer rates in the future [5, p.47S]. It would appear that China has much to gain both medically and economically by dramatically expanding the use of Natural Family Planning.

Costa Rica: Dr. Nancy Lee et al noted that, "by 1981, 11% of married women in Costa Rica ages 20-49 had used depot-medroxyprogesterone acetate (DMPA) and 58% had used oral contraceptives." [19, p.1247]. DMPA is the active ingredient in Depo-Provera. She also found that women who had taken it in that country had a 2.6-fold risk (1.4-4.7) of developing breast cancer despite the fact that her study had a severe stack effect and death effect, both of which serve to underestimate the relative risks she found. Women who had more than a 10-year time span since they first used DMPA had a 4.0-fold (1.5-10.3) risk. Both the high use of OCPs and the noted risk for DMPA in Costa Rica put its women at increased risk for breast cancer.

Cuba: Cuba had one of the highest abortion rates in the world in the early 1970s which puts its women at an increased risk for developing breast cancer [20, p.19].

Denmark: The researcher Marianne Ewertz noted that: "In Denmark, oral contraceptives were released for general usage in 1966" [21, p.1176]. In addition, Denmark has a fairly high rate of induced abortion performed early in a woman's reproductive life — higher than England, Finland, and Norway [20, p.46]. As of the early 1980s, over

90% of Denmark's youngest women (ie, 13- and 14-year-olds) and over 65% of its 17 to 18 year olds chose abortion over delivery when becoming pregnant [12]. In addition, over 86% of women born after 1950 in Denmark have used OCPs according to Ewertz et al [5, p.36S]. Both of these factors put Denmark's women at increased risk for breast and cervical cancer.

Eastern European countries: Almost all other "Eastern European countries" which have followed Russia's example of legalizing abortion in the 1950s, are at risk and will be at even higher risk should their women begin to use synthetic contraceptives. Hungary and Bulgaria had abortion rates that were even higher than those of the U.S. in the 1970s. Hungary was noted for having a high rate of abortion in its *younger* women [20, p.39]. Czechoslovakia (ie, the former Czech Republic and Slovakia) also has a very high rate of abortion in women under the age of 24. Czechoslovakia and Hungary are also at special risk because of their high rate of abortions done in women over the age of 35 [20, p.46].

England: Two separate large English studies have noted that between 82 to 93% of English women born after 1950 have used OCPs, putting this subset of young women at great risk [5, p.36S]. In addition, English women have one of the highest rates of OCP use in women under the age of 20, which also places them at high risk [5, p.40S].

France: France has the distinction of having one of the highest rates of chemical abortion in the world (ie, via RU-486) as well as a high rate of OCP use in its younger women, with Lé et al estimating that 86% of "controls" born since 1950 had used OCPs [5, p.36S; 216]. Ironically, France's own government, which controls the stockholder rights to RU-486, mandated the legality of this drug in spite of public opposition [14].

Germany: The Federal Republic of Germany (previously West Germany) had the fourth highest cumulative amount of OCP use when measured in total number of prescriptions filled in a given country [10] placing its women at increased risk for breast and cervical cancer. German women have also had one of the lowest birth rates in the world, thus putting its women at even higher risk for breast cancer.

Greece: This country had the second highest cumulative amount of OCP use when measured in total number of prescriptions used in a given country [10]. Its women should be carefully screened for breast, cervical, and liver cancer.

Iceland: Tomasson et al from Iceland published a prospective study on the risks of OCP use in that country, which showed no overall risk. However, they took data from as early as 1965 which virtually invalidates their results because the researchers were collecting data on women with breast cancer before oral contraceptives even came to Iceland (ie, OCPs have been available in Iceland since 1967) [22, p.158]. They also failed to provide any data on risk of OCP use before a FFTP. In a better designed study, Tryggvadottir et al found that young women (ie, those born after 1953) who had more than 4 years of OCP use, sustained a 2.2 (1.0-4.7) RR of developing breast cancer. Tryggvadottir noted that early use of OCPs in Iceland has risen dramatically In women born between 1945 and 1947 only 20% used OCPs prior to the age of 20, whereas 82% of women born between 1963 and 1967 had used OCPs before the age of 20. He summarized by noting: "In this study, a significant association was detected between breast cancer and exposure to oral contraceptives at young age in women born after 1950, whereas no association was evident in the older cohorts, and the association was not detectable after mixing of the younger and the older cohort. The results support the findings in several recent studies of an association between oral contraceptive use and breast cancer in young women, and they stress the importance of doing separate analyses on groups with different possibilities of exposure at young age." [23, p.142]. According to Tryggvadottir's analysis and that of Romieu et al [24], at least 82% of Iceland's young female population should be extremely concerned.

India: The "birth control vaccine" is being studied by Talmar et al in India, supported by the World Health Organization[26]. Because this "vaccine" works by causing early abortion(s) and *attacking one of the most important hormones that protects against breast cancer* (ie, *hCG*), should its use become widespread, millions of Indian women could be at risk for a higher incidence of breast cancer. Cervical cancer and breast cancer are two of the most prevalent types of cancer in India [15].

Israel: Data from the WHO trial has estimated that about 50% of Israeli women born since 1950 have used OCPs. This is a lower rate than most European countries, but its women are still at increased risk for breast cancer, especially because Jewish people in general have a higher baseline rate of breast cancer than most of the rest of the world. It was noted earlier that Jewish women have a higher frequency of a defect in the BRCA1 gene. This has special implications given that if two groups of women both had a mutation of the BRCA gene, and if one group used OCPs for 4 years or more before their first birth, that group would have a 680% increased risk of getting breast cancer [25].

Italy: A number of studies have been done in Italy, usually under the guidance of La Vecchia. Unfortunately, many of these studies suffer from a number of weaknesses, especially low statistical power in analyzing younger aged women. In 1986, La Vecchia et al [27] published a study, funded in part by Wyeth pharmaceutical laboratories, which showed a 1.13 (0.81-1.52) multivariate relative risk of breast cancer for "ever/never" use of OCPs. In addition to the obvious conflict of interest as regards the drug company which helped sponsor the study, La Vecchia only provided data for women who were age 60 and under, thereby failing to analyze the one group that would have had a reasonable latent period and the possibility of using OCPs at an early age — that is, women under the age of 45 on or before 1995. He did note an increased risk after 10 years since first use in these elderly women: 1.45 (1.01-2.08).

A later study published in 1995 [28] suffered from a large stack effect (ie, 4.2% of "cases" vs. 7.1% of "controls" under the age of 35). It noted a 1.3 RR (0.9-1.9) in women who took OCPs prior to their FFTP. The authors did provide a table [28, p.166] that showed that risk for OCP use increased in the younger aged groups (ie, women under the age of 45). For example, women aged 35 to 44 years old who took OCPs for fewer than 10 years had a 1.9 RR (1.2-2.9). Italy's young women reportedly have a lower rate of OCP use than countries such as France, former West Germany, and the U.S. [5, p.36S].

Japan: Japan has traditionally had a lower breast cancer rate than the rest of the world, but it has been increasing dramatically in the last few years (see Chapter 1). This may increase if Japanese women begin to use oral contraceptives as women in Western countries do.

Middle Eastern countries: Little data has been published on countries in the Middle East, especially those with a Muslim majority such as Iran, Egypt, Syria, Morroco, and Iraq. If the women of these countries refrain from abortion and hormonal contraceptive use as has been reported, they would be one of the few populations in the world which would be spared from the increased risks of breast, cervical, and liver cancer.

Netherlands: Rookus noted that women under the age of 36 who used OCPs prior to the age of 20 had a 1.44 RR per year of use ($p=0.04$) [29]. He also noted that as of 1994, when the paper was written, 14%, 3%, and < 1% of those women who were 36 years old or less, 36 to 40, 41 to 45, respectively, had used OCPs for 2 or more years prior to their FFTP. This would indicate that young women who live in the Netherlands today face a far higher increased risk of developing breast cancer than their elderly compatriots because the younger women would be more likely to have used OCPs for longer times before their FFTP. Because about 19 out of 20 women born since 1950 in the Netherlands have used OCPs, Dutch women will be at increased risk especially after the year 2000 [5, p.36S].

New Zealand: Women in New Zealand have used DMPA (depot-medroxypro-gesterone acetate) extensively [6]. If these same women used DMPA for significant periods before their FFTP or before the age of 25, they are at increased risk according to the WHO and New Zealand trials. *Skegg* et al [7] pooled the results of the WHO and New Zealand studies and found that women who had taken DMPA for between 2 and 3 years before the age of 25 had a 310% statistically significant risk of getting breast cancer [RR=4.1 (1.6-10.90)] whereas women who had taken DMPA for more than 3 years prior to the age of 25 had at least a 190% increased risk that was also significant (2.9: [1.2-7.1]).

In addition, New Zealand has a high rate of early OCP use: "New Zealand women actually reported a higher prevalence of early use of the pill than the Californian population studied by Pike et al. Of our control population under 37, 30% had used oral contraceptives for 4 years or longer before the age of 25, compared with 11% in the California study" [30, p.725]. Finally, Paul et al noted that over 90% of women born since 1950 have used OCPs in New Zealand [5, p.36S].

Norway: As of the early 1980s, over 90% of Norway's youngest women (ie, 13- and 14-year-olds) chose abortion over delivery when becoming pregnant [12], putting these women at especially high risk in the future.

Russia: Russia is a country in which abortion has been legal since 1955; it has an especially high frequency of elective abortion. "For many years after legalization in 1955, the number of abortions (roughly 7 million annually in the mid-1980s) has been exceeding the number of live births (about 5.5 million)." [31, p.506, 140]. By 1986, Henshaw estimated that Russia performed 11 million abortions annually [12, p.250]. This puts this country's women at high risk for developing breast cancer. Remennick [31] has noted that there is a statistically significant correlation between the percentage of abortions in primagravidas (ie, women who aborted their first child) and the crude breast cancer rate (r =0.62; p<0.05) (the higher the "r value," the higher the correlation, with 1.00 representing a perfect correlation). It should be noted that Russian women have not used oral contraceptives widely nor have they had widescale access to artificial hormones such as Norplant or Depo-Provera. Should Russian women start to use oral contraceptives or artificial progestins such as Depo-Provera in the future, they will be at even higher risk than they are currently for both breast and cervical cancer.

Singapore: This country has one of the highest rates of early and late abortions compared to the rest of the world — putting its women at high risk for the development of breast cancer in the future [20, p.47].

South Africa: A study performed on South African women in 1997 found that 72% of *black women* had used an injectable progestin contraceptive and that 30% of women had used one for 5 years or more [32]. The progestin used most often was either DMPA or norethisterone and these injectable hormones have been used there since the mid 1960s. The study noted that *white South African women* had a far lower use of these progestin hormones. *It must be noted that using DMPA for more than 2 years before the age of 25 has been noted to cause at least a 190% increased risk in breast cancer according to Skegg et al. [7].* In addition, in a large study, Herrero et al [33] found that women who had received injectable progestins (ie, usually DMPA [depot-medroxyprogesterone] or norethisterone enanthate) for at least 5 years and who had used them at least 5 years ago, suffered a 430% increased risk of developing cervical cancer [RR=5.3 (1.1-10.0)]. These two citations should alarm women from South Africa who have taken Depo-Provera because cervical cancer and breast cancer are the most common female cancers in that country respectively.

Sweden: Meirik et al noted that: "The high prevalence of long-term (oral contraceptive) use that is found for Swedish women is in good accordance with the findings in the Swedish fertility survey in 1981, in which 30% of women aged 26 to 45 years reported that they had used OCPs for

5 years or more. . . To our knowledge, the proportion of long-term users in Swedish women exceeds that reported from other countries." [34, p.653]. The same study found a 4.4 (1.2-15.5) relative risk in women who took OCPs for more than 8 years [34, p.652]. Of note, at least 87% of Swedish women born after 1950 have used OCPs according to one study [5, 36S].

In another notable Swedish study, Olsson et al [35] found a 2-fold relative risk in premenopausal women who had taken OCPs for 4 years or more prior to their FFTP. Olsson noted that 33% of the "controls" and 47% of the "cases" took OCPs before their FFTP, which is especially worrisome when one considers that he also found that women who took them before the age of 20 had a 5.8 *RR* (2.6-12.8), and that women who took them for more than 5 years before the age of 25 had a 5.3 RR (2.1-13.2). The author of this study warned: "The present findings, together with those of other studies on the biology of breast tumors in early users of OCPs, raise great concern about early use of OCPs." [35, p.1004]

In addition to this, Sweden had the highest abortion rate per pregnancy of any country in the world in women under the age of 18 in the late 1970s and early 1980s [20, p.40]. This is especially dangerous because Daling et al [36] have noted that women under the age of 18 who had an induced abortion had 150% increased risk of developing breast cancer. As of the early 1980s, over 90% of Sweden's youngest women (ie, 13 and 14 year olds) and over 65% of its 17 to 18 year olds chose abortion over delivery when becoming pregnant [12].

United States: Women in the U.S. may have the highest increased risk of developing breast cancer. They have one of the highest rates of abortion in young women, which is an especially high risk age group [20, p.39]. Of special note is that nulliparous women in the U.S. had the highest rate of abortions per 100 pregnancies. Tietze pointed out that while every country in the world had an abortion rate of less than 30 per 1,000 in women under the age of 19 in the early 1980s, the U.S. had a rate of 44.4 per 1,000! In addition, the U.S. has the "distinction" of having more than 3 times the rate of abortions compared to any other country in the world, in young women aged 13 or 14 years old [12, p.252]. States whose women might be expected to be at particularly high risk because they have high rates of abortion include: California, New York, Nevada, Massachusetts, New Jersey, Florida, and especially the District of Columbia [37, p.5].

The U.S. has the highest cumulative amount of OCP use when measured in total number of prescriptions written in a given country [10]. Even in the early 1980s, more than 84% of women born after 1950 had taken OCPs (as per the CASH study), and this figure has reached 90% according to a later study by Daling et al [5, p.36S]. In addition, Brinton et al, in one of the largest and most recent studies to date, noted that 72.6% of parous women had used OCPs prior to their FFTP and that 30% of parous women had taken OCPs for 4 years or more prior to their FFTP [38, p.832].

Other countries:

"Greece, Portugal, Spain, Taiwan, and Turkey all relaxed their abortion laws in the early 1980s" [12]. This implies that they will all be at increased risk in the future. It should also be noted that women who are childless and have abortions are at especially high risk. "Childless women have constituted the majority of all abortion patients in recent years in Canada, England and Wales, Finland, the Netherlands, New Zealand, Scotland, and the U.S. and they have represented the single largest subgroup in Denmark, Sweden and West Germany. In contrast, women with two previous births have represented the largest subgroup in Czechoslovakia, Hungary and Italy" [12, p.253].

References:

1. Kenya PR. Oral contraceptive use and liver tumours: a review. *East African Medical Journal.* 1990; 67:146-153.

2. Marx PA, et al. Progesterone implants enhance SIV vaginal transmission and early virus load. *Nature Medicine*. 1996; 2: 1084-1089.

3. Rohan T, McMichael A. Oral contraceptive agents and breast cancer: a population-based case-control study. *The Medical Journal of Australia*. 1988; 149: 520-526.

4. Ellery C, MacLennan R, et al. A case-control study of breast cancer in relation to the use of steroid contraceptive agents. *The Medical Journal of Australia*. 1986; 144: 173-176.

5. Collaborative Group on Hormonal Factors in Breast Cancer. Breast cancer and hormonal contraceptives: further results. *Contraception*. 1996; 34: S1-S106.

6. Kaunitz A. Long-acting injectable Contraception with depot medroxyprogesterone acetate. *Am J Obstet Gynecol*. 1994; 170: 1543-1549.

7. Skegg DCG, Noonan EA, et al. Depot medroxyprogesterone acetate and breast cancer [A pooled analysis of the World Health Organization and New Zealand studies]. 1995; *JAMA*: 799-804.

8. Brind J. ABC down under. *Abortion Breast Cancer Quarterly Update*. Summer, 1997.

9. Howe H, et al. Early abortion and breast cancer risk among women under age 40. *Int J Epidemiol*. 1989; 18: 300-304.

10. Anonymous. Oral contraceptives in the 1980s. *Population Reports*. May-June 1982. X: A189-A222.

11. Gomes L, Guimaraes M, et al. A case-control study of risk factors for breast cancer in Brazil, 1978-1987. *Int J Epidemiol*. 1995; 24: 292-299.

12. Henshaw SK. Induced abortion: a worldwide perspective. *Family Planning Perspectives*. 1986; 18: 250-254.

13. Nullis C. WHO OKs birth control injections. *Pittsburgh Post-Gazette*. 6/5/93.

14. Davies Matthew. RU-486 and Post Coital Contraception. Lecture at Hershey Medical Center, 11/13/97.

15. Parkin et al. Estimates of the worldwide frequency of sixteen major cancers in1980. *Int J Cancer*. 1988; 41: 184-197.

16. Lee HP, Gourley L, et al. Risk factors for breast cancer by age and menopausal status: a case-control study in Singapore. *Cancer Causes and Control*. 1992; 3: 313-322.

17. Wang Q, Ross R, et al. A case-control study of breast cancer in Tianjin, China. *Cancer Epidemiology*. 1992; 1: 435-439.

18. Yuan J, Yu M, et al. Risk factors for breast cancer in Chinese women in Shanghai. *Cancer Research*. 1988; 48: 1949-1953.

19. Lee NC, Rosero-Bixby L, et al. A case-control study of breast cancer and hormonal Contraception in Costa Rica. *J Natl Cancer Inst*. 1987; 6: 1247-1254.

20. Tietze C. *Induced Abortion: A World Review*. 5th ed. Population Council; 1983.

21.   Ewertz M. Oral contraceptives and breast cancer risk in Denmark. *Eur J Cancer.* 1992; 28A: 1176-1181.

22.   Tomasson H, et al. Oral contraceptives and risk of breast cancer: [A historical prospective case-control study]. *Acta Obstet Gynecol Scand.* 1996; 75: 157-161.

23.   Tryggvadottir L, et al. Oral contraceptive use at a young age and the risk of breast cancer: an Icelandic, population-bases cohort study of the effect of birth year. *Br J Cancer.* 1997; 75: 139-143.

24.   Romieu I, Berlin J, et al. Oral contraceptives and breast cancer. Review and meta-Analysis. *Cancer.* 1990; 66: 2253-2263.

25.   Ursin G, et al. Does oral contraceptive use increase the risk of breast cancer in women with BRCA1/BRCA2 mutations more than in other women? *Cancer Research.* 1997; 57: 3678-3681.

26.   Talwar, et al. Phase I clinical trials with three formulations of anti-human Chorionic Gonadotropin vaccine. *Contraception,* 1990; 41: 301-316.

27.   La Vecchia C, Decarli A, et al. Oral contraceptives and cancers of the breast and of the female genital tract. Interim results from a case-control study. *Br J Cancer.* 1986; 54: 311-317.

28.   La Vecchia C, Negri E, et al. Oral contraceptives and breast cancer: A cooperative Italian study. *Int J Cancer.* 1995; 60: 163-167.

29.   Rookus MA, Leeuwen FE. Oral contraceptives and risk of breast cancer in women ages 20-54 years. *The Lancet.* 1994; 344: 844-851.

30.   Paul C, Skegg DC, et al. Oral contraceptives and breast cancer: a national study. *Br Med J.* 1986; 293: 723-726.

31.   Remennick L. Reproductive patterns and cancer incidence in women: a population-based correlation study in the USSR. *Int J Epidemiol.* 1989; 18: 498-510.

32.   Bailie R, et al. A case-control study of breast cancer risk and exposure to injectable progestin contraceptives. *S Afr Med J.* 1997; 87: 302-305.

33.   Herrero, et al. Injectable contraceptives and risk of invasive cervical cancer: evidence of an association. *Int J Cancer.* 1990; 46: 5-7.

34.   Meirik O, Lund E, Adami HO, et al. Oral contraceptive use and breast cancer in young women. *The Lancet.* Sept. 20, 1986: 650-653.

35.   Olsson H, Moller TR, Ranstam J. Early contraceptive use and breast cancer among premenopausal women: Final report from a study in southern Sweden. *J Natl Cancer Inst.* 1989; 81: 1000-1004.

36.   Daling J, Malone K, et al. Risk of breast cancer among young women: relationship to induced abortion. *J Natl Cancer Inst.* 1994; 86: 1584-1592.

37.   Henshaw SK, O'Reilly K. Characteristics of abortion patients in the U.S., 1979 and 1980. *Family Planning Perspectives.* 1983; 15: 5-16.

38.   Brinton LA, Daling JR, et al. Oral contraceptives and breast cancer risk among younger women. *J Natl Cancer Inst.* 6/7/1995; 87: 827-835.

Chapter 16:
Anticipated Objections

Q-16A: Rushton et al [1] confined their analysis to studies published between 1980 and 1989 and noted that the overall relative risk of developing breast cancer in women less than the age of 45 who had used OCPs was only 1.16 (1.07-1.25). Is this accurate?

It would appear to be accurate but two important items must be considered. *First, Rushton gave no statistics for OCP use prior to a first full-term pregnancy (FFTP). Second, although Rushton took his information from studies that were published between 1980 and 1989, this is not the same as taking your data from studies whose data were collected after 1980. For example, the data from some of the studies that Rushton examined came from as far back as the 1960s and early 1970s and would fail to have allowed for a latent period that would have been long enough to reflect an accurate relative risk [1, p.240].* This is the same weakness from which the Oxford study suffered [2].

Q-16B: What groups or people might be expected to disagree with the findings of this book?

There is certainly a large amount of information in this book and there will be those who disagree with particular points. This author welcomes their input and opinions. As people start to become informed about the content and implications of this material, intense resistance from several groups is expected.

1) *Pharmaceutical companies*: The conflict of interest and the risk of potential litigation for specific companies

that produce oral contraceptives or injectable progestins, or chemical abortifacients (eg, RU-486) are obvious. They have billions of dollars at stake — expect fierce resistance from them.

2) *Physicians*: Although this author would hope that most physicians would be receptive to the findings in this book, many of them will feel pressured by their respective medical organizations to "play down the findings." Fortunately, many physicians are still fairly independent and many have lost respect for such "collective" medical organizations as the AMA (American Medical Association), the AAP (American Academy of Pediatrics), and the ACOG (American College of Obstetricians and Gynecologists). These organizations often seem more concerned about protecting their hierarchy than about doing what is right for patients. It should be noted that any physician who recommends abortion and/or distributes hormonal contraceptives to his or her patients and chooses to withhold the findings in the literature, especially after being shown the evidence by the laity and/or other colleagues, could be at risk for litigation.

3) *Medical journals (many but not all)*: It was already written that all three of the national medical organizations have endorsed abortion and certainly favor OCP use for young women who are sexually active. But the AAP, the ACOG, and the AMA also have a tremendous influence on the literature, because they control three large and respected journals, specifically the journal of *Pediatrics*, the journal of *Obstetrics and Gynecology,* and *JAMA (the Journal of the American Medical Association).* Unfortunately, a reasonable response to this book may be more likely to appear in the foreign journals, such as the British literature which has been less biased in its presentation of "politically incorrect" medical findings.

4) *Groups that promote abortion and early OCP use, and also receive federal funds*: One would hope that groups like Planned Parenthood and the World Health Organization would mention the findings of this book to the mil-

lions of women who are currently at risk. Until now, they have failed to do so.

Q-16C: What if a researcher disagrees with the findings in this book?

Legitimate arguments are welcome, but it must be remembered that many of the researchers in the U.S. survive on grants which are almost all decided and distributed by federal agencies. It should also be remembered that a conflict of interest is inherent in a government that openly spends hundreds of millions of dollars on hormonal contraceptives and funds agencies which perform thousands of abortions each year (eg, Planned Parenthood). *Therefore, the opinion of most researchers in the U.S. who rely on federal grants must be considered in light of the inherent conflict of interest which places a great deal of pressure on them.* The sad truth is that the U.S. Federal Government has become so "politically correct" that researchers often fear losing their funding.

Q-16D: Why have so few researchers and physicians spoken out about the critical risks of OCP use and abortion performed early in a woman's reproductive life?

A major problem is that although a limited number of researchers and/or other sources have noted the dangers of early OCP use, most have underemphasized them or failed to mention them at all. Among the few researchers who have made some "warning statements" are: Miller and Rosenberg et al who wrote: "Oral contraceptive use is common enough to anticipate that a resulting increase in risk of breast cancer among young women might be reflected in rising incidence rates. In that regard, the recent increase in breast cancer incidence and mortality among women under age 50 years in the U.S. is of concern." [3, p.279] In addition Hawley et al [4] performed a meta-analysis in 1990 and concluded that: "This meta-analysis suggests a possible increased risk for breast cancer in women who use oral contraceptives before a first full-term pregnancy. The data, however are confounded by studies that are generally of low quality." [4, p.123].

Another honest comment was found in the 1995 *Lancet.* "Several studies, including a multi-country study from the WHO, suggest that oral contraceptives (used by 61 million women worldwide) are associated with a relative risk of 1.3 to 1.5 for breast cancer that will be diagnosed before age 40-45." [5, p.883]. It is alarming that statements like these fail to generate any true warnings to patients from their physicians. As was noted with DES, the dangerous assumption that the risks of OCPs will not extend to women as they reach their 50s and 60s was made once in our history. The most commonly used text used by internists, *Harrison's Principles of Internal Medicine* noted: "The use of oral contraceptives for durations in excess of 4 years prior to first full-term pregnancy has been reported to increase the relative risk of breast cancer at an early age to as high as 1.7." (ie, 70%) [6]. Finally, Staffa et al [7] did comment on the risks of DMPA (ie, the hormone in Depo-Provera) noting that "two potential high-risk groups were suggested: women who used depo-MPA at least 2 years prior to age 25 and long-term users. . ."

Unfortunately others have taken the "hide and seek" approach. At a London-based meeting in which the risks of breast cancer and OCPs were discussed, "Professor Michael Baum was anxious that cancer warnings could be counterproductive since they might frighten patients" [8, p.286]. Other researchers have erroneously and prematurely commented that abortion performed early in a woman's reproductive life and early OCP use carries no real risk. In 1982 Vessey et al wrote: " A recent publication from California (ie, Pike et al) in this journal has suggested that both prolonged oral contraceptive use and abortion before first term pregnancy increase the risk of breast cancer in young women. Data are presented on 1176 women aged 16 to 50 years old with breast cancer interviewed in London or in Oxford, together with a like number of matched control women. The results are entirely reassuring, being in fact more compatible with protective effects than the reverse." [9, p.327]. These premature comments, made despite the authors' failure to separate induced and spontaneous abortion (ie, miscarriage), and despite a failure to allow an adequate latent period to pass, *may well have given false assurance to thousands of women who now have breast cancer that may have been preventable had they been properly warned.* Finally, the American Cancer Society's "Facts and Figures-1996" booklet does not specifically mention early OCP use as a risk factor and briefly comments that abortion is a risk factor that is "currently under study." [10, p.12].

Q-16E: Will it be argued that this author's views colored the findings in this book?

There is no article or book that is written without being "colored by an author's views." However, it is the cited scientific and medical documentation in this book that is the legitimate subject of discussion. Personal attacks, if they come, are an admission of an inability to argue on the basis of the facts contained within the literature.

References:

1. Rushton L, et al. Oral contraceptive use and breast cancer risk: a meta-analysis of variations with age at diagnosis, parity and total duration of oral contraceptive use. *Br J Obstet Gynaecol.* 1992; 99: 239-246.

2. Collaborative Group on Hormonal Factors in Breast Cancer. Breast cancer and hormonal contraceptives: further results. *Contraception.* 1996; 34: S1-S106.

3. Miller D, Rosenberg L, et al. Breast cancer before age 45 and oral contraceptive use: new findings. *Am J Epidemiol.* 1989; 129: 269-279.

4. Hawley W, Nuovo J, et al. Do oral contraceptive agents affect the risk of breast cancer?: A meta-analysis of the case-control reports. *J Am Board Fam Pract.* 1993; 6: 123-135.

5. Hulka B, Stark A. Breast cancer: cause and prevention. *The Lancet.* Sept. 30, 1995; 346: 883-887.

6. Fauci AS, et al. *Harrison's: Principle of Internal Medicine.* 14th ed. New York: McGraw Hill; 1998.

7. Staffa JA, Newschaffer CJ, et al. Progestins and breast cancer: an epidemiologic review. *Fertility and Sterility.* 1992; 57: 473-491.

8. Brahams D. What must women be told about the pill? *The Lancet.* July 129; 1989: 285.

9. Vessey MP, McPherson K, et al. Oral contraceptive use and abortion before first term pregnancy in relation breast cancer risk. *Br J Cancer.* 1982; 45: 327-331.

10. Cancer Facts & Figures-1996. American Cancer Society, 1996.

Chapter 17:
Conclusions and Recommendations

Conclusions:

Breast cancer is the most prevalent cancer in women world-wide and is the most common cause of cancer death for U.S. women ages 20 to 59 years old. This book has shown that both induced abortion and oral contraceptive use, especially at a young age, markedly increase a woman's risk for developing breast cancer. A review of the major findings contained within this book follows.

General Risk Factors:

Breast cancer risk factors in addition to induced abortion and oral contraceptives include:

- family history of breast cancer
- increased age
- nulliparity (never having given birth)
- total estrogen exposure and/or progestin exposure
- late menopause
- early menarche (early onset of menses)
- greater age at first birth
- some types of fibrocystic breast disease
- a previous occurrence of breast cancer
- postmenopausal hormone use
- a defective BRCA1 or BRCA2 gene
- moderate to high alcohol consumption
- obesity in postmenopausal women

- radiation exposure
- exposure to diethylstilbestrol (DES).

Other possible risk factors include:

- breast status characterized by a "dense" mammogram
- history of having other cancers
- miscarriage prior to first full-term pregnancy.

A number of specific findings are listed below along with the section of the book where more detailed information and references may be found.

Breast Cancer in General

1. In the U.S. more than 43,000 women die from   Intro.
   breast cancer yearly. It is the most common cause
   of cancer death for women ages 20 to 59 years old.

2. The U.S. has one of the highest rates of induced   Ch. 15
   abortion and oral contraceptive use in the world,
   especially in its young women. These factors will
   likely result in an even higher increase in the
   incidence of breast cancer once the latent period
   has passed.

3. Many of the published studies on the relation   Ch. 2
   of breast cancer to hormonal contraceptive use   Ch. 3
   and/or abortion contain design errors resulting in an   Ch. 5
   underestimation of the risk of breast cancer.

4. Breast cancer in the U.S. is more prevalent   Ch. 11
   in young black women than in white women of
   equivalent age, and is the second leading cause of
   cancer death (after lung cancer) among black
   women. This may be a consequence of more
   extensive hormonal contraceptive use (eg, Depo-
   Provera) and/or a greater prevalence of abortion
   among young black women. Black women who
   develop breast cancer generally have more aggressive cancers resulting in a shortened life expectancy.

5. Studies of animals demonstrate that rats that   Ch. 2
   undergo an induced abortion have an increased   Ch. 3
   risk of developing breast cancer compared with

rats that bear their pups (Russo and Russo, 1980). Animal studies of monkeys, dogs and rodents show that all have an increased risk of developing breast cancer when they receive hormonal contraceptives.

Breast Cancer and Abortion

6. The most meticulous and comprehensive meta-analysis to date on the relation of breast cancer to induced abortion (Brind, 1996) concludes that women who have an abortion prior to their <u>first full-term pregnancy</u> (FFTP) have a 50% increased risk of developing breast cancer whereas those who have an abortion after their FFTP have a 30% increased risk.   Q-2C

7. As of January 1999, 11 out of 12 epidemiological studies in the U.S. and 25 out of 31 studies worldwide showed that women who elect to have an induced abortion have an elevated risk of developing breast cancer (Brind, 1999).   Q-6B

8. Daling noted in 1994 that women younger than 18 who had an abortion experienced a 150% increased risk of developing breast cancer. This risk increased to 800% if they had their abortions between the 9th and 24th week of pregnancy.   Q-2C, Q-7C

9. Women who have a family history of breast cancer and choose to have an abortion are at very high risk of developing breast cancer. Andrieu et al (1994) found that women who have a family history of breast cancer and who had two or more induced abortions have a 7-fold risk of breast cancer as compared to the rest of the population. Daling et al (1994) noted that women who had an abortion prior to the age of 18 and had a positive family history of breast cancer had an *infinitely* increased risk of developing breast cancer compared to young women who had a family history of breast cancer and had not had an abortion. She also noted that women who were 30 years old or older at the time of their abortion and had breast cancer in their family history had a 270% increased risk.   Q-7M

10. A woman diagnosed with breast cancer while   Q-7S
    pregnant has a longer life expectancy if she gives
    birth rather than aborts. Clarck and Chua (1989)
    found that of the women who had breast cancer
    while pregnant and had an abortion, none were
    alive after 11 years whereas 20% of the women
    who had breast cancer and chose to deliver their
    babies were alive after 20 years.

11. Calculations based on the available studies indicate   Q-7E
    that induced abortion may result in over 46,800
    additional "cases" of breast cancer in the U.S.
    annually.

12. If one considers the increased risk of breast cancer   Q-7F
    and suicide due to an induced abortion, and the
    decreased risk of ovarian cancer with a full-term
    pregnancy, abortion is many times more hazard-
    ous in the long run than carrying a child to term.

Breast Cancer and the Pill

13. If a woman takes the oral contraceptive pill (OCP)   Q-3O
    before her first full-term pregnancy (FFTP), she
    suffers a 40% increased risk of developing breast
    cancer. If she takes oral contraceptive pills for 4
    years or more prior to her FFTP, she suffers
    between a 44% to 72% increased risk of develop-
    ing breast cancer (Thomas, 1991; Romieu, 1990).

14. Eighteen out of 20 studies performed since 1980   Q-9D
    have shown that women who take oral contracep-   Q-9H
    tives prior to their FFTP have an increased risk
    of developing breast cancer. Eighteen out of 21
    studies show an increased risk when comparing
    women who ever had used contraceptive pills
    with women who had never done so.

15. Women who took oral contraceptive pills early in   Q-9V
    their lives and who develop breast cancer gener-
    ally develop more aggressive breast cancer and
    have a poorer prognosis.

16. Each of four large studies that examined breast   Q-9N
    cancer risk due to oral contraceptive pill use in
    young women found statistically significant
    increases in breast cancer risk of 90% or higher
    almost 20 years after initial exposure.

17. Available studies of women who used DMPA   Q-12H
    (Depo-Provera) show a 190% increased risk of   Q-12K
    breast cancer in women who used it for 2 or more
    years prior to the age of 25. Young black women
    in the U.S. are at higher risk of breast cancer
    because they use Depo-Provera far more fre-
    quently than white women.

18. Women who have the defective BRCA gene, which   Q-9X
    is more common in Jewish women, have a 680%
    increased risk of developing breast cancer if they
    take the oral contraceptive pill for more than 4
    years prior to their FFTP (Ursin, 1997).

Other Health Consequences of the Pill

19. Oral contraceptive pill use decreases the risk of   Q-14M
    uterine and ovarian cancer, but increases the risk
    of cervical and liver cancer in addition to breast
    cancer. It is estimated that between 42,000 to
    80,000 "cases" of cancer will occur in the U.S.
    annually when the cumulative effect of oral
    contraceptive use on all cancers is considered.

20. Several studies in animals and humans indicate   Q-12U
    that oral contraceptive and injectable   Q-14Q
    progestin use facilitate transmission of HIV.

21. A summary of studies examining the effect of oral   Q-13C
    contraceptive use on invasive cervical cancer
    shows the following increased risks: for any use
    (30%); long- term use (62%); use before the age of
    25 (65%); use before the age of 20 (80%).

22. Oral contraceptive use has not been proven to   Q-14P
    protect against osteoporosis.

Control Factors for Cancer Risk

23. Of the many identified risks of breast cancer,   Q-1D
    several are controllable by behavior: hormone
    treatment (including hormonal contraceptives),
    abortion, number of births, age at first child-
    birth, length of breastfeeding, degree of alcohol
    use, obesity, and radiation exposure.

24. A major study (Clarck and Chua, 1989) showed that   Q-7T
    women who had multiple pregnancies *after* being
    treated for breast cancer had a better 5-year

survival rate (96%) than women who had a single pregnancy (73%).

25. Natural Family Planning (NFP) methods have been shown to be more effective and far safer than oral contraceptives. Couples who use NFP can accurately determine the days of a woman's menstrual cycle in which she is or is not capable of conceiving. This is done by observations of cervical mucus and/or (for some NFP methods) by measuring basal body temperature and tracking other symptoms. Natural Family Planning methods may also be used to diagnose and treat a variety of female reproductive system disorders including infertility.   Q-3U

26. Common medical conditions such as menstrual cramps can be treated with more natural methods such as magnesium and calcium supplements that involve less toxicity than oral contraceptives.   Q-3S

27. Women who have an induced abortion and also use oral contraceptives have a "multiplied risk" of developing breast cancer. For example, Daling noted that women who have an induced abortion prior to the age of 18 have a 150% increased risk of developing breast cancer, whereas Romieu et al noted that women who use oral contraceptives for 4 or more years prior to their first full-term pregnancy (FFTP) have a 72% increased risk. According to the multiplier effect, women who are in both of these categories would have a relative risk of: 2.5 x 1.72 = 4.3. This is a 330% increased risk.   Q-7M

Recommendations:
For Prevention of Breast Cancer:

A major educational effort is needed to raise awareness in physicians, pharmacists, nurses, and especially the laity regarding controllable risk factors as well as protective factors for breast cancer and the other diseases noted above. Women must be informed of the risks of both hormonal contraceptives and induced abortion especially when they have additional risk factors such as a family history of breast cancer, being less than 18 years of age, or being a black American.

Women need to be told about Natural Family Planning methods, none of which increase cancer risk. Women must be informed of practices that reduce breast cancer risk such as long-term breastfeeding, bearing a child at a young age, and bearing more than one child. The use of Vitamin A may be of benefit, though this should be avoided by women who could become pregnant as it may (rarely) cause birth defects.

For Women with Identified Breast Cancer Risks:

Women who have had induced abortions and/or used oral contraceptive pills, especially at an early age, need lifetime physician monitoring. They (and all women) should consistently perform self-breast exams. They should also seriously consider protective strategies such as extended breastfeeding and/or use of Vitamin A. Tamoxifen and drugs similar to it have been found to decrease the risk of breast cancer in certain groups of women. A report by the Eli Lilly company stated that Evista (raloxifene), an artificial hormone given to some postmenopausal women to prevent osteoporosis, may reduce breast cancer risk (Company Press Release, Eli Lilly manufacturer, 12/11/98). Neither drug should be given to pre- or peri-menopausal women who might conceive. Additional exposure to risk factors such as repeat abortion or additional hormone (eg, contraceptive) use should be avoided.

For Women with Breast Cancer:

Women who already have breast cancer should be treated with the appropriate combination of surgery and/or radiation and/or chemotherapy and/or hormonal therapy. They should ask their physicians about the effectiveness of Vitamin A, and should be encouraged to ask about new treatments such as "virus infecting tumor cells," which are currently being studied, as well as new medicines which target specific proteins or genes that a breast cancer cell may produce (eg, the drug Herceptin). Herceptin has been used to treat a type of breast cancer known as HER-2/neu, which is more common in women who have used oral contraceptive pills at an early age (Ranstam, 1992). If the patient with breast cancer is pregnant, the baby *should not be aborted* as abortion markedly reduces the mother's life expectancy (Clarck and Chua, 1989).

Public Policy:

Breast cancer and other medical problems caused by hormonal contraceptives and/or induced abortion represent a serious and growing health problem. The government, health professionals as a body and the research establishment have not responded well to this situation, in which millions of lives are at stake. It is critical that the responsible parties address this pressing crisis. Eventually public opinion and/or court action will make this unavoidable.

Current U.S. domestic and foreign policy which promotes hormonal contraceptive use and induced abortion must be reversed in light of the drastic effects these risks have on the lives of women. The long-term effects of each risk factor have likely not yet been realized because the full latent period has not passed. As the health consequences of hormonal contraceptive use and induced abortion become evident to the citizens of the affected countries, the good will of the major promoters will be questioned and their credibility undermined. It is time for a major reassessment and restructuring of our policy on these matters. An apology to the affected countries and their people is also long overdue.

For Individual Women:

Because the government, the media, the medical establishment, and the research community have failed to educate women about the health risks identified here, it is necessary for individual women to inform themselves of the pertinent risks. It is possible that women can blunt or even reverse the epidemic of breast and other cancers that currently threaten them by avoiding the hazardous risks of induced abortion and hormonal contraception and by instead adopting natural means of spacing children and other strategies which lower breast cancer risk. Although this would involve a definite cultural shift, there is little doubt that thousands of lives would be saved in the long run.

Appendix 1:
The Age Factor
(a detailed analysis)

This section is challenging, but an understanding of why age plays such an important role in the field of breast cancer is crucial. Proper age-matching between the "cases" and "controls" is among the most important factor that must be accounted for, and yet many research articles have failed to properly adjust for either the average age or the distribution of age.

Figure A1A shows how rapidly the rates of breast cancer rise as women grow older. (Data taken from *SEER Cancer Statistics* from the years 1988-1992) [1, p.122]

Figure A1A:
BREAST CANCER INCIDENCE AMONG WOMEN OF DIFFERENT AGE GROUPS IN THE U.S.

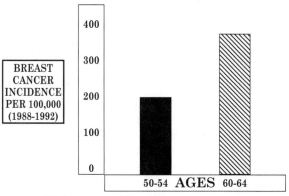

What would happen if one were to compare women with breast cancer (the "case group") with the "control

265

group" if the "cases" have an average age that is 5 years older than the "control group"? We can see from the graph that the rate of breast cancer per 100,000 women is about 230 for a 52-year-old woman but jumps to about 340 for a 62-year-old woman. Note that a 10-year age difference has resulted in a 48% increased rate of breast cancer between 52- and 62-year-old women or about a 5% increase for each year.

If one were performing a prospective study and the women who had abortions performed at a young age (ie, the "cohort") were 5 years older than the women who did not have an abortion performed at a young age (ie, "the controls"), one might "fail to find" the risk of the abortion performed at a young age because the "cohorts" would tend to have a higher incidence of breast cancer due to their older age.

What about retrospective studies — does an age difference have an effect? It certainly does. Let us look again at the situation in which we have a 5-year age difference between the groups, specifically when the "cases" (ie, women with breast cancer) are 5 years older than the "controls." The main problem with this type of set-up is that, as a general rule, women who are in the younger group (and researchers in this field almost always pick the "controls" to be the younger group) will have had more exposure to abortions performed at a young age and early oral contraceptive pill (OCP) use because both of these activities have increased dramatically in younger women since the late 1960s. [2, Table 14]. McPherson et al noted this in 1987 when he wrote that OCP use before a first live birth was markedly different in the groups of women who were over the age of 45 compared to those under the age of 45. "Among the older group barely 3% had any OCP use before first term pregnancy, while in the younger group around 25% reported such use" [3]. It is obvious that when comparing the two groups — women with and without breast cancer — the latter (ie, the "controls") may have had significantly more early OCP use and/or abortions if they are even one or two years younger than the "case group." This effect could easily be responsible for the Bostonian researcher Lynn Rosenberg's "statistically borderline" finding of a relative risk of 1.4 (1.0-1.9) for breast cancer from an abortion performed at a young age. In her study [4], the mean age for the "cases" was 52 years old, whereas that of the "controls" was 40!

In another example concerning the area of OCPs and breast cancer, Paul's New Zealand study suffered from a large age difference with the "cases" being almost 4 years older than the "controls."* [5]. This study may well have shown a larger relative risk, which might have been statistically significant, had she matched the "cases" and "controls" properly. Unfortunately, the researcher who claims to find "no difference" between two groups when failing to match subjects for age at the beginning of the study may well be masking the real cause/effect relationship.

*Calculations made from weighted estimate of raw data given in journal article [5, p.368].

The stack effect:

This section is fairly technical. The reader may be better off going to the end of the chapter for a simpler explanation, but *see Figure A2B and read its explanation* before going to the example at the end of the chapter entitled: A Practical example: The Stack Effect in a Day Care Setting.

What if the "cases" and "controls" have the same average age but a different distribution of age. This is called the "stack effect" because the subjects are "stacked" at both the young and old ends of the age curve — as seen in Figure A1B — instead of being evenly distributed!

Figure A1B: THE STACK EFFECT

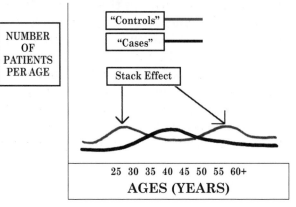

NUMBER OF PATIENTS PER AGE

"Controls"

"Cases"

Stack Effect

25 30 35 40 45 50 55 60+
AGES (YEARS)

Researchers often study a limited number of younger women with breast cancer (ie, the "cases" less than age 35) because of the low prevalence of breast cancer in younger aged women. *Often they "overmatch" these younger groups with excessive young "controls" of the same age in an attempt to "increase the statistical stability" of any findings in these lower age groups.* Dr. Newcomb noted this in her 1996 study on the risks of OCP use in the U.S.: "The controls were selected at random to have an age distribution similar to that of the cases, but were oversampled in younger age strata in the New England states to increase statistical power" [6, p.526]. Unfortunately, this attempt to "overmatch" young "cases" among "the controls" *has led to one of the largest and least acknowledged flaws in a number of major research studies* — one on which very few researchers, such as Pike and Bernstein [7, 8], and Olsson [9] have commented.

What effect does "stacking the data" have on the relative risks of a particular risk factor such as abortion performed at a young age and/or OCP use? When researchers "stack" a study by oversampling the "controls" in the younger age groups, they end up underestimating the relative risk for early OCP use and/or abortion performed at a young age. Why? It was noted that women in the late 1970s and the 1980s used OCPs far earlier and longer and had more abortions performed at a young age than women did in the late 1960s and early 1970s [2, p.9S]. Thus, if the younger aged "controls" (eg, those women under the age of 35) are oversampled compared to the younger "cases," the "control group" will be much more likely to have women in it who had early OCP use and/or an abortion performed at a young age, and this will artificially inflate the risks in this group. *But artificially inflating the "control group's" risk is another way of saying that one has artificially deflated the "case group's" risks. In other words, when the control group is stacked, one ends up underestimating the risks of abortion performed at a young age and/or early OCP use.*

Dr. McPherson, from Oxford, came close to describing this effect, without naming it as such, more than 10 years ago in the *British Medical Journal* in 1986 where two different studies were compared [10]: "On the other hand, the Swedish study [by Olsson et al, 11] matched the controls with the cases very closely. In the New Zealand study [Paul et al] the controls were not matched at all: adjustments were made in the analysis, and this may not be adequate when one is concerned with a rapidly changing exposure rate. In studies of this kind age is a crucial confounding variable because it influences not only the risk of breast cancer but also the risk of exposure to oral contraceptives. The popularity of oral contraceptives among young women has dramatically changed over a short time, and in current studies older women are much less likely than younger women to have been exposed to oral contraceptives at an early age. Because the patterns of pill use have changed so quickly adjustment within five-year intervals, as was done in the New Zealand study, may be inadequate. In the Swedish study controls were the same age as each case to within a single month."

Obviously the "stack effect" is critical if the "control group" has a larger percentage of subjects in the lowest aged brackets as noted again in Figure A1B. A difference of 1 or 2% between two different group's population distribution in the younger age brackets can alter the outcome of an entire study. It means that a study whose results claimed to show "no real risk" may in fact "have a real risk" (ie, a false negative) and those studies which showed a real risk may well have shown a greater risk if stacking had been avoided when the study was designed. In other words, when the "control group" is stacked, it generally means that the risks of early OCP use and/or an abortion performed at a young age are even greater than those stated in the paper. Unfortunately, some of the best known studies in both the fields of breast cancer/early abortion, and breast cancer/early OCP use, are riddled with this effect.

In regard to the abortion/breast cancer studies, we find this effect in Janet Daling's 1994 study (17% "controls" vs.

8% "cases" in the 21-30 age bracket) and again in the 1996 study: (19.7% "controls" vs. 14.6% "cases" in the ages 20-34). Both show a large stack effect. In spite of the noted positive findings for abortion as a risk factor in these studies, the results may well have shown abortion performed early in a woman's reproductive life to be even riskier and with stronger statistical significance if this effect had been eliminated by proper age-distribution matching from the onset.

The stack effect is even more prevalent in the OCP/breast cancer literature; some of the most prominent studies show this. The CASH study (Cancer and Steroid Hormone Study) [12] noted that 3.9% of the "controls" versus 0.5% of the "cases" were in the youngest age bracket of 20 to 24 year olds, and 24.8% of the "controls" versus 16.2% of the "cases" were less than the age of 35; the WHO (World Health Organization) study by Thomas [13] showed that 35.8% of the "controls" were younger than the age of 35 whereas only 14.2% of the "cases" were; Paul's New Zealand study [5] had 21.7% of the "controls" in the youngest age bracket of 25 to 34 year-olds, versus only 7.2% of the "cases"; Emily White's large study [14] in the *Journal of the National Cancer Institute* in 1994 showed that "controls" comprised 17% of the 21 to 30 year-old age bracket versus 9% of the "cases." The Italian researcher La Vecchia [15] noted that 11.3% of the "controls" versus 6% of the "cases" were younger than 35 years of age; the French researchers Clavel and Andrieu's study had 6.1% of the premenopausal "controls" in the less than 30 year-old age bracket versus 3.4% of the "cases"; Dr. Lee, in her study of OCPs and Depo-Provera in Costa Rica [16], noted that the "controls" comprised 37.3% of the youngest age bracket (25-34) whereas the "cases" comprised only 9.9%.

Fortunately, as noted earlier, some researchers have astutely commented on this effect, especially in regard to the CASH study. For example, Pike and Bernstein wrote: "but in the CASH study, where the age distributions of cases and controls differ so much, adjustments are important. . . In neither of the CASH papers are the adjustments for age or the rationale for lack of adjustment for region described in detail, but it does not seem that the required finely stratified age-adjusted analysis were made." [8, p.615]. Later in the July 15, 1989 *The Lancet*, Pike and Bernstein again took issue with the stack effect in CASH; "In the footnote to their Table 1, however, they (ie, the authors of CASH) stated that, in a logistic regression analysis, age (and hence cohort) is adjusted for as a continuous variable. This is inadequate; as we stated previously, 'in data on OCP use where there are striking changes by birth cohort and by single years of age, adjustment needs to be made in single years for both birth cohort and age.'" [7, p.158]

Finally, *Olsson summarized the stack effect most concisely* in his response to the CASH study (commenting on Dr. Stadel's work, who was involved with the CASH study): "Sir, — In view of the high relative risks found in our study of oral contraceptives (OC) and breast cancer, we were surprised by the negative findings of Dr. Stadel and colleagues. The seemingly contradictory results between the two studies may be explicable by a flaw in Stadel's statistical analysis. As your Nov. 2 editorial notes, there is a strong time trend in the exposure to OC in young ages. The Stadel study design does not seem to take this effect into account. *This could imply that the young OC starters among the controls represent women born recently and thus having short latency times. The relative risk would be biased downward because of interactions bias from the shorter latency times for this young group. Adjusting for age alone will thus (not) eliminate such a bias."* (emphasis added) [9, p.1181]

Q-A1A: Is there a way to prevent or work around the "stack effect?" Can this be done by making adjustments in the statistical package that is used in a computer to help analyze the data?

Researchers have often "stacked" the "control group" at the younger ages in order to increase the stability of the statistics at the lower ages because there are usually so few "cases" at the younger spectrum of the age curve. It would be far better, however, to totally avoid the "stack effect" by making sure that the "controls" and the "cases" have not only a similar average age, but a similar distribution of subjects at the various age levels. A computer's statistical program cannot simply adjust for the stack effect. *This is because the prevalence rates of early OCP use in any given year are usually rather crude.*

A way to counter for this effect in studies that already have a stacked "control group" would be to compare the results for the respective age groups; that is, by comparing women who had abortions prior to their first full-term pregnancy who are currently in the same age bracket: for example, those between 25 and 29 years of age, those between 30 and 34, those between 35 and 39. . . Both Miller and Rosenberg [17, p.272] and Melbye in 1997 [18] subdivided women into specific age groups, however, each study failed to look at early OCP use, or abortion *prior to* a first full-term pregnancy (FFTP), in a similar manner. Although one could partially correct for the stack effect, it is disappointing to note how widespread it has been in even the most prominent papers, and how little it has been acknowledged. It may certainly make the difference between finding a significant cause and effect relationship and not finding one.

Q-A1B: Do prospective studies suffer from a type of "stack effect" which may be termed as a "prospective follow-up differential?"

Yes, although it appears to be severely under-acknowledged. In order to answer this, one must explain more about prospective studies. As noted previously, in a prospective study, one follows a group of women with a particular risk factor (ie, the "cohort") who are matched against a number of women who do not have the risk factor (ie, the "controls"). Let us take the example of women who have had abortions performed at a young age compared to those who have not. One takes a sample of 100,000 women who had abortions before their first full-term pregnancy (ie, the "cohort") and matches them against 100,000 women who did not have an abortion. Now the researcher follows both groups through time over the next 30 years. (For simplicity, we assume that no women drop out). If the groups were otherwise perfectly matched, and one found that 6000 of the women in the "cohort group" developed breast cancer, whereas only 3,000 of the "controls" did, one could conclude that having an abortion at a young age would appear to confer a 2-fold risk of getting breast cancer within the next 30 years. Researchers frequently measure how long the "cohort" group and "control group" are followed up in "women-years" or "person-years." Note that in this example, each group was followed for 3 million woman-years (ie, 30 years x 100,000 women).

Now what is the *prospective follow-up differential?*" In the example noted above, the "cohort group" was followed for the same length of time as the controls. However, frequently when researchers perform a prospective study, the "cohort" and the "control group" will have *different lengths of follow-up time* although the total number of "woman-years" of follow-up may be identical between the two groups. In effect, one ends up following the "cohort group" for significantly shorter periods of time than the "control group" so it is no surprise when the risk factor of the "cohort group" fails to show up as a risk factor.

For instance, in the example cited previously, if the cohort group had been followed for 15 years and the "controls" were followed for a full 30 years, it would surprise few if out of the original group of "cohorts" only 2,500 women developed breast cancer. Note that this group of women would have been followed for 1.5 million woman-years. If the researcher would now claim that there is no difference between the groups, it would obviously be erroneous, because a significant follow-up differential exists.

Regrettably, distinguished researchers have published studies that *have allowed huge follow-up differentials* between the "cohorts" and the "controls," and have still claimed that their study failed to identify that the risk factor was significant! Unfortunately, few epidemiologists in the OCP/abortion/breast cancer debate have pointed this out. (This author has found only one who has done so (ie, V. M. Chinchilli [19]).

Q-A1C: Can you give an example of a prospective study that points out the "prospective stack effect"?

In early 1997, Melbye et al [18] published a study which specifically claimed that "induced abortions have no overall effect on the risk of breast cancer." This bold and presumptuous claim was based upon a study that followed the "cohort group" (ie, women who had abortions) for a significantly shorter period of time than the "control group." Melbye noted that the 280,965 women who had abortions were followed for 2,697,000 person-years, which comes to an average follow-up time of 9.6 years per woman who had an abortion (ie, 2,697,000/280,965). But the "controls" were followed for a much longer period of time. The 1,248,547 women who did not have abortions were followed for an average of 25,850,000 person-years which comes to a follow-up time of 20.7 years per woman in the "control group." *Melbye's study failed to allow a significant latent period for the "cohorts" in addition to the large difference of follow-up time periods between the two groups.*

If you understood this appendix well there is no need to read the following example, but for those who wish to get a more practical grasp of this important phenomenon, the following example is provided:

A Practical Example: The Stack Effect in a Day Care Setting:

Suppose one were studying the relationship between the time that a toddler spent at a daycare center (the suspected cause) and the frequency of colds that he or she contracts (the effect). Let's assume that a state has a law that permits only 2- and 3-year-olds to participate in daycare centers. Let's also divide "the effect" into those children who get 2 or fewer colds per year (see Group B in Table A1A below) and those who get more than 2 colds per year (see Group A in Table A1A). Note that starting at the age of 4 and older, none of the children spent time in day care as the state law in this case required.

Table A1A:

AGE →	2 years	3 years	4 years	5 years	6 years	7 years
Group A						
Number of children with more than 2 colds/year	10	10	10	10	10	10
months in day care	6/child = 60 total	6/child = 60 total	0	0	0	0
Group B						
Number of children with 2 or fewer colds/year	10	10	10	10	10	10
months in day care	4/child = 40 total	4/child = 40 total	0	0	0	0

We see that in Group A, for children who had more than 2 colds per year, the total number of months spent in day care was 60+60 = 120 months. Thus, 120 months divided by 60 children (ie, the sum of *all children ages 2-7 years old*) shows us that those children who had more than 2 colds per year spent an average of 2 months per child in a daycare center each year.

What about Group B? As noted above, the children who got 2 or fewer colds per year spent a total of 40+40 = 80 months in day care giving us: 80/60 or 1.25 months in day care per child each year for this group. Thus children who had more colds were noted to have spent more time in day care on average. This might seem like an obvious result to mothers and fathers who have a child in a daycare center. Note that the average age of the children in both groups is 4.5 years old.

Now what would happen if we "stack the data"? Let us now take Group B — those children who had 2 or fewer colds per year and choose only very young and older children (ie, those who are 2, 3, 6, or 7 years old) and less "middle-aged" children (ie, those who are 4 or 5 years old). This would give us Group C as shown in Table A1B:

Table A1B:

AGE →	2 years	3 years	4 years	5 years	6 years	7 years
Group C						
Number of children with 2 or fewer colds/year	15	15	0	0	15	15
months in day care	4/child = 60 total	4/child = 60 total	0	0	0	0

Note what has now happened! By stacking the data on both ends of the age scale, that is by adding 2, 3, 6 and 7 year olds and taking away 4 and 5 year olds, the average age of the children is still 4.5 years. But if we look carefully, we see that now this group spent a total of 120 months in day care and if we divide this by 60 students we find that the average student spent 120/60= 2 months in day care. *See what happened? By stacking the data, despite having a similar average age for Groups A and B, Group C's results were made to look just like Group A's!* That is, by stacking the data in Group C, we "failed to find" the real result, namely that having your child at day care increased his or her risk of having more colds each year. If one takes two groups which have the same average age but a different age distribution of subjects (ie, Groups B and C) one can arrive at totally different results — so different that they can easily hide the effect of the real risk factor.

References:

1. National Cancer Institute. *SEER Cancer Statistics Review.* 1973-1992: Tables and Graphs. Bethesda, Maryland.
2. Collaborative Group on Hormonal Factors in Breast Cancer. Breast cancer and hormonal contraceptives: further results. *Contraception.* 1996; 34: S1-S106.
3. McPherson K, Vessey MP, et al. Early oral contraceptive use and breast cancer: Results of another case-control study. *Br J Cancer.* 1987; 56: 653-660.
4. Rosenberg L, Palmer JR, et al. Breast cancer in relation to the occurrence and time of induced and spontaneous abortion. *Am J Epidemiol.* 1988; 127: 981-989.
5. Paul C, Skegg DC, et al. Oral contraceptives and risk of breast cancer. *Int J Cancer.* 1990; 46: 366-373.

6. Newcomb PA, Longnecker MP, et al. Recent oral contraceptive use and risk of breast cancer (United States). *Cancer Causes and Control.* 1996; 7: 525-532.

7. Pike MC, Bernstein L. Oral contraceptives and breast cancer. *The Lancet.* July 15, 1989: 158.

8. Pike MC, Bernstein L. Oral contraceptives and breast cancer. *The Lancet.* March 18, 1989: 615-616.

9. Olsson H, Ranstam J, et al. (Letter on CASH) *The Lancet.* November 23, 1985: 1181.

10. McPherson K. The pill and breast cancer: why the uncertainty? *Br Med J.* Sept. 20, 1986; 293: 709-710.

11. Olsson H, Moller TR, Ranstam J. Early contraceptive use and breast cancer among premenopausal women: Final report from a study in southern Sweden. *J Natl Cancer Inst.* 1989; 81: 1000-1004.

12. Stadel BV, Lai S, et al. Oral contraceptives and premenopausal breast cancer in nulliparous women. *Contraception.* 1988; 38: 287-299.

13. Thomas DB. Oral contraceptives and breast cancer. *J Natl Cancer Inst.* 1993; 85: 359-364.

14. White E, Malone K, Weiss N, Daling J. Breast cancer among young U.S. women in relation to oral contraceptive use. *J Natl Cancer Inst.* 1994; 86: 505-514.

15. La Vecchia C, et al. Breast cancer and combined oral contraceptives: an Italian case-control study. *Eur J Cancer.* 25 11-G: 1613-1618.

16. Lee NC, Rosero-Bixby L, et al. A case-control study of breast cancer and hormonal Contraception in Costa Rica. *J Natl Cancer Inst.* 1987; 6: 1247-1254.

17. Miller D, Rosenberg L, et al. Breast cancer before age 45 and oral contraceptive use: new findings. *Am J Epidemiol.* 1989; 129: 269-279.

18. Melbye M, Wohlfahrt J, et al. Induced abortion and the risk of breast cancer. *N Engl J Med.* 1997; 336: 81-85.

19. Brind J, et al. Induced abortion and the risk of breast cancer. *N Engl J Med.* 1997; 336: 1834.

Appendix 2:
The Bias Factor
(a detailed analysis)

The term "bias" is often referred to in studies concerning abortion, breast cancer, and the oral contraceptive pill (OCP). What does it mean? There are two main types of bias. The first has to do with the author(s)' own bias (referred to as "author's bias" or simply "bias"). The second phenomenon is referred to as "recall bias." Recall bias refers to "a bias in recall" by patients either in the "control group" or the "case group." That is, if a study has recall bias it means that one group or the other recalled their history of experience in, or of, a particular risk factor (eg, OCP use or abortion) more accurately than the other group.

There are many reasons for "author's bias." Almost every author has an opinion of the way he or she wants the results to turn out, and if that opinion is stronger than his or her desire to let the final results speak for themselves, the study may be subtly undermined by either failing to present the significant findings (ie, the "reverse file drawer" phenomenon mentioned in Chapter 5), or by presenting the data in such a skewed fashion so as to mask or grossly diminish or augment the main findings.

A second source of author's bias revolves around the issue of money. Researchers survive by obtaining grants for their studies. There may be a conflict of interest between the grantor and the grantee as noted previously. This is obvious when the grantor is a drug company and the grantee is the researcher.

Another factor which may influence the researcher concerns the special interests of other grantors. For example, many studies have been supported by the World Health Organization (WHO) [1,2,3], or the Family Health International [3, 4, 5], or USAID (United States Agency for International Development) [4]. As noted previously in Chapter 5, these organizations have either openly funded studies favoring abortion or are financially and philosophically committed to widespread use of hormonal contraception and/or abortion — hardly an atmosphere of impartiality.

A fourth type of influence which could bias the researcher revolves around the issue of "medical correctness" as concerns the medical establishment's endorsement of induced abortion and contraception. Three of the main organizations in the medical field include the AMA (American Medical Association), the AAP (American Academy of Pediatrics), and the ACOG (American College of Obstetricians and Gynecologists). Each of them plays a dominant role in its respective branch of medicine, especially because each one publishes a journal *which cannot fail to be controlled by them.* It was noted previously that the AMA publishes *JAMA*, the AAP publishes the journal of *Pediatrics,* and the ACOG publishes the journal of *Obstetrics and Gynecology.* For those familiar with the medical world, it comes as no surprise that the influence of these journals on physicians, nurses, and other medical professionals is enormous. Obviously, the position taken on issues such as induced abortion and oral contraception, especially in regard to young women, is critical in gaining an understanding of the general atmosphere of this entire debate. What are these professional organizations' respective positions? An insight can be gained from the following quotation taken from the 1996 journal of *Pediatrics* [6, p.746]: "The American Medical Association, the Society for Adolescent Medicine, the American Public Health Association, the American College of Obstetricians and Gynecologists, the (AAP) American Academy of Pediatrics, and other health professional organizations have reached the consensus that minors should not be compelled or required to involve their parents in their decisions to obtain abortions. . ."

"Journal bias" has become so obvious that even the secular press has started commenting on the ability (or lack thereof) of different medical journals to report unbiased results. In December, 1996, the editors (ie, Douglas L. Weed and Barnett S. Kramer) of the prominent journal put out by the National Cancer Institute called the *Journal of the National Cancer Institute*, actually stated their own opinion on the abortion/breast cancer link: "We believe that there is as yet insufficient evidence to claim that a true association exists between induced abortion and breast cancer." [7, p.1699] (Note: Editors of medical journals are not supposed to be interjecting their opinions. They are supposed to let the results speak for themselves and/or allow the actual researcher to comment.) *A strong opinion by an editor leaves the reader and other researchers little doubt as to which way their journal will lean in the future, and to which way the researcher who has his or her study published by the journal is "expected to lean."* John McGinnis, commenting in the *Wall Street Journal* wrote: "There's one more question that needs further study: Why are the *Journal of the National Cancer Institute* and the *New England Journal of Medicine* departing from the scientific method when it comes to breast cancer risks? Given the lessons of the past, women ought to demand better treatment. 'If politics gets involved in science' said Dr. Daling, 'it will really hold back the progress we make.'" [8].

No researcher can fail to notice the "*tone*" of the aforementioned medical groups and named journals. Unfortunately, this atmosphere certainly puts pressure on a researcher to subjugate his or her work to the current "medically correct" philosophy instead of allowing an open presentation of the data.

Recall Bias:

The second type of bias that has cropped into the breast cancer/abortion/OCP debate is the following: Some researchers are postulating and even claiming to prove that women who have breast cancer answer more honestly than women who do not have breast cancer to the following question: "Did you ever have an induced abortion?" This is the so-called "recall bias."

There are two main studies which claimed to show evidence for recall bias regarding having an abortion at a young age and/or early OCP use. The first is a study in 1991, funded by Family Health International and conducted by researchers Lindefors-Harris and Meirik from Sweden. They gave their thoughts on recall bias: "We hypothesized that a woman who had recently been given a diagnosis of a malignant disease, contemplating causes of her illness, would remember and report an induced abortion more consistently than would a healthy control" [3, p.1003]. The immediate question which may enter the medical mind is: "Why was this the working hypothesis instead of its direct counterpart?" That is, why did these authors not originally hypothesize that a woman who has breast cancer might be less candid about her recall of abortion? After all, *denial* is one of the first reactions that patients have. When a woman is told that she has breast cancer, it is not uncommon to deny to herself that she really has it. *It would seem just as logical to think that such women would be more likely to deny factors that may have contributed to the breast cancer such as abortion and/or early oral contraceptive use.*

In addition, if Lindefors-Harris' hypothesis was correct, it would mean that thousands of other studies in medicine might now be deemed "worthless." Every time one had a disease or "effect" that was caused by a controversial risk factor (ie, one of the causes), the study might be considered invalid based upon "recall bias." Studies on "suicide attempts and a history of child abuse" or "cervical cancer and the number of sexual partners a woman has had" or "the diagnosis of AIDS and the number of homosexual encounters a man has had," are all examples of an *effect that is associated with a controversial cause. Accepting the Lindefors-Harris hypothesis implies that all these studies* — and thousands of others — are possibly compromised as they all could suffer from recall bias because a controversial risk factor was involved after a patient received news of severe disease.

In any case, Dr. Lindefors-Harris noted that in Sweden all abortions are supposedly reported to the Swedish National Board of Health and Welfare. Almost every national registry has inaccuracies in reporting, so it is difficult to assess how accurate the Swedish registry is, given the fact that many women wish to have as few people learn of their abortion as possible. The information from Tables A2A and A2B of the Lindefors-Harris study [3, p.1005] comparing register data to interview responses for both "cases" and "controls" follows:

Table A2A:
DATA FROM THE LINDEFORS-HARRIS STUDY
Responses from *women with breast cancer* to the question of whether they had an induced abortion in the past:

	Answered yes (based on register)	Answered no (based on register)	
Answered yes (based on interview)	19	7	26 = total yes's from interview
Answered no (based on interview)	5	286	291 = total no's from interview
	24 = total Yes from register	293 = total No from register	317 = total overall responses

Table A2B:
Responses from *women without breast cancer* to the question of whether they had an induced abortion in the past:

	Answered yes (based on register)	Answered no (based on register)	
Answered yes (based on interview)	43	1	44 = total yes's from interview
Answered no (based on interview)	16	452	468 = total no's from interview
	59 = total Yes from register	453 = total No from register	512 = total overall responses

In Table A2A one notes that although the register stated that 24 women had abortions, only 19 of them, or 79.2% stated that they had an abortion when asked in the interview. In the "control group" 43 women stated that they had an abortion whereas the register noted that 59 were recorded as having one, for a total of 72.9%. According to these figures, women with breast cancer had "more accurate" recall than the "controls," although the literal difference between them is less than 7% (ie, 72.8% - 79.2%). It is difficult to build a case based on this small difference.

There is another problem with the results in Table A3A and A3B. *Here we see that the authors of the paper noted that 7 out of the 26 "cases" who stated that they had an induced abortion at a young age, actually did not, according to the national register.* What does this mean? In short, this implies that out of the 26 women with breast cancer who stated that they had an abortion, 7 of them (or 27%) "lied." That is, 27% of the women with breast cancer actually stated that they had an abortion at a young age when the national register noted that they did not! Only 2.2% of the "controls" "lied." Now this is rather bizarre!! *Are we to believe that 27% of the women with breast cancer actually "made up" the "fact" that they had an abortion when they did not?* Dr. Daling, another prominent researcher, later commented directly on this in her study in 1994: "However, we believe it is reasonable to assume that virtually no women who truly did not have an abortion would claim to have had one. . ." [9, p.1590].

Q-A2A: If the data are as noted, how and why did Lindefors-Harris and Meirik claim that their study showed recall bias which inflated their study's risk by 50%?

When Lindefors-Harris and Meirik calculated the estimated (RR) of abortion based on interview response (see Tables A3A and A3B) they noted a risk of 0.95: (26/292 divided by 44/468). When the same calculation was performed using the register's responses, the RR was 0.63 (24/293 divided by 59/453). They claimed that the difference (about 50%) was due to recall bias. There are two major problems with their claim however. First, they were assuming that the national register is the "gold standard", which is a faulty assumption to which Meirik even admitted [10]. Second, in using the register's data, the authors were not only measuring the effect of "recall bias," they were also measuring "*recall confabulation.*" That is, the authors were using data that artificially inflated the "interview relative risk" because they used the data from 7 out of the 26 women who reportedly "*confabulated*" (ie, "made up the idea") that they had an abortion when the register stated that they did not. *In other words, the 50% increase in the RR due to "recall bias" would be due to both "recall bias*" (ie, "cases" remembering better than "controls"), and "*recall confabulation*" (ie, "cases" confabulating better than "controls"). Because almost no one places any merit on the latter item, the "50% figure" is in fact an inflated *statistic based on a failure to distinguish two separate phenomenon* as researcher Daling aptly noted. It should be pointed out that if neither the "cases" nor the "controls" had "confabulated," the "recall bias" phenomenon could have been measured more accurately. When this calculation was performed by separating out the "recall confabulation bias," *the effect of "recall bias" in their study turned out to be about 16%* — a statistic which is the same as that which Janet Daling calculated in 1994 [9] (see end of this appendix for details.)

The fact that the Lindefors-Harris' study was funded by Family Health International, showed a 16% difference in recall (and this is based on an "*accurate*" Swedish register), claimed to show that "women with breast cancer confabulate 27% of the time," and was openly critiqued by a prominent epidemiologist, all serve to make one openly wonder why this study has received so much attention. It hardly qualifies as a "landmark study" and offers little concrete evidence for the "hypothesis" of "recall bias."

The second major study which claimed to support the theory of recall bias was published by Rookus and van Leeuwen in 1996 [11]. They noted that there was a greater percentage (63%) of Roman Catholic women living in the southeast portion of the Netherlands than in the west, which has a 28% Roman Catholic population. They predicted that this would render the southeastern Netherlands more morally conservative than the western section.

The paper noted that in the western regions, the relative risk (RR) of breast cancer when a woman had an abortion was 1.2, whereas in the southeastern section the RR was 14.6. The authors took this to implicate recall bias as a major factor in this discrepancy, implying that conservative Catholic "controls" would be less truthful about their abortion histories than the rest of the population.

This conclusion, however, offers little proof that recall bias is the culprit. First, one must note that being a "Roman Catholic" may have little to do with one's moral values. For example, the Netherlands is widely known as a country with extremely liberal views on euthanasia, widespread birth control, and sex-education. As Rookus himself wrote: "This lower rate (of abortion) in The Netherlands is attributable to the wide availability of oral contraceptives and the 'morning-after' pill, open sex education. . ." (11, p.1762]. It is quite probable that the "average Roman Catholic" in the Netherlands is far more liberal than, for example, a Catholic who resides in Ireland or Poland. To claim that the "Catholic factor" is responsible for the difference in RR between the west and the southeast is one step short of conjecture. There certainly could be many other factors which explain the difference among the regions and it cannot simply be "assigned" to "the Catholic factor." Even if this factor played any role, however, it would still make it difficult to explain why a 12.2-fold difference between the west and the southeast regions (ie, 14.6 divided by 1.2), could be explained by only a 2.3-fold difference in their respective Catholic populations. An additional critique is that the RR for abortion in the southeast Netherlands was based on only 13 subjects — a very small sample size.

Finally, it should be noted again that Rookus et al found that women who had an abortion in the southeastern regions had a 14.6 or 1360% increased rate of breast cancer. Note that in claiming that this result is due to "extreme recall bias" *the authors are now placing an addition on the old recall bias theory*. In effect they are saying: "In comparing women with breast cancer and more *conserva-*

tive moral values to morally *conservative* women without breast cancer, the degree of recall bias will be even greater than that of morally *liberal* women who have and do not have breast cancer. *"But should the "degree of recall not increase or decrease proportionately for both the "morally conservative cases and controls" and the "liberal cases and controls?" In other words, whereas the old recall bias theory hypothesized that a woman's response would be affected by whether or not she had cancer, the "Rookus bias theory" adds to this and postulates that religious values now also play a role in the recall bias phenomenon.* This is amazing! Rookus et al apparently felt justified in arbitrarily expanding a totally unproved theory. Perhaps the saddest commentary is that so few even challenged this highly speculative gesture, indicating perhaps the degree of intimidation or carelessness that exists in the research world.

In regard to recall bias and the OCP/breast cancer debate, Rookus et al claimed support for the theory when commenting on the following table which reported oral contraceptive use in the Netherlands: [the numbers in the table are the number of months of discrepancy between how long a woman states she was taking oral contraceptive pills (OCPs) compared to how many months the office medical records stated she was taking them. A number such as (-3.0) for example, would mean that a woman might have stated that she was taking OCPs for 15 months whereas the office records showed that she took them for 18 months.]

Table A2C:
DATA FROM THE ROOKUS STUDY

	Difference in reporting by "cases"	Difference in "controls"
Western region	-3.0	-0.5
Southeastern region	-2.3	-6.8

Rookus and van Leeuwen stated: "...control subjects in the southeastern regions underreported the duration of their oral contraceptive use by 6.3 months more than control subjects in the western regions." (11, p.1761). Although this statement is true, the authors failed to note another very important fact. In the *western* Netherlands (reportedly more liberal) *the "cases" had a greater difference of recall (ie, -3.0 months) than did the "controls" (-0.5 months). This flies directly against the recall bias theory which would predict that "controls" would recall "less accurately" than "cases."*

In summary, it should be noted that the "proof" for recall bias in the OCP/abortion and breast cancer research debate has little solid support and seems to be based more on various author's "hypotheses" than on solid documentation. Nevertheless, the physician, nurse, or lay reader need not continue to speculate about recall bias because there are two fairly direct ways to deal with this unproved hypothesis. How can this be done?

The first approach is to let the laity "decide for themselves." For example, Dr. Joel Brind, in a comprehensive meta-analysis regarding abortion and breast cancer [12], noted that the relative risk of breast cancer in women who had an abortion at a young age (before their first full-term pregnancy [FFTP]) was 50%. If recall bias had played a role, for example, if the "control" group had admitted to having abortion half as often as the "case" group, then the relative risk of 50% might not be a real relative risk. The real question to the laity is: "Do you really believe this?" That is, does anyone really believe that women without breast cancer would really be "50% as candid" as women with breast cancer? Would not most members of the laity and the medical community have a difficult time believing that a significant number of women would lie when asked "Did you have an induced abortion or use OCPs prior to your FFTP?" Even fewer would believe that the diagnosis of breast cancer would suddenly cause the patient to be more candid about her past medical history. If one really believes the Lindefors-Harris presumption, one would have to believe the following example: A 47-year-old woman walks into the office and is asked if she ever had an abortion. The next year she is diagnosed as having breast cancer. If you ask her the same question after she is diagnosed she will be 50% more likely to tell you the truth. Why not let the laity "decide this question for themselves?"

But ironically, it is Dr. Rookus himself who provides a far superior solution. Rookus noted in 1994 [13] that there was a relative risk (RR) for breast cancer in women under the age of 36, of 1.44 for each year of OCP use before the age of 20. In commenting on his results [13, p.849] he noted that when he measured the degree of "differential misclassification bias" — that is "recall bias" by comparing interview responses directly to information from the patient's prescribers (doctor's records) *there was only a 2% difference!* In other words, the recall bias was only 2% in this study. To strengthen the argument, Rookus even went as far as referencing two other classic papers, both of which went back and measured recall bias between "cases" and "controls" when asked about OCP use. The UK National study published in *The Lancet* concluded that: "moreover, this bias is reduced to 1% when all data from all sources are used" [14, p.980]; the other study from the WHO, showed only a 0.6 month (ie, about a 20 day [probably less than 3%]) difference in recall between the "cases" and the "controls" regarding their oral contraceptive histories.

What does this tell us? It certainly shows that if one compares office records to interview responses, the recall bias phenomenon is less than 3% in these three different studies. These results are important for two reasons. First, they offer strong reassurance that the recall bias hypothesis as concerns the OCP debate has little support — especially in the three alluded to papers that measured it. This should satisfy critics who "chanted the recall bias mantra," such as Clavel and Andrieu, who "hypothesized" in their study of women in France [15, p.37], that "recall bias is probable because the name and pattern of use of the oral contraceptive is less readily forgotten by women with breast cancer. . ." Second, and perhaps even more important, *it gives researchers a way to measure the degree of recall bias in any study.* We have seen that researchers were able to go back to the office records and compare physician notes on

OCP use to patient's interview responses; from that, the researchers could calculate any degree of recall bias. The same principle can and should be applied to the abortion/breast cancer studies. *That is, if one can calculate the degree of recall bias for the OCP studies by going back to a woman's medical records, one can do the same thing for a woman's abortion history.*

How would one go about doing this? To do this the researcher would need to get permission to review the obstetrical and gynecologic medical records of both the "cases" and the "controls." *A well-trained obstetrician or gynecologist* * *will record how many abortions a patient has had* — in his or her history and physical — and what type they were; that is, were they "spontaneous abortions" (ie, miscarriages) or were they induced abortions. A researcher could then compare both the "case group's" and the "control group's" interview responses with the office records. One would soon discover how "real" the recall bias is in this area of research. One has to wonder why such a basic procedure has never been done in the abortion/breast cancer studies, because it would enable one to measure the degree of recall bias in any study and factor it into the calculated results. Let us hope that the "hypothesis of recall bias" will be put to rest once and for all by conducting studies which accurately measure its influence — if it has any at all — by comparing actual interview responses to office record responses.

*When this author writes of a trained obstetrician or gynecologist, this does not refer to the man or woman who performed the abortion, especially if this occurred in an abortion clinic. Rather, it refers to a woman's personal obstetrician/gynecologist who has or had followed the patient over the long-term. Thus, the medical data would be obtained from one who was removed from the actual performing of the abortion and would be less subject to bias.

Addendum:
Details on the recall bias phenomenon:

If neither the "cases" nor the "controls" had "confabulated" that they had an abortion when the register stated that they did not, the Lindefors-Harris study would have yielded the following data:

Table A2D:
HYPOTHETICAL DATA WITHOUT CONFABULATION EFFECT

	RESPONSES FROM REGISTER	
(INTERVIEW RESPONSE)	HAD AN ABORTION	NO ABORTION
"Cases" with abortion	26	0
"Cases" without abortion	5	286
Totals	31	286
"Controls" with abortion	44	0
"Controls" without abortion	16	452
Totals	60	452

Note that the RR based on the interview response would have still been 0.95 (26/291 divided by 44/468), but the RR based on the register would now be 0.82 (31/286 divided by 60/452). But the ratio of these odds ratios is 0.95/0.82 which is 1.16 or a 16% difference. In other words when one separates out the "confabulation effect," which few people believe, the "recall bias" effect in the Lindefors study comes to about 16% (exactly the figure that Daling et al calculated [9, p.1590]).

References:

1. Paul C, Skegg DC, et al. Oral contraceptives and risk of breast cancer. *Int J Cancer.* 1990; 46: 366-373.

2. Thomas DB, Noonan EA. Breast cancer and combined oral contraceptives: results from a multinational study [The WHO collaborative study of Neoplasia and steroid contraceptives]. *Br J Cancer.* 1990; 61: 110-119.

3. Lindefors-Harris BM, Eklund G, et al. Response bias in a case-control study: analysis utilizing comparative data concerning legal abortions from two independent Swedish studies. *Am J Epidemiol.* 1991; 134: 1003-1008.

4. Lee NC, Rosero-Bixby L, et al. A case-control study of breast cancer and hormonal Contraception in Costa Rica. *J Natl Cancer Inst.* 1987; 6: 1247-1254.

5. Lin TM, Chen KP, MacMahon B. Epidemiologic characteristics of cancer of the breast in Taiwan. *Cancer.* 1971; 27: 1497-1504.

6. American Academy of Pediatrics. The adolescent's right to confidential care when considering abortion. *Pediatrics.* 1996; 97: 746-751.

7. Weed D, Kramer B. Induced abortion, bias, and breast cancer: why epidemiology hasn't reached its limit. *J Natl Cancer Inst.* 1996; 88: 1698-1699.

8. McGinnis J. The politics of Cancer research. *The Wall Street Journal.* February 28, 1997.

9. Daling J, Malone K, et al. Risk of breast cancer among young women: relationship to induced abortion. *J Natl Cancer Inst.* 1994; 86: 1584-1592.

10. Meirik, et al. Relationship between induced abortion and breast cancer. *J Epidemiol Community Health.* 1998; 52.

11. Rookus M, Leeuwen F. Induced abortion and risk for breast cancer: reporting (recall) bias in a Dutch case-control study. *J Natl Cancer Inst.* 1996; 88: 1759-1764.

12. Brind J, Chinchilli M, et al. Induced abortion as an independent risk factor for breast cancer: a comprehensive review and meta-analysis. *J Epidemiol Community Health.* 10/ 1996; 50: 481-496.

13. Rookus MA, Leeuwen FE. Oral contraceptives and risk of breast cancer in women ages 20-54 years. *The Lancet.* 1994; 344: 844-851.

14. Chilvers C, McPherson K, et al. Oral contraceptive use and breast cancer risk in young women (UK National Case-Control Study Group). *The Lancet.* May 6, 1989: 973-982.

15. Clavel F, Andrieu N, et al. Oral contraceptives and breast cancer: A French case-control study. *Int J Epidemiol.* 1991; 20: 32-38.

Appendix 3:
The Chickenpox Vaccine (a lesson in bias)

A look at the history of the chickenpox vaccine provides a useful illustration of how research bias can enter the scientific debate, be it over childhood illness or the rising problem of breast cancer among women. The first section contains information concerning the efficacy of the chickenpox vaccine (ie, varicella vaccine) and is technical. For the reader who is interested in the information regarding research bias and the pharmaceutical industry, please skip down to the mid-section of this appendix labeled: "Bias and the Chickenpox Vaccine."

On March 17, 1995 the FDA approved the use of Varivax, the varicella vaccine (ie, chickenpox vaccine) made by Merck, for use in healthy young children. A number of concerns still remain.

First, there is the issue of efficacy — will the vaccine work or will it offer "attenuated immunity?" Specifically, will adults who have been vaccinated be at increased risk as the immunity fades? In adults the chickenpox virus carries 35 times the morbidity and 20 times the mortality compared to youngsters. Although Merck's literature and that of various other researchers note that antibody to the varicella zoster virus (VZV) remains high even 20 years after vaccination, almost all openly admit that this is due to a booster effect from subclinical re-infection occurring (years) after vaccination, and from being exposed to children who have naturally acquired chickenpox. This means that when one gets the vaccine and then is later exposed to a child who has a real case of the chickenpox, this exposure serves to "boost the immune system" of the child who originally received the vaccine. Unfortunately, in the future, if the incidence of chickenpox decreases, subclinical re-infection (ie, the "booster phenomenon") will become more rare, and one will have to rely solely on the vaccination's immunity. The literature, however, clearly notes that vaccine-induced immunity fades with time when the booster effect is absent. Both humoral immunity [1,2] and cell mediated immunity (CMI) [3] either drop dramatically or give far lower levels of protection than natural varicella infection when measured months after vaccination instead of years. For example, Bogger [2] noted that the antibody level following natural infection was more than 25 times as high as that found in vaccinated individuals when measured 14 months after exposure. He also noted that antibody levels fell more than 8-fold within a 14-month time period, whether one had acquired natural varicella or whether one had been vaccinated, thus giving a strong indication of what can be expected once the booster effect diminishes. Gershon [3] noted that the stimulation index (SI) — the measure of cell mediated immunity — is over 4-fold greater in adults after natural infection than adults who received the vaccination. What happens if vaccinated adults are found to be susceptible? Researchers for Merck claim that they could be revaccinated, but this may not be so simple. As family practitioners and internists know, most adults never get their 10-year tetanus updates — compliance may be a problem and travelers will have to make sure they are "up-to-date" when flying to any country in which they might be exposed to the virus.

Another potentially serious problem concerns the newborn child of the vaccinated mother. Normally, about 95% of U.S. born mothers have been exposed to the varicella virus and pass the antibodies on to their newborn babies before birth, which gives them protection for the first $5^1/_2$

months of life. Newborns who get the varicella virus with-out having maternal antibody protection are known to be at high risk for mortality (31%) [4]. *Will the newborn baby who is born to the mother who was vaccinated as a child still receive enough (any?) antibody, and will he or she now be vulnerable to the virus at this critical stage when the baby's immune system may not be able to fight the virus? This question has never been answered, let alone asked, by the medical establishment.*

Bias and the Chickenpox Vaccine:

The second point is the presence of an overt bias which appears in a number of papers concerning the costs/ben-efits of the chicken pox vaccine (made by Merck). It is true that 60 to 90 people die each year from the virus; about 40% of these are adults and 25% are immunocompromised children. As noted, we really do not know if the long-term mortality will decrease with mass vaccination although it would appear that some reduction is likely over the next few years. Merck is estimated to receive $150 million an-nually from sales [5], which American families will fund either through higher taxes or via higher insurance premi-ums.

Of note, each year 2000 youngsters die in drownings and 600 die in bicycle accidents. Is it not likely that if we were to spend $150 million annually in safety programs and radio and television awareness ads that less young-sters would die from these causes as well? Perhaps in an-ticipation to arguments like these or others, some re-searchers have noted the "savings to society" that Varivax (the chicken pox vaccine) would bring because mothers would have to take less time off to care for their sick chil-dren. In one study *funded by Merck* and published in the *Journal of Pediatrics*, Daniel M. Huse [6] noted how he es-timates the value of a typical day of lost wages for the woman who takes care of her sick child: "Finally our esti-mate that the value of a day lost from work would be $103 was based on one-fifth of the 1991 average weekly earnings for U.S. women." There is, however, one major problem with this "economic analysis." Mr. Huse has missed the obvious and *has failed to attach any economic value to the time which mothers spend with their sick children. Of note, these mothers must deem the time they spend with their sick children to be worth more than a day's wages or they would not be taking off in the first place.* By failing to take into account the economic worth of the mother's time with her sick child, *the authors seem to imply a rather shallow assumption* — namely, *that the time these women gave up is "valueless"*!

Third, it is a bit disconcerting to note that 11 out of 26 papers that this author reviewed concerning the varicella vaccine had been *funded by Merck.* This is an obvious conflict of interest as is the case when Merck funded its own cost/benefit analysis [6]. Neither can one take comfort when one notes that in the paper entitled "Recommendations for the Use of Live Attenuated Varicella Vaccine" [7], the recommendation committee members of the American Academy of Pediatrics are listed at the end of the paper: Two of the authors might catch one's attention — *one is a member of the Food and Drug Administration and the other has previously published a paper that was funded by Merck!* This hardly makes for an independent process. *Members of the FDA, Merck, and the American Academy of Pediatrics are not supposed to be offering collaborative opinions in a process that ought to involve an independent evaluation.*

Finally, an ethical controversy has started regarding the source of the cell line in which the vaccine is currently grown (MRC-5). Pro-life groups have taken note that this cell line (MRC-5) was derived from an aborted child: "Fetal lung tissue taken from a 14-week-old male fetus removed for psychiatric reasons from a 27-year-old woman. . ."[8]* Merck freely admits that vaccinated children will receive DNA from this very same cell line: the vaccine contains

*This same ethical concern applies to the rubella vaccine, which was developed from an aborted baby. Likewise, women making choices about OCP use, other hormonal contraceptives and abortion should make an informed decision, understanding (as this book illustrates) the impact of research bias and the suppression of cautionary data.

"residual components of the MRC-5 cell line including DNA and protein." [9] Which patients are ever told that the vaccine their children are about to receive contains DNA and/or protein that was derived from a surgically aborted baby?

In summary, at a time in which the U.S. is involved in a massive program of childhood vaccination, it would appear that there are a number of concerns that have not been resolved. The vaccine may well prove beneficial in terms of decreasing morbidity and mortality, but before embarking on a venture of this magnitude *the ethical problems* (eg, especially the MRC-5 cell line and another named WI 38) must be resolved (ie, use/develop an alternate cell line(s)-[see Hoskins [10] below]). The *major efficacy concerns* (ie, the neonatal immunity question) must be addressed as well. Although the vaccine may decrease morbidity and mortality in the short run, the long run effects are simply not known. *Parents* should make an informed decision for their children based upon a knowledge of all of the current facts.

References:

1. Asano Yoshizo, et al. Clinical and serologic testing of a live Varicella Vaccine and two-year follow-up for immunity of the vaccinated children. *Journal of Pediatrics.* 1977; 5: 60.

2. Bogger-Goren S. Antibody response to Varicella-Zoster Virus after natural or vaccine-induced infection. *J Infect Dis.* 1982; 146: 260.

3. Gershon, Anne, A. Live attenuated Varicella Vaccine: protection in healthy adults compared with leukemic children. *J Infect Dis.* 1990; 161: 661-666.

4. Preblud Stephen. Varicella: complications and costs. *Journal of Pediatrics.* Supplement 1986; 78: 728.

5. Severyn, Kristine. Children to be used as guinea pigs for drug company profits. Ohio Parents for Vaccine Safety: May 10, 1995. [251 West Ridgeway Drive, Dayton, Ohio 45459].

6. Huse Daniel. Childhood Vaccination Against Chickenpox: An Analysis of Benefits and Costs. *Journal of Pediatrics.* June, 1994; 124: 869-873.

7. Hall Caroline B. Recommendations for the use of live attenuated varicella vaccine. *Journal of Pediatrics.* 1995; 95: 791.

8. Jacobs Patrick, Jones C.M., Baille J.P. Characteristics of human diploid cell designated MRC-5. *Nature.* 1970; 227: 168-170.

9.   Merck: Drug insert of VARIVAX, 1995.

10. Hoskins J.M., Plotkin S.A. Behaviour of Rubella Virus in Human Diploid Strains. Wistar Institute of Anatomy and Biology, Philadelphia, PA. Jan 16, 1967. [The authors describe two cell lines, one developed from spontaneous abortions and one from induced abortions. Both were capable of sustaining growth of the rubella virus.]

Appendix 4:

Commentary on the Oxford Meta-analysis on Oral Contraceptives and Breast Cancer

The Oxford meta-analysis, published in complete form in the journal of *Contraception* [1] and in summary form in *The Lancet* [2], is the largest meta-analysis done to date regarding the various studies concerning oral contraceptive use and the consequent risk of breast cancer. It combines data from 54 separate studies from 26 countries, and studies 53,297 "cases" and 100,239 "controls." It was performed by a group called the Collaborative Group on Hormonal Factors in Breast Cancer, and relied on input from top researchers from around the world. One major strength of this meta-analysis is that it provides the reader with a historical bibliography of almost every study available concerning OCPs and breast cancer; nearly every prospective and retrospective study is referenced. It contains some of the best and most exhaustive information in the world and yet it contains some glaring deficiencies which cannot go uncontested. A critique/analysis follows: (All journal references to data and tables come from the *Contraception* article [1]).

Q-A4A: Does the meta-analysis suffer from the stack effect?

Yes. The authors noted [1, Table 2] that 12% of the "controls" and 9% of the "cases" were less than 34 years old, and that 2% of the "controls" and 1% of the "cases" were less than 25 years old. Because the authors combined the information of many studies which themselves had a stack effect, it is no surprise that the summary of the data of those studies would result in a cumulative stack effect.

Q-A4B: What effect does a "cumulative stack effect" have?

It has the same effect that a stack effect would have in any study which looks at early OCP use — it "waters down" the relative risk. Why? Because if the "control" group in this meta-analysis is "stacked" — that is, if it has a disproportionate number of young women (ie, under the age of 34), it now contains the one group of women who are at a very high risk for having used OCPs early in life and for longer periods of time (ie, young women in the 1980s and 1990s), but who are at a relatively low risk of developing breast cancer because they are still fairly young. Thus, the stacked group (ie, the "controls") will have an artificially inflated rate of early OCP use which means that the "cases" will have an artificially reduced rate of early OCP use. This results in *underestimating* the relative risk of OCP use and its effect upon developing breast cancer.

Q-A4C: Does the Oxford study show any data which support the statement that young women have a higher rate of oral contraceptive use at early ages compared to older women?

Table A4A:

ORAL CONTRACEPTIVE USE
FOR VARIOUS AGE GROUPS

AGE→	<35	35-44	45-54	55+
FIRST USE AT AGE:				
<20	42%	16%	1%	0%
20-24	43%	42%	15%	1%
25-29	13%	25%	29%	7%
30-34	2%	12%	28%	24%

Yes it does. Table A4A, whose information was taken from the Oxford trial and published in *Contraception* [1, p.9S], clearly shows that the younger women (those under the age of 35) *have a far higher rate of early oral contraceptive use* (ie, before the age of 20) than any other age group. Naturally, any group which has a disproportionate percentage of these younger women, (ie, the "controls") will have an artificially inflated rate of early OCP use compared to the other group.

Q-A4D: The Oxford study noted that there is no evidence of an increase in the risk (of breast cancer) more than 10 years after stopping use (of OCPs). Is this a fair statement?

Absolutely not. It must be remembered that the Oxford study included data from older studies and that *more than 60% of the women in the Oxford study started using OCPs before 1970* [1, p.7S]. But as the Oxford study noted: "Reporting of use for short durations is common, especially among women whose last use of oral contraceptives was long ago: the proportion of users whose total duration of use was reported to be 12 months or less was 17% for women who stopped use less than 10 years ago, 35% for women who stopped use 10 to 19 years ago, and 62% for women who stopped use more than 20 years ago" [1, p.13S]. Thus, women in the 1960s and early 1970s took OCPs for far shorter periods of time and at later ages (according to Table A4A), than women of the late 1970s and 1980s. The authors of the Oxford study even admitted this in their results section: "For example, women who had stopped use long ago would not have had the opportunity to have taken oral contraceptives for long durations" [1, p.7S]. *When the Oxford study examined women who had stopped using OCPs at least 10 years ago, it ended up placing the bulk of its emphasis on women who used OCPs for shorter periods of time and those who had used them at a later age in life* — thus, having a greater probability of using them after their first full-term pregnancy (FFTP). If the Oxford collaborators had limited themselves to looking at those studies in which women developed breast cancer in the 1980s and 1990s, they would have concluded that women who had stopped taking OCPs more than 10 years ago would have shown an increased risk of breast cancer as noted in Table A4B which examines the few studies which took the bulk of their data after 1980 and followed women up to 20 years after their first use of OCPs.

Table A4B:
RISKS OF BREAST CANCER TO WOMEN WHO TOOK OCPS 10-20 YEARS AGO

STUDY→	BRINTON [3]: WOMEN LESS THAN AGE 35	PALMER [4]*** BLACK WOMEN LESS THAN 45	MILLER [5]** WOMEN LESS THAN 45	ROSENBERG (6): WOMEN AGED 25-34
YEAR OF INTERVIEW	1990-1992	1977-1992	1983-1986	1977-1992
INTERVAL SINCE FIRST USE OF OCP				
< 10 YEARS				1.6 (1.1-2.3) = 60%
10-14 YEARS	1.63 (1.1-2.5) = 63%			1.8 (1.3-2.6) = 80%
15-19 YEARS	2.02 (1.2-3.4) = 102%	2.6 (1.5-4.6) = 160%		1.9 (1.0-3.5) = 90%*
>= 20 YEARS	3.01 (0.3-34.9) = 201%*	2.0 (1.0-4.3) = 100%*	6.0 (1.6-22) = 500%	

*This result reflects a trend toward an increased or decreased risk but does not attain statistical significance.

**In women who used OCPs for more than 5 years.

***In women who used OCPs for more than 3 years.

Q-A4E: The previous answer implies that OCP use might result in an increased risk of breast cancer 10 to 15 or even 20 years after first use — is this possible?

Yes, it's very possible. No one knows how long the latent period is between early OCP use and breast cancer. It could be anywhere from 5 to 30 years or more. As researcher David Thomas observed: "The Institute of Medicine report notes that studies will have to be continued for the next 20-40 years to assess the long-term effects of prolonged early (OCP) use. . ." [7, p.362].

Q-A4F: If the latent period turns out to be 10 years, does this mean that "the worst is over" regarding the likelihood of early OCP use to cause an increase in breast cancer?

Table A4C:
EXAMPLE OF DES AND A PROPER LATENT PERIOD

TIME SINCE EXPOSURE	RELATIVE RISK
0-9 years	13% increase: RR=1.13 (0.38-3.37)
10-19 years	13% increase: RR=1.13 (0.70-1.81)
20-29 years	36% increase: RR=1.36 (0.93-1.99)
30 or more years	33% increase: RR=1.33 (0.95-1.87)

Absolutely not. One can see from Table A4C that DES showed a 13% statistically insignificant increased risk for causing breast cancer within the first 10 years of use and from the time period of 10 to 19 years after first use. It was only after 20 years, however, that the increase was noted to rise to 36% and DES continued to cause cancer even 30 years after use.

Q-A4G: The Oxford study used data from older studies which were noted to have "watered down" the usefulness of this meta-analysis as regards the category of women who last took OCPs more than 10 years ago. Does the inclusion of older data affect other subgroups as well?

Absolutely. For example, what if one were to ask the question: What is the overall risk of breast cancer in women under the age of 45 who used OCPs before their first pregnancy or in women who had used them in any manner at all?

Obviously, the inclusion of older studies as part of the meta-analysis will have the effect of including many studies that have a relatively short latent period, and thus will fail to pick up the effect of OCPs in that they have a latent period of 10 or 15 years or more. Table A4D gives a specific example in which the results of three different groups of women with imaginary data taken from 1960, 1970, and 1990 are shown.

Table A4D:
AN EXAMPLE OF WHAT HAPPENS
WHEN USING OLDER DATA

YEAR→	1960		1970		1990	
	"Cases"	"Controls"	"Cases"	"Controls"	"Cases"	Controls
Women studied	1000	1000	1000	1000	1000	1000
Took DES?	22	20	22	24	75	50

If one were to calculate the estimated relative risk or odds ratio (OR) of DES exposure based on the data from only the 1990 study one would obtain an OR of 1.5 or a 50% increased risk (75/1000 x 1000/50). But look what happens when one adds in the data from the earlier studies. Because the latent period between DES and the causation of breast cancer is most elevated after 20 years, it is no surprise that the studies from 1960 and 1970 show little effect. Combining the data from all three of the studies we now get a OR of only 1.27: (119/3000 x 3000/94) or a 27% increased risk.

The same principle applies to the OCP/breast cancer issue. For example, if the question were asked: "Does early OCP use prior to a FFTP (first full-term pregnancy) effect the risk of breast cancer?" Data from the studies before 1980 would be unlikely to show much risk because the latent period is too short and because few women used OCPs for significant periods of time prior to their FFTPs in the late 1960s and early 1970s compared to women in the late 1970s and 1980s. Unfortunately, more than 60% of the Oxford study's data comes from women who first started using OCPs before 1970 [1, p.7S] and the median age when women began using OCPs was 26 [1, p.6S] — an age that is certainly higher than the median age of woman who took OCPs in the 1980s and 1990s.

Q-A4H: Could the researchers of the Oxford study have overcome the "older data" effect?

Yes. They could perform a meta-analysis on the studies whose "cases" developed breast cancer after 1985. According to the Oxford study's data [1, Table 1], about 50% of the study's data comes from research which was taken after 1985 — this would be more than enough to yield some credible results.

Q-A4I: Why do some researchers believe that OCP use will cause no long-term risk of breast cancer — only a short-term risk?

Some researchers fail to see the lack of discretion in the Oxford meta-analysis, but most are more cautious and realize that Oxford said nothing about the long-term effects of OCP use prior to a FFTP. Other researchers have theorized that OCPs act like promoters and not initiators, hypothesizing that OCP use basically "increases the speed of development" of tumors that would have shown up eventually anyway. They theorize that long-term OCP use will result in a decrease in the rate of breast cancer as women grow older, because the early OCP use resulted in detection of cancers that would have appeared anyway some time later in a woman's life.

There are, however, some profound problems with this type of reasoning. To begin with, no one is sure exactly how or why OCP use prior to a FFTP results in an increase in breast cancer. Anderson et al [8] have shown that OCP use certainly speeds up the rate of breast cell division in the nulliparous woman (ie, women without children), and cells that are induced to divide more rapidly are certainly more vulnerable to becoming cancerous. Thus, OCP use creates an environment that is ripe for carcinogenesis and may be acting as an initiator, or a factor that facilitates initiation, and/or a promoter. *If this is true, the largest increase in breast cancer from early OCP use may be yet to come, just as occurred with DES.* In addition, it has been noted earlier that OCP use prior to a FFTP has resulted in the development of more aggressive breast cancers, which have a higher percentage of being estrogen and progesterone negative, as well as being associated with a far lower rate of survival [9, 10]. If OCPs were "simple promoters" one would *not expect* them to create a disproportionate number of aggressive breast cancers that are estrogen receptor negative and yet that is exactly what Olsson et al found [11].

The truth is that no one really knows what will happen when the data from OCP use prior to a FFTP comes in, for those women 20 to 25 years after their first OCP use, especially if OCPs were used prior to their FFTP. It should be stressed that for over 25 years researchers claimed that DES caused little risk in breast cancer elevation — must we make the same mistake twice?

Q-A4J: Is there any other reason why the first 10 years after OCP use seem to show an especially high risk?

The answer to this is almost the converse of a previous answer. Just as women who took OCPs more than 10 years ago are likely to belong to a group of women who took them in the 1960s and 1970s for short periods of time, women who used OCPs within the last 10 years are more likely to have been those women who used them in the late 1970s and 1980s — a time in which they would have been more likely to use them for longer periods of time and at earlier times in their lives (thus, more likely to have used them before their FFTP). It is no surprise that this combination (ie, early and long OCP use) would cause an increased risk of breast cancer that researchers have identified.

Q-A4K: What should doctors be telling their patients regarding the long-term risks of OCP use in young women (under the age of 35)?

At this point doctors need to inform their patients that the studies which looked at the risk of OCP use even after almost 20 years since first use, found statistically significant risk increases of *over 90%*.

Q-A4L: Did the researchers who coordinated the Oxford study examine the effect of oral contraceptive use prior to a FFTP?

The Oxford study contains 80 appendices which contain some of the most detailed data presented on the subject of OCPs and breast cancer in an elaborate display of charts and tables for variously selected subgroups. However, in spite of this, *the authors failed to include a single table or chart concerning the risk of oral contraceptives before a premenopausal woman's first full-term pregnancy*

(FFTP)! This is a truly stunning omission, because millions of young women are now using OCPs prior to their FFTP and are doing so for far longer periods of time than they did in the 1960 and 1970s.

Figure 5 in the *Lancet* reference [2] does list the risk of OCP use in parous women who took them prior to FFTP, but failed to limit itself to premenopausal women and also included data from studies which took their data prior to 1980, thus including those with an inadequate latent period. However, a number of tables do show data on women who took OCPs prior to the age of 20, but this is no substitute for the question of risk of OCP use prior to a FFTP — (see Appendices 33 35, 36, 41, 44, 46, 49, 52, and 63 in source [1]). Another table (ie, appendix 34) did look at women who took OCPs within 5 years of menarche, but, unfortunately, few had a latent period of more than 10 years since last use of OCPs (ie, a total of 326 "cases" from the entire meta-analysis). Also, as has been noted earlier, the women who took OCPs within 5 years of menarche and took them at least 10 years ago, often were those who took OCPs in the 1960s, and thus had far shorter lengths of OCP use than do today's women. The authors do give one statistic that is pertinent. In Appendix 28 of their paper they noted that women who took OCPs on or before the age of 17 and had used them for the last time at least 15 years ago, had a 1.24 (0.96-1.52) increased risk.

In summary, it is difficult to imagine why the authors of the Oxford study failed to include data on the risk of OCP use before a FFTP because that is the group that is at most risk today, given today's pattern of OCP use in young women. In addition, had the authors done so, the results would surely have been significant if they limited themselves to studies which took their data after 1985 (see Table 9B, Chapter 9).

Q-A4M: Did the Oxford study measure the effect of long-term OCP use before a FFTP?

One of the biggest problems with the Oxford study is that it failed to ask the question of what the risk of OCP use was prior to a FFTP. Another major weakness is that *the study failed to ask the question of what the risk of long-term OCP use (eg, greater than 4 years) before a FFTP was.* This is especially important because today's women are using OCPs for far longer periods of time than women did in the 1960s and early 1970s. The failure to address this question is a gross inadequacy. Hopefully, some researchers will have the courage to ask the question: What is the risk of breast cancer to women under the age of 45 who used OCPs for 4 or more years prior to their FFTP, when confined to the studies that obtained their data after 1985?

Q-A4N: The researchers of the Oxford study performed their meta-analysis by using the "99% confidence limits" — was this fair?

The writers of the Oxford study chose to analyze their data by subjecting it to a 99% probability of statistical certainty. Almost all of the medical studies upon which the Oxford study draws its information required only a 95% confidence interval. Why did the authors increase it to 99%? The authors wrote: "Due to the large number of estimates involved, 99% confidence limits are used." In effect, by increasing the confidence limits to 99%, they made it less likely that trends of increased risk due to OCP use would be registered as "statistically significant." Thus, many of the tables that would have shown results that were statistically significant at the 95% confidence level, now fail to do so at the 99% level. The trained researcher would realize this — *the lay person might not.*

Q-A4O: Does the Oxford study suffer from the death factor?

Yes. It should be noted again that because the Oxford study is an accumulation and summary of many other studies — many of which have a significant death effect — it too suffers from the death effect.

As noted in Chapter 5, the death effect occurs when a small percentage of the women who have been diagnosed with breast cancer cannot be interviewed because they have become too sick or have died before the interview process begins. If early OCP use and having an induced abortion at a young age truly lead to more aggressive cancer as Olsson indicated [11], then the death factor would result in an underestimate of the risk of early OCP use and/or abortion, because women who die early from their aggressive breast cancer will not live long enough to be interviewed, thereby decreasing the study's relative risks of OCP/abortion.

Q-A4P: The authors of the Oxford study make the statement that: ". . .cancers diagnosed in ever users tend to be less advanced clinically than the cancers diagnosed in never users." Is this a misleading statement?

It can be, depending on the reader's familiarity with the subject. Why? The authors of the Oxford study present their data in bar graph form [1, p.19S]. Data from the first graph show that women who took OCPs have a higher rate of local breast cancer (ie, breast cancer that is confined to the breast at presentation) than do women who did not use OCPs. The next graph notes that women who took OCPs have a statistically insignificant increase in distal breast cancer if the cancer was diagnosed within 4 years of last OCP use, and a statistically insignificant decrease in distal breast cancer cases (as compared to never users) if they used OCPs more than 4 years ago. Thus, although the authors' statement contains a partial truth — namely, that distal disease is decreased in women who took OCPs more than 4 years ago as compared to women who did not take OCPs, they fail to stress or mention two key pieces of information, namely:

1) As mentioned, distal breast cancer disease is increased in women who used OCPs within the last 4 years [1, p.82S];

2) *The authors mention little* about the risk of *early OCP use* in their discussion whereas their table notes that there was a statistically significant increase in both local and distal breast cancer in women who had used OCPs within the last 5 years and before the age of 20 [1, p.83S].

This is "a little less than fair," because Olsson et al [11] have clearly noted that women who use OCPs *at an early age* (ie, before the age of 20) are at especially high risk of developing more aggressive cancers and have a far poorer survival rate. "A high proliferation rate, a large proportion DNA aneuploidy, and amplification of the proto-oncogene HER-2/neu appeared to be related to OCPs when used during adolescence but not to OCP usage at higher ages." [12, p.705C]. It has been noted previously that women today are using OCPs far more often prior to their FFTP than in the 1960s and 1970s — hence, today's women are at high risk for developing aggressive breast cancer, yet the Oxford study completely fails to comment on this subset of women. Would the reader consider this misleading?

Q-A4Q: Are there any problems with the way the Oxford researchers presented the data on women who took the all progestin "minipill" or on those women who were injected with long acting progestins?

Yes, there certainly are problems which are similar in type to those discussed regarding the Oxford study's treatment of OCP use, for example the "mixing of the older data effect." The data which is presented does not look at *early* use of progestins for longer time periods, thus many of the women ended up taking the oral or injectable progestins *after* their FFTP — a time in which they would theoretically be at less risk for breast cancer formation. The Oxford authors also presented data in a table which showed that women who took oral progestins more than 15 years ago had no overall increased risk — this result means little because the reader has no idea if this group of women took the oral progestins before a FFTP and how long they took them. Chapter 12 addressed the studies on injectable progestins and showed that they were noted to be even more dangerous than OCPs when taken for prolonged times at an early age [13].

Q-A4R: If the Oxford researchers perform a "re-analysis" of their data, or a future meta-analysis, are there any specific data/results that should be presented?

One would hope that a future analysis would certainly address the question of OCP use before a FFTP and limit its participants to women the age of 45 or under — as of the year 1995 — with corresponding adjustments as time goes by (ie, limit to the age of 50 and under by the year 2000, 55 by the year 2005, etc.). It would also be hoped that *studies whose data come from after 1985* be used. Any future analysis should also specifically measure the effect of OCP use in parous women who took OCPs prior to their FFTP because this is the cohort that most young women under the age of 45 are likely to be in.

Q-A4S: Would any other parameters be useful in their presentation of the data/results?

Yes, it would be good to see the corresponding risk of OCP use in women who had used them for various lengths of time prior to their FFTP. It would also be useful to measure the risks at different latent periods, such as 10, 15, 20, 25, and 30 years after "first use of OCPs prior to a FFTP," as Colton did in his DES analysis [14]. Last, in order to overcome the stack effect, it would be hoped that the authors would present the risk data for specific age groups (ie, 25-29, 30-34,. . .) as well as the more general "under the age of 45 or under the age of 50" category.

Q-A4T: The writers of the Oxford study published several tables which noted the cumulative number of projected new "cases" of breast cancer. For example, they estimated that for every 10,000 women who used OCPs between the ages of 25 and 29, a total of about 4 new cases of breast cancer will be found before the age of 50, for an increased rate of only 0.04% [1, p.24S]. Is this an accurate estimate?

No. First, it must be remembered that it is an estimate — no one really knows how dangerous the long-term effect of early OCP use will be 20 years after having taken them. It must be remembered that the researchers are making their projections based on the results of their data — *data which fail to selectively study the effect of OCP use prior to a FFTP in women under the age of 45.* If we study women who have taken OCPs for prolonged periods of time before their FFTP, the estimates would be far different. As Chapter 13 noted, over 97,000 women would be expected to get breast cancer from the use of early extended OCP use if the risk used by Romieu (ie, 72% increased risk for 4 or more years of OCP use prior to a FFTP [RR=1.72 (1.36-2.19)]) continues to apply as women grow older. This is an extremely conservative risk, because women who have used OCPs who are nulliparous, or those who used them for less than 4 years prior to a FFTP, or those who used them after the age of 25, have not been factored in. As breast cancer rates continue to increase around the world, must the research world continue to deny that the noted "new risk factors" play a significant role?

References:

1. Collaborative Group on Hormonal Factors in Breast Cancer. Breast cancer and hormonal contraceptives: further results. *Contraception.* 1996; 34: S1-S106.

2. Collaborative Group on Hormonal Factors in Breast Cancer. Breast cancer and hormonal contraceptives: collaborative reanalysis of individual data on 53,297 women with breast cancer and 100,239 women without breast cancer from 54 epidemiological studies. *The Lancet.* 1996; 347: 1713-1727.

3. Brinton LA, Daling JR, et al. Oral contraceptives and breast cancer risk among younger women. *J Natl Cancer Inst.* 6/7/1995; 87: 827-835.

4. Palmer J, Rosenberg L, et al. Oral contraceptives use and breast cancer risk among African-American women. *Cancer Causes and Control.* 1995; 6: 321-331.

5. Miller D, Rosenberg L, et al. Breast cancer before age 45 and oral contraceptive use: new findings. *Am J Epidemiol.* 1989; 129: 269-279.

6. Rosenberg L, Palmer JR, et al. Case-control study of oral contraceptive use and risk of breast cancer. *Am J Epidemiol.* 1996; 143: 25-37.

7. Thomas DB. Oral contraceptives and breast cancer. *J Natl Cancer Inst.* 1993; 85: 359-364.

8. Anderson TJ, Battersby S, et al. Oral contraceptive use influences resting breast proliferation. *Hum Pathol.* 1989; 20: 1139-1144.

9. Ranstam J, Olsson H, et al. Survival in breast cancer and age at start of oral contraceptive usage. *AntiCancer Research.* 1991; 11: 2043-2046.

10. Olsson H, Ranstam J, et al. Proliferation and DNA ploidy in malignant breast tumors in relation to early contraceptive use and early abortions. *Cancer.* 1991; 67: 1285-1290.

11. Olsson H, Borg A, et al. Early oral contraceptive use and premenopausal breast cancer-A review of studies performed in southern Sweden. *Cancer Detection and Prevention*. 1991; 15: 265-271.
12. Ranstam J, et al. Oral contraceptives and breast cancer. *Dissertation Abstracts International*. 1992; 53: 705C.
13. Skegg DCG, Noonan EA, et al. Depot medroxyprogesterone acetate and breast cancer [A pooled analysis of the World Health Organization and New Zealand studies]. *JAMA*. 1995: 799-804.
14. Colton T, Greenberg ER, et al. Breast cancer in mothers prescribed diethylstilbestrol in pregnancy. *JAMA*. 1993; 269: 2096-3000.

Appendix 5:
How Do the Pill and Other Contraceptives Work?

<u>Part A</u>

The oral contraceptive pill, also known as the birth control pill, is currently being used by over 10 million women in the U.S. [1]. A number of physicians and researchers have noted that the oral contraceptive pill (OCP) is actually an abortifacient (ie, an agent that causes an early abortion; specifically, any agent that causes death of the zygote, embryo, or fetus after conception has occurred). Others have stated that they do not believe the OCP is an abortifacient as noted in the recent publication (1998), written by several physicians entitled: *Hormonal Contraceptives: Are they Abortifacients?* [2]

The ethical question of whether contraception is morally permissible has varied between the Catholic Church and the Protestant churches. Both agreed on the "sin of contraception" before 1930 [3], whereas both differ in general on the issue today. This appendix will focus on the medical and technical aspects concerning the cited questions regarding the pill's abortifacient qualities.

In order to answer the question of whether the OCP causes early abortions, a number of basic questions need to be answered such as:

Q-A5A: What is an oral contraceptive pill (OCP) and how does it work?

Normally, as shown in diagram A, the pituitary gland produces two hormones called FSH (Follicle Stimulating

Hormone) and LH (Luteinizing Hormone). These hormones serve to stimulate the ovary to produce an egg each month (ie, to ovulate). The ovary is the site of production of the woman's two central female hormones, *estradiol* (EST), a type of estrogen, and *progesterone* (PRO), a type of progestin. Oral contraceptive pills (OCPs) are a combination of *synthetic* estrogen and progestin. Oral contraceptives "fool" the pituitary gland so that it produces less follicle stimulating hormone and luteinizing hormone. These two hormones are needed for ovulation to occur, therefore, OCPs suppress, *but do not eliminate* ovulation.

Diagram A:

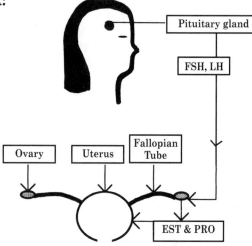

Oral contraceptives have two other main effects:

1) They thin the inner lining of the uterus (called the endometrium), depleting it of glycogen (ie, a type of sugar), and decreasing its thickness. A thinner endometrium has a decreased blood supply.

2) They may thicken the cervical mucus, making it more difficult for the sperm to travel up through the cervix. The evidence for this is weak [4,5] and not strongly supported by the rabbit model [6].

Of course, OCP use could not cause abortions if it always stopped ovulation so this needs to be the first issue that is raised. A clear proof of the occurrence of ovulation is provided by noting what the drug companies which manufacture OCPs state. If one opens up the *PDR* (*Physician's Desk Reference, ©1998*) one will find a table describing the "efficacy rate" of the OCP. In every table listed under each OCP one notes a "typical failure rate" of 3%. The *PDR* defines this as the rate of annual pregnancy occurrence noted in "typical couples who initiate use of a method (not necessarily for the first time) and who use it consistently and correctly during the first year if they do not stop for any other reason." This means that even couples who used the pill consistently over the course of a year had a pregnancy rate of 3%. A 1996 paper by Potter [7] gave an excellent overview of the matter. She noted that the most recent data point to a rate of pregnancy for "typical use" as being 7%, which is probably the more accurate statistic given the immediacy of her research and the fact that today's OCPs are lower dose ones, theoretically permitting a higher rate of breakthrough ovulation. From these estimates of OCP failure and the common experience of on-pill pregnancies, it is clear that both ovulation and conception occur in couples who use OCPs.

Q-A5B: Could you present the evidence that some physicians and researchers give to support their claim that the OCP indeed acts as an abortifacient?

Before presenting the evidence, the normal anatomy and *histology* (ie, the study of the body's tissues on a microscopic level) of the inner lining of the uterus, (ie, the *endometrium*) need to be explained (see Diagram B).

Diagram B:

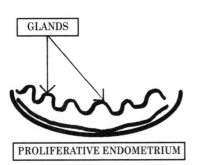

PROLIFERATIVE ENDOMETRIUM

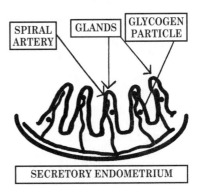

SECRETORY ENDOMETRIUM

The endometrium slowly gets built up *before ovulation* (the *proliferative phase*) and then reaches its peak in the *secretory phase* (shortly after ovulation [and conception if it has occurred]). The endometrium is *"ready for the newly conceived child to implant"* when it reaches its peak in the secretory phase a few days after ovulation. The blood flow, specifically the oxygen and nutrients to the glandular cells of the endometrium, increases through the cycle as the *spiral arteries* enlarge during the secretory phase. The size of the *endometrial glands* also enlarge in the secretory phase. The glands contain important nutritional building blocks for the unborn child who is about to implant, including *glycogen* (a type of sugar), mucopolysaccharides (building blocks for a cell's growth), and lipids (fats) [8].

Q-A5C: What does the phrase "ready for implantation" mean?

The author of a histology text designed for medical students noted: "Thus, the various changes that take place in the endometrium during the second half of the menstrual cycle may be regarded as preparing the uterine lining for the nourishment and reception of the fertilized ovum (blastocyst)" [8]. It would appear that God perfectly designed a woman's body and the lining of her uterus to be "optimal for implantation" a few days after ovulation and conception have occurred.

Q-A5D: Does OCP use cause changes in the lining of the uterus that could be detrimental to the newly conceived child's ability to implant himself or herself?

It would appear so. Because we know that use of the oral contraceptive pill (OCP) allows ovulation and conception to occur at times, if OCP use causes unfavorable changes in the endometrium it would make it difficult for the unborn child to implant, and would support the conclusion that it acts as an abortifacient.

Q-A5E: What are some of those changes?

The first change that use of the OCP makes is to *markedly decrease the thickness of a woman's endometrial lin-*

ing. Women who take OCPs know this because *they can tell you* that the volume of menstrual contents lost in their monthly cycles significantly decreases once they start taking OCPs. *Obviously if a woman is losing less menstrual contents each month, the layer of endometrium that is being shed must be thinner and less well developed.*

Q-A5F: Is there a technical or quantitative way to measure how much thinner a woman's endometrium becomes when she uses OCPs?

Yes, in 1991 researchers in the U.S. performed MRI scans (Magnetic Resonance Imaging) on the uteri of women, some of whom were taking OCPs and some of whom were not [9]. The OCP users had endometrial linings that were almost 2 millimeters thinner than that of the nonusers. Although this may sound like a small difference, it represented a 57% reduction in the thickness of the endometrial lining in women who used OCPs in this study.

Q-A5G: But is there really any evidence that a thinner endometrium makes it more difficult for implantation to occur?

Yes. A number of different research papers have studied this issue and it has been widely described in the medical literature concerning in vitro fertilization where it has been noted that the newly conceived child is much less likely to implant on a thinner uterine lining than a thicker one. Originally an older smaller study (Fleisher et al [10], 1985) did not find that the thickness of the endometrium played an important role in in vitro implantation rates, however, other studies have found a positive trend (Rabinowitz et al, 1986 [11]; Ueno et al, 1991 [12]) or a statistically significant effect (Glissant et al, 1985 [13]) of the decreasing thickness of the endometrium in relationship to a decreased likelihood of implantation. Larger and more recent studies (Abdalla et al, 1984 [14]; Dickey et al, 1993 [15]; Gonen et al, 1989 [16]; Schwartz et al, 1997 [17]; Shoham et al, 1991 [18]) have reaffirmed this important connection. Most studies have found that a decrease of even 1 millimeter in thickness yields a substantial decrease in the rate of implantation. In two studies, when the endometrial lining became too thin, no implantations occurred (Abdalla [14]; Dickey [15]).

Q-A5H: What happens to the actual endometrial lining in women who take OCPs when one looks at it under a microscope?

As we saw in Diagram B, the uterine lining is at an "optimal state for implantation" when the glands and uterine arteries are at their maximal size. This makes intuitive sense because at this point the blood supply and glycogen and lipid levels that the tiny unborn child needs to survive are at their maximal state. It has already been stated that it becomes significantly thinner but what does it look like on the microscopic level?

Researchers who study the histology of the endometrium find that OCP use causes a number of effects. First, *the spiral arteries regress significantly,* becoming much smaller and even difficult to find when one looks under a microscope [19-22]. This of course is important, because an adequate blood supply is critical to the existence of the implanting unborn child. A loss of blood flow means a drastic curtailment in the food and oxygen supply that the child needs to survive. The blood flow to the endometrium is so important that in 1996 one researcher wrote directly about it as concerns its relationship to an unborn child's likelihood of implantation [23]. She first discovered that the blood flow through the spiral arteries peaks at day 16 to 18 of the menstrual cycle and then noted that: "It seems that endometrial perfusion presents more accurate noninvasive assay of uterine receptivity than uterine artery perfusion alone. Therefore, *blood flow velocity waveform changes of spiral arteries may be used to predict implantation success rate* to reveal unexplained infertility problems and to select patients for correction of endometrial perfusion abnormalities. . ." [23] (emphasis added). In layman's language, Kupesic is stating that the efficacy of implantation correlates with the blood flow through the spiral arteries.

Q-A5I: Are there any other changes on the microscopic level in addition to the reduced blood supply from the spiral arteries?

Yes, the second prominent effect is that *the endometrial glands become much smaller* and the "mitotic rate" (rate of cell division) of the cells of the glands decreases [19-22]. Obviously, if the glands which supply the glycogen (sugar), mucopolysaccharides, or lipids (fats) are compromised, the preborn child who needs those nutrients will have a more difficult time implanting and/or surviving.

Q-A5J: Many of the studies that examined the endometrial lining are older and were performed when OCPs contained a much higher level of estrogen content (100 micrograms or more). Would the same effect be occurring with more recent OCPs?

Yes. First it should be mentioned that if you ask a woman who is taking lower dose OCPs about the amount of monthly menstrual contents that she loses, she will note that she loses significantly less after she starts taking the OCP. Obviously, if she is losing less menstrual contents then she is shedding less each month because the lining of the uterus has become thinner. But what about at the histologic level? Even studies which looked at OCPs that contained 50 micrograms of estrogen (a medium dose) and 0.5 mg of a progestin (eg, norgestrel) found that the spiral arteries and the endometrial glands "shrivel up." [20,21].

Q-A5K: Some researchers [24] have argued that if a breakthrough cycle does occur while a woman is taking OCPs, her endometrial lining would become similar to that of the non-OCP user for that cycle. Is this an accurate statement?

To the best of this author's knowledge, that statement has no support in the literature. If the above statement were true, it would mean that each time a woman had a breakthrough cycle while taking the OCP (if she does not become pregnant), she should experience as heavy a cycle as if she were not taking OCPs. This phenomenon has not been described in the medical literature either.

Q-A5L: Is there any other new evidence that supports the argument that OCPs act by causing an early abortion?

Yes. In 1996 a researcher names Stephen Somkuti published an article concerning the endometrium and a group of molecules called "integrins." [25] *Integrins* are a group of adhesion molecules that have been implicated as playing an important role in the area of fertilization and implantation. There are different types of integrins and it is believed that the endometrium is most receptive to implantation when it expresses certain types of integrins. Oral contraceptive pills change the type of integrins that the endometrial lining produces theoretically making it more difficult for the unborn child to implant. In the words of Dr. Somkuti: "These alterations in epithelial and stromal integrin expression suggest that impaired uterine receptivity is one mechanism whereby OCs exert their contraceptive action." [25]

Q-A5M: Has anyone proven that OCP use causes early abortions?

In order to prove if and how often women are having abortions while taking OCPs one needs to be able to measure how often women become pregnant while taking them. But early pregnancy tests are currently not accurate enough to confirm pregnancy within the first week (although some researchers have been able to detect the hormonal changes in pregnancy as early as 4 days after conception [26,27]). Until a very early test is developed that can detect pregnancy in women in spite of being on OCPs, or until researchers physically measure how many abortions are occurring in women who take OCPs, one cannot state with absolute certainty how often OCPs cause early abortions. New ultrasound technology, which is capable of detecting ovulation, may give new insights in the future (see answer to question O). As of today, the most accurate description of the current evidence is as follows:

All of the evidence on a microscopic, a macroscopic and an immunological level strongly support the argument that OCP use causes an early abortion at times. Until further studies are done, we should take heed and act upon the current data.

Q-A5N: Recently a group of physicians, many of whom are experienced Ob/Gyns, wrote a booklet entitled: Hormonal Contraceptives: Are They Abortifacients? **[2] In it they wrote: "The 'hormonal contraception is abortifacient' theory is not established scientific fact. It is speculation. . ." Could you comment on why a group of physicians would hold this view and on the nature of their arguments?**

An overview and rebuttal to the arguments cited in the booklet entitled *"Hormonal Contraceptives: Are They Abortifacients?"* is found in the Addendum to this appendix. This author believes that some of their own arguments can be shown to actually support the argument that OCP use is abortifacient.

Part B: Questions Regarding other Contraceptives

Q-A5O: How frequently does OCP use cause an early abortion?

At this point, no one knows. There are many factors which influence the answer to this question and it is possible that as technology improves, an accurate estimate will be made. One of the determining factors is how often OCP use allows ovulation to occur. If the rate of ovulation is documented to be substantially higher than the pregnancy rate, then one could start to make an estimate of the frequency of abortion in women who take the OCP.

Measuring a woman's ability to ovulate is difficult. Researchers measure ovulation rates in women who are taking the pill by using several parameters including:

1) Ultrasound measurements of the ovary, specifically the size of the largest (dominant) follicle (which contains the egg or oocyte), and 2) hormonal assays of progesterone and estradiol levels. Until now, many researchers have arbitrarily accepted that a pregnancy has occurred when the

progesterone levels reaches a certain height, but it is possible that OCP use depresses the ovary's ability to produce progesterone despite pregnancy as noted as early as 1962 by Holmes et al [28]. It would seem more accurate to measure ovulation rates based on daily pelvic or vaginal ultrasound exams. In 1985, Ritchie [29] wrote in his review of the role of ultrasound in the evaluation of normal and induced ovulation that: "With daily scanning, ovulation can be demonstrated in >80% of cases." This statistic can only improve as technology moves forward.

There are a number of other reasons why determining the frequency of ovulation by such a method is important. First, studies of women who take OCPs often show a high rate of "ovarian activity" in their dominant follicles which may reach a size that is consistent with those seen in non-OCP users who ovulate. In other words, the ultrasound measurements indicate that these women (ie, the OCP users) are about to ovulate. But these same studies often conclude that ovulation has not occurred because the progesterone level has not reached a critical level [eg, 30, 31]. This is somewhat counter-intuitive in light of a recent study [31] that found: "Patients using the lower-dose monophasic and multiphasic pills had follicular activity similar to that of those using nonsteroidal contraception, with the important exception that ovulation rarely occurred." This study, as almost all others, used the criteria that ovulation is confirmed when progesterone levels reach a certain level. This may not be accurate.

High-tech ultrasound may reveal that ovulation rates are higher than today's commonly quoted rates of 3 to 5% [29]. The two reasons for this are that today's OCPs contain far less estrogen and progestin than the early OCPs did and therefore suppress ovarian activity less often. Second, many studies have examined the rate of breakthrough ovulation *in women who have recently started taking OCPs* but the question that must be asked is: "Does the rate of ovulation go up in women who have taken OCPs for more than a year?" This phenomenon occurs with

Norplant, where it was noted that the breakthrough ovulation rate in the first year was only 11%, but increased dramatically after that year, so that a 7-year average yielded an annual breakthrough ovulation rate of 44% [32] (although part of the reason for this increase may have been declining Norplant hormone levels over time). But could a woman's pituitary gland "compensate" or "reset itself" to adjust for the presence of the hormones in the OCP so that ovulation occurs more frequently with time? If so, future trials may show that the rate of breakthrough ovulation increases in women who take the low dose OCP for longer periods of time.

It seems likely that a study will be done in the future that measures the rate of ovulation based on serial ultrasounds (although some may claim that such a study might be unethical, it might be possible to avoid the ethical questions by studying women who are taking OCPs but are not sexually active). If such a study is performed in women who have been taking *low dose* OCPs *for longer than a year*, it could yield information that leads to a more credible estimate of the abortion rate for women taking OCPs.

Q-A5P: Does use of the intrauterine device (IUD) cause abortion?

Yes, use of the IUD does not prevent ovulation [33] and works by changing the inner lining of a woman's uterus so that the newly conceived child cannot implant in the womb.

Q-A5Q: Do groups who favor abortion admit that OCPs and the IUD work by causing early abortions?

The abortifacient nature of OCP and IUD use is openly admitted by the most ardent pro-abortion supporters. In his arguments before the Supreme Court in 1989, in a case that received worldwide publicity — the case of Webster versus Reproductive Health Services — Mr. Frank Susman, arguing for the pro-abortion side spoke to Justice Anthony Scalia and stated: "If I may suggest the reasons in response to your question, Justice Scalia. The most common forms of what we generally in common parlance call contraception today, IUD's, and low-dose birth control pills, which are the safest type of birth control pills available, act as abortifacients. They are correctly labeled as both." (*The New York Times, 1989*: [34])

Q-A5R: Does use of other hormonal contraceptives such as the long acting progestins cause early abortions?

Norplant, manufactured by Wyeth-Ayerst, and Depo-Provera, made by Pharmacia-Upjohn, are made of artificial *progestins*. Norplant is composed of *levonorgestrel* and Depo-Provera of *medroxyprogesterone*. Depo-Provera is a long-acting progestin that is injected every 3 months intramuscularly — it is used worldwide despite the fact that studies have shown that it increases the risk of breast cancer by at least 190% in women who take it for more than 2 years before the age of 25! [35] Norplant is an artificial progestin that consists of a series of Silastic (ie, rubber-like) strips which are filled with levonorgestrel and are implanted under the skin of a woman's upper arm, slowly releasing the progestin into the woman's body over a 5-year time period.

Use of Norplant has been noted to allow breakthrough ovulation in over 44% of a woman's monthly cycles [32]. In addition, a study in rabbits conducted by a researcher named Chang [6] has shown that sperm freely reached the rabbits' fallopian tubes — even when the rabbits were given high doses of synthetic progestin. The combination of a high rate of breakthrough ovulation and documented sperm migration to the fallopian tubes (in animals) implies that use of progestins such as Norplant and Depo-Provera allow a high rate of abortion — most likely, higher than the rate with OCP use.

Q-A5S: Does use of "the morning after pill" cause an early abortion?

The "morning after pill" consists of a series of high dose OCPs which some women have taken 1 or 2 days after thinking that they have conceived. These high dose hormones act as abortifacients at times by unfavorably altering the lining of the uterus, thus preventing the newly conceived child from implanting. The animal model described by Castro-Vazquez in 1971 demonstrated this effect in rats [36]. In addition, the *Medical Letter* stated that some studies suggest — and some do not — that Preven (the emergency contraceptive hormone kit) may work at times by interfering with implantation. [37]

Q-A5T: Some emergency rooms give "hormones" to women who have recently been raped. Can use of these cause an early abortion?

Yes. The woman who has been raped within a few hours of going to the emergency room, may or may not have already conceived. Some emergency rooms will give such a woman high dose estrogen and progestin hormones very similar to the "morning after pill" (the exception is often found in Catholic hospitals whose physicians are not supposed to give the "post-rape pill"). Even if the woman is near the time of ovulation, the hormones do not consistently stop ovulation. Therefore, informed practicing Christian physicians will not give the "post-rape pill" in any circumstances.

Q-A5U: Does artificial fertilization cause early abortion(s).

Every method of artificial fertilization that this author is aware of, whether it be in vitro fertilization, or ZIFT (zygote intrafallopian transfer) or GIFT (Gamete intrafallopian transfer) involves the death of many unborn children during the process. Fewer than 1 out of 20 conceived children "survive" the process of in vitro fertilization. Even GIFT involves the exposure of more than one egg to multiple sperm — a situation in which multiple early abortions are extremely likely to occur. In addition to these methods, it is possible that women who take fertility pills such as Clomid® (which work by causing the ovaries to "super-ovulate") may be experiencing early abortion(s) because some studies [38-41], but not all [15], indicate that this drug thins the lining of the uterus, theoretically making it more difficult for the conceived child(ren) to implant.

Q-A5V: Can the estrogens that women take "after menopause" cause an early abortion?

Often women are started on estrogen replacement near the time of menopause. This usually has a beneficial effect of reducing the risk of osteoporosis while increasing the risk of uterine and breast cancer. Unfortunately, many women are now starting estrogen replacement before they have completely stopped their cycles — that is, they are not always in true menopause, but are still having occasional cycles. If a woman were to start estrogen at a time in which she were still having an occasional cycle, she could still conceive and have an early abortion. This is something to be aware of and women who wish to avoid this effect should not start hormonal replacement therapy until they have not had a cycle for a 1-year period.

Q-A5W: Why was the term "contraceptive" placed in quotations when referring to the various artificial hormones?

Oral contraceptives, Norplant, Depo-Provera, the IUD, the "morning after pill," the "post-rape pill," all work by causing an early abortion at least part of the time. The word "contraceptive" was consistently placed in quotations because all of the evidence points to these hormones or procedures as being abortifacient — that is, their use causes an early abortion either some or part of the time. Contraception technically means "to prevent conception" — clearly use of the hormones which were alluded to cause the deaths of unborn children after conception and cannot accurately be solely called "contraceptive."

Addendum: Response to the arguments put forth in the brochure entitled: *Hormonal Contraceptives: Are they Abortifacients?*

Introduction: In January, 1998, a group of 22 physicians (almost all are Ob/Gyns) wrote a collaborative report addressing the question of the abortifacient nature of the oral contraceptive pill (OCP) [2]. Their three main arguments (found on page 7 in their booklet) are presented here, with a corresponding rebuttal to each by Dr. Kahlenborn:

1: *They write:* "We know of no existing scientific studies that validate the 'hormonal contraception is partly abortifacient' theory. 'On-pill' pregnancy rates roughly parallel 'on-pill' ovulation rates (about 3-5% on 35 mcg pill). Increased spontaneous abortion of "on-pill" pregnancies is not noted."

Response: (Here, the term "pregnancy rate" refers to the rate of pregnancy as confirmed by a positive pregnancy test, while acknowledging that a woman is actually pregnant before one can measure it [ie, directly after conception]).

The claim that "on-pill" pregnancy rates roughly parallel "on-pill" ovulation rates may appear to be a satisfying argument, but on closer examination this contention actually bolsters the argument in favor of the OCP acting as an abortifacient. Why?

If a woman is taking the OCP she will experience an artificially regulated cycle that lasts 28 days, so she will have about 13 cycles per year (365 days divided by 28). Thus a group of 100 women would be expected to have a total of 1300 cycles per year. If women taking the OCP experience a breakthrough ovulation rate (ie, "on-pill" ovulation rate) of between 3% to 5%, a group of 100 women would be expected to have between 39 to 65 breakthrough cycles in one year (1300 x 3% - 5%). *William's Obstetrics* notes that the average woman has a "natural fecundibility rate" of 28 percent.[33] ("Natural Fecundiblity rate," perhaps more accurately called the *fertility rate*, is defined in this section of *William's Obstetrics* as *liveborn infants per ovarian cycle*).

But *William's Obstetrics* also notes that for every 600 live-born children, 279 embryos or fetuses are miscarried, 176 of them after a positive pregnancy test and 103 of them prior to being able to detect that a woman is pregnant. This means that the average couple will actually have a detectable pregnancy rate of: 28% + (176/600 x 28%) = 36.2%.* So a group of 100 woman who are sexually active and using the oral contraceptive pill, might expect between 14 and 24 detectable pregnancies per year: (ie from 36.2% x 39 to 36.2% x 65). But the *PDR* (*Physician's Desk Reference*) notes that a group of 100 women who are using OCPs in a consistent manner will have about 3 pregnancies per year [42] and a 1996 study by Potter [7] yielded an updated statistic of 7 pregnancies per year. In other words, if the *condition* that "on-pill" pregnancy rates roughly parallel "on-pill" ovulation rates *is true*, then *the conclusion* that the *OCP does not act as an abortifacient is highly suspect.* This is because if the ovulation rate is 3% to 5%, we might expect the pregnancy rate to be 14% to 24% — that is, far higher than the ovulation rate. Because we do not see this clinically, we must ask*: why is the clinically measurable pregnancy rate far lower than the theoretical rate based on the rate of breakthrough ovulation?* A number of explanations exist including the failure of sperm to reach the egg due to thicker cervical mucus or a change in motility within the fallopian tubes which OCP use may cause. But one must also recognize that the difference in rates may be due to a failure of the zygote/embryo to implant due to effects of OCP use on the endometrial lining. In short, the observation that "on-pill" pregnancy rates roughly parallel "on-pill" ovulation rates, serves, if anything, to give evidence in favor of the argument that the OCP acts as an abortifacient.

*The *total pregnancy rate* (detectable and non-detectable pregnancies) would be the total number of pregnancies per cycle in the average woman: 28% + (279/600 x 28%) = 41.0%.

2: *They write:* "There is regular successful implantation of the invasive blastocyst on surfaces a great deal more 'hostile' than 'hostile endometrium' (eg, fallopian tube lining). 'Hostile endometrium' is not a demonstrated clinical reality."

Response: It has already been stated in the answers to questions B-K that the sum of the evidence — both recent and old — supports the argument that OCPs change the lining of the endometrium in a fashion unfavorable for implantation. The fact that the unborn child may attach him or herself to a structure such as the fallopian tube lining has little to do with the previous arguments. Although one can make the argument that a rare occurrence or an exception disproves a theory, one cannot deduce the converse, namely, that the exception proves the theory. That is, noting that some unborn children do implant in the fallopian tube, or for that matter in the peritoneal cavity, merely *proves that it is possible for this event to occur.* But *it offers no evidence* that justifies the claim that a favorable implantation site *is just as good as* an unfavorable one.

3: *They write:* "The extremely rare reporting of ectopic pregnancies associated with hormonal contraception would indicate the rarity of actual conception by patients using these modalities."

Response: Once again these physicians apparently were unaware that their statement *serves the purpose of supporting the action of OCPs as abortifacient.* Women who take OCPs and those who do not, can and do become pregnant. The pregnancy can be an extrauterine pregnancy (EUP) (ie, usually a tubal pregnancy) or an intrauterine pregnancy (IUP) (ie, the normal type of pregnancy). One can measure the ratio of EUP to IUP in either group. What should happen to this ratio (ie, EUP/IUP) if one compares women who are not taking OCPs to those who are?

The Ob/Gyns would argue that this *ratio should remain* constant and if the reporting of ectopic pregnancy was *"practically unreported,"* as the Ob/Gyns wrote, one might even expect *the ratio to decrease,* because the numerator would become smaller. On the contrary, if OCP use caused more early abortions (ie, less intrauterine pregnancies), one would expect the number of intrauterine pregnancies (IUPs) to decrease in comparison to the number of extrauterine pregnancies (EUPs) and thus the *ratio should increase*. What does the literature say?

The studies to date note that women who take OCPs have *an increased ratio* of EUP to IUP. They note that women who take OCPs are far more likely to experience more EUP's per IUP than women who do not take OCPs, which supports the argument that the OCP acts as an abortifacient. The odds ratio (eg, an odds ratio of 2.0 is the same as saying a 2-fold risk) of the increased risk of EUP/IUP in women taking OCPs compared to women who were not taking OCPs were as follows: 1) WHO [43] found an odds ratio of 1.7 (1.1-2.5); 2) Mol et al [44] found an odds ratio of 1.8 (0.9-3.4); 3) Job-Spira et al [45] found an odds ratio of 4.3 (1.5-12.6); 4) Thorburn et al [46] found an odds ratio of 4.5 (2.1-9.6); and 5) Coste et al [47] found an odds ratio of 13.9 (1.8-108.3). These clinical studies once again contain evidence which suggests that the OCP acts as an abortifacient.

In conclusion, the arguments presented by the 22 physicians in the booklet entitled *Hormonal Contraceptives: Are they Abortifacients?* lack substance and actually serve to bolster the evidence that use of oral contraceptive pills causes early abortions. (An excellent overview of the histologic and immunologic evidence is given in great detail by Larimore and Stanford in the February, 2000 edition of the *Archives of Family Medicine* [48].)

References:

1. Faust JM. Image change for condoms. ABC News Report. [Internet Website]. 6/8/97.

2. DeCook JL, McIlhaney J, et al. *Hormonal Contraceptives: Are they Abortifacients:* 1998; Frontlines publishing. Sparta, MI. For contact information call 1-616-887-6256. Email: order@frontlines.org

3. Smith, Janet. *Contraception, Why Not?* ©One More Soul. Dayton, OH (513-279-5433)

4. Elstein M, et al. Studies on low dose oral contraceptives: cervical and plasma hormone changes in relation to circulating d-norgestrel and 17alpha-ethyniyl estradiol concentrations. *Fertility and Sterility.* 27; 1976: 892-899.

5. Wolf DP, et al. Human cervical mucus v. oral contraceptives and mucus rheologic properties. *Fertility and Sterility.* 32; 1979: 166-169.

6. Chang MC, Hunt DM. Effects of various progestins and estrogen on the gamete transport and fertilization in the rabbit. *Fertility and Sterility.* 1970; 21: 683-686.

7. Potter LA. How effective are contraceptives? The determination and measurement of pregnancy rates. *Obstet Gynecol.* 1996; 88: 13S-23S.

8. Snell, Richard. *Clinical and Functional Histology for the Medical Student.* Little, Brown & Co. Boston; © 1984, 586-591.

9. Brown HK, et al. Uterine junctional zone: Correlation between histologic findings and MR Imaging. *Radiology.* 1991; 1798: 409-413.

10. Fleischer AC, et al. Sonography of the endometrium during conception and nonception cycles of in vitro fertilization and embryo transfer. *Fertility and Sterility.* 1986; 46: 442-447.

11. Rabinowitz R, et al. The value of ultrasonographic endometrial measurement in the prediction of pregnancy following in vitro fertilization. *Fertility and Sterility.* 1986; 45: 824-826.

12. Ueno J, et al. Ultrasonographic appearance of the endometrium in natural and stimulated in-vitro fertilization cycles and its correlation with outcome. *Hum Reprod.* 1991; 6: 901-904.

13. Glissant A, et al. Ultrasound study of the endometrium during in vitro fertilization cycles. *Fertility and Sterility.* 1985; 44: 786-789.

14. Abdalla HI, et al. Endometrial thickness: a predictor of implantation in ovum recipients? *Hum Reprod.* 1994; 9: 363-365.

15. Dickey RP, et al. Relationship of endometrial thickness and pattern to fecundity in ovulation induction cycles: effect of clomiphene citrate alone and with human menopausal gonadotropin. *Fertility and Sterility.* 1993; 59: 756-760.

16. Gonen Y, et al. Endometrial thickness and growth during ovarian stimulation: a possible predictor of implantation in in-vitro fertilization. *Fertility and Sterility.* 1989; 52: 446-450.

17. Schwartz LB, et al. The embryo versus endometrium controversy revisited as it relates to predicting pregnancy outcome in in-vitro fertilization-embryo transfer cycles. *Hum Reprod.* 1997; 12: 45-50.

18. Shoham Z, et al. Is it possible to run a succesful ovulation induction program based solely on ultrasound monitoring: The importance of endometrial measurements. *Fertility and Sterility.* 1991; 56: 836-841.

19. Hilliard George D, Norris HJ. *Pathologic effects of oral contraceptives.* Recent Results in *Cancer Research.* 1979; 66: 49-71.

20. Ober WB. The effects of oral and intrauterine administration of contraceptives on the uterus. *Hum Pathol.* 1977; 8: 513-527.

21. Ober WB. Synthetic progestagen-oestrogen preparations and endometrial morphology. *J Clin Pathol.* 1966; 19: 138.

22. Roland M, et al. Sequential endometrial alterations during one cycle of treatment with synthetic progestagen-estrogen compounds. *Fertility and Sterility.* 1966; 17: 339.

23. Kupesic S. The first three weeks assessed by transvaginal color doppler. *J Perinat Med.* 1996; 24: 301-317.

24. DeCook J, et al. *Hormonal Contraceptives, Controversies and Clarification.* February, 1999. Pro-Life Obstetrician. PO Box 81, Fennville, MI 49408.

25. Somkuti SG, et al. The effect of oral contraceptive pills on markers of endometrial receptivity. *Fertility and Sterility.* 1996; 65; 484-488.

26. Witt B, Wolf G, et al. Relaxin, CA-125, progesterone, estradiol, Schwangerschaft protein, and human Chorionic Gonadotropin as predictors of outcome in threatened and nonthreatened pregnancies. *Fertility and Sterility.* 1990; 53: 1029-1036.

27. Norman RJ, et al. Inhibin and relaxin concentration in early singleton, multiple, and failing pregnancy: relationship to gonadotropin and steroid profiles. *Fertility and Sterility.* 1993; 59: 130-137.

28. Holmes, et al. Oral contraceptives: An assessment of their mode of action. *The Lancet.* June 2, 1962: 1174-1178.

29. Ritchie WGM. Ultrasound in the evaluation of normal and induced ovulation. *Fertility and Sterility.* 1985; 43: 167-181.

30. Van der Vange N. Ovarian activity during low dose oral contraceptives. *Contemporary Obstetrics and Gynecology.* G. Chamberlain, London, Butterworths; 1988: 315-326.

31. Grimes DA, et al. Ovulation and follicular development associated with three low dose oral contraceptives: A randomized controlled trial. *Obstet Gynecol.* 1994; 83: 29-34.

32. Croxatto HB, Diaz S, et al. Plasma progesterone levels during long-term treatment with levonorgestrel silastic implants. *Acta Endocrinologica.* 1982; 101: 307-311.

33. Cunningham, et al. *Williams Obstetrics.* 20th ed. Stanford, CT: Appleton and Lange; 1997: 580-581.

34. Alderson Reporting Company. Transcripts of oral arguments before court on abortion case. *The New York Times.* April 27, 1989: B12.

35. Skegg DCG, Noonan EA, et al. Depot medroxyprogesterone acetate and breast cancer [A pooled analysis of the World Health Organization and New Zealand studies]. 1995; *JAMA:* 799-804.

36. Castro-Vazquez. Macome JC, et al. On the mechanism of action of oral contraceptives. Effect of Lynestrenol on ovum implantation and oviductal morphology in the rat. *Fertility and Sterility.* 1971; 22: 741-744.

37. An Emergency contraceptive kit. *The Medical Letter.* October 23, 1998; 40: 102-103.

38. Eden JA, et al. The effect of Clomiphene citrate on follicular phase increase in endometrial thickness and uterine volume. *Obstet Gynecol.* 1989; 73: 187-190.

39. Yagel S, et al. The effect of ethinyl estradiol on endometrial thickness and uterine volume during ovulation induction by clomiphene citrate. *Fertility and Sterility.* 1992; 57: 33-36.

40. Fleischer AC, et al. Sonographic depiction of endometrial changes occurring with ovulation induction. *J Ultrasound Med.* 1984; 3: 341-346.

41. Imoedemhe DA, et al. Ultrasound measurement of endometrial thickness on different ovarian simulation regimens during in vitro fertilization. *Hum Reprod*. 1987; 2: 545-547.

42. *Physicians' Desk Reference*: 1997 (The noted information can be found when looking up any oral contraceptive. Failure rate for "typical use" is noted to be 3 percent.)

43. The WHO Task Force on intrauterine devices for fertility regulation. A multinational case-control study of ectopic pregnancy. *Clin Reprod Fertil*. 1985; 3:131-143.

44. Mol BWJ, Ankum WM, Bossuyt PMM, and Van der Veen F. Contraception and the risk of ectopic pregnancy: a meta analysis. *Contraception*. 1995; 52:337-341.

45. Job Spira N, Fernandez H, Coste J, Papiernik E, Spira A. Risk of Chlamydia PID and oral contraceptives. *JAMA*. 1990; 264: 2072-2074.

46. Thorburn J, Berntsson C, Philipson M, Lindbolm B. Background factors of ectopic pregnancy. I. Frequency distribution in a case-control study. *Eur J Obstet Gynecol*. 1986;23:321-331.

47. Coste J, Job-Spira N, Fernandez H, Papiernik E, Spira A. Risk factors for ectopic pregnancy: a case-control study in France, with special focus on infectious factors. *Am J Epidemiol*. 1991; 133: 839-849.

48. Larimore WL, Stanford J. Postfertilization effects of oral contraceptives and their relationship to informed consent. *Arch Fam Med*. 9; 2000: 126-133.

Appendix 6:
Further Research

During this review of the risks connected to oral contraceptive pills and abortion, a number of other important questions have surfaced. As researchers address these questions it is crucial to avoid the traps that weakened so many of the studies referred to in this book, notably the stack effect, the death effect, and the failure to allow for a proper latency period.

Some questions to be answered by further research:

Does having a miscarriage before a first full-term pregnancy increase the risk of breast cancer?

It was noted in Chapter 3 that 6 out of 8 studies showed an increased risk of breast cancer for women who have a miscarriage before their first full-term pregnancy (FFTP). A meta-analysis is needed to answer this question.

Do the quoted benefits of oral contraceptive pill (OCP) use in the prevention of ovarian and uterine cancer hold true in light of the evidence that low-dose oral contraceptive pill use allows more breakthrough ovulation?

As noted in Chapter 14, low-dose oral contraceptive pill use allows a higher frequency of breakthrough ovulation and theoretically yields less protection against ovarian and uterine cancer. Goldzieher stated in 1994 that, ". . .the protection against these types of reproductive cancers (ie, ovarian and endometrial) have been shown repeatedly with high-dose oral contraceptives but not, to date, with lower-dose oral contraceptives."

Does long-term oral contraceptive pill use result in an increased risk of developing liver carcinoma and/ or malignant melanoma?

Data presented in Chapter 14 implicated long-term (more than 5 years) oral contraceptive use as a risk factor for these cancers, and warrants a meta-analysis to answer these questions.

Does use of Norplant increase a woman's risk of developing breast cancer as much as Depo-Provera?

The evidence presented in Chapter 12 showed that use of Depo-Provera increases a woman's risk of breast cancer by 190% if she takes it for 2 or more years prior to the age of 25 (Skegg, 1995). Use of Norplant may be just as dangerous but no good studies have been performed examining its risk for breast cancer.

Does use of the intrauterine device or having chemical abortions (eg RU-486 or Methotrexate/Cytotec abortions) increase the risk of breast cancer?

Because use of the intrauterine device causes multiple early abortions it would be appropriate to explore its effect on breast cancer. Chemical abortions theoretically carry at least as high a risk as surgical abortions.

Does having an induced abortion increase the risk of cervical cancer?

Some studies (Thomas, 1996; Parrazini, 1988; Molina, 1988), but not all (Daling, 1994; Zondervan, 1996) indicated an association. Additional research is needed.

Will the daughters and sons of women who become pregnant while taking the oral contraceptives pill develop cancers, as did the daughters of the women who took DES?

Potter (1996) calculated that women who take OCPs have an actual method-related failure rate of 7%. Thus, over 700,000 women in the U.S. alone become pregnant each year while taking OCPs. This means that hundreds of thousands of babies are being exposed to significant levels of artificial hormones while in utero. Could this result in an increased risk of cancers of the reproductive organs in the children who were exposed, such as testicular cancer which has increased by 50% in the last 25 years? The answer is unknown but research in these areas must be done as soon as possible.

Is total body hyperthermia a possible treatment for breast cancer?

This author has come across no article examining the effect of total body hyperthermia in the treatment of breast cancer. However, the author has a personal interest in discovering any new research in this area because some types of cancer cells appear to be more heat sensitive than the original cells from which they mutated.

Table of Abbreviations

Abbreviation	Title
Acta Obstet Gynecol Scand	*Acta Obstetrica et Gynecologica Scandinavica*
Acta Pathol Microbio Immunol Scand Supplement	*Acta Pathologica, Microbiologica, et Immunologica Scandinavica, Supplement*
Am J Epidemiol	*American Journal of Epidemiology*
Am J Obstet Gynecol	*American Journal of Obstetrics and Gynecology*
Am J Pathol	*American Journal of Pathology*
Am J Public Health	*American Journal of Public Health*
Ann Epidemiol	*Annals of Epidemiology*
Ann Intern Med	*Annals of Internal Medicine*
Arch Gynecol Obstet	*Archives of Gynecology and Obstetrics*
Arch Intern Med	*Archives of Internal Medicine*
Biomed Pharmacotherapy	*Biomedicine and Pharmacotherapy*
Br J Cancer	*British Journal of Cancer*
Br J Hosp Med	*British Journal of Hospital Medicine*
Br J Obstet Gynaecol	*British Journal of Obstetrics and Gynaecology*
Br J Rheumatol	*British Journal of Rheumatology*
Br Med J	*British Medical Journal*

Abbreviation	Title
Bull World Health Org	*Bulletin of the World Health Organization*
CA Cancer J Clin	*CA — A Cancer Journal for Clinicians*
Clin Reprod Fertil	*Clinical Reproduction and Fertility*
Eur J Cancer	*European Journal of Cancer*
Eur J Clin Onc	*European Journal of Clinical Oncology*
Eur J Epidemiol	*European Journal of Epidemiology.*
Eur J Obstet Gynecol	*European Journal of Obstetrics, Gynecology and Reproductive Biology*
Genet Epidemiol	*Genetic Epidemiology*
Hum Pathol	*Human Pathology*
Hum Reprod	*Human Reproduction*
IARC Sci Pub	*IARC Science Publications*
Int J Cancer	*International Journal of Cancer*
Int J Epidemiol	*International Journal of Epidemiology*
Int J Fertility	*International Journal of Fertility*
Int J Gynecol Obstet	*International Journal of Gynecology and Obstetrics*
J Ac Immune Defic Syn Hum Retro	*Journal of Acquired Immune Deficiency Syndromes and Human Retrovirology*
J Am Board Fam Pract	*Journal of the American Board of Family Practice*
J Biosoc Sci	*Journal of Biosocial Science*
J Chron Dis	*Journal of Chronic Diseases*
J Clin Endocrinol Metab	*Journal of Clinical Endocrinology and Metabolism*
J Clin Epidemiol	*Journal of Clinical Epidemiology*

Abbreviation	Title
J Clin Oncol	Journal of Clinical Oncology
J Clin Pathol	Journal of Clinical Pathology
J Epidemiol Community Health	Journal of Epidemiology and Community Health
J Gyncol Obstet	Journal de Gynocologie, Obstetrique et Biologie de la Reproduction
J Infect Dis	The Journal of Infectious Diseases
J Natl Cancer Inst	Journal of the National Cancer Institute
J Perinat Med	Journal of Perinatal Medicine
J Reprod Med	Journal of Reproductive Medicine
J Steroid Biochem Mol Biol	Journal of Steroid Biochemistry and Molecular Biology
J Toxicol Environ Health	Journal of Toxicology and Environmental Health
J Ultrasound Med	Journal of Ultrasound in Medicine
Japanese J Cancer Research	Japanese Journal of Cancer Research
Life Sci	Life Sciences
Med Oncol Tumor Phamacother	Medical Oncology and Tumor Pharmacotherapy
N Engl J Med	New England Journal of Medicine
Natl Cancer Inst Monogr	National Cancer Institute Monographs
Obstet Gynecol	Obstetrics and Gynecology
Oncol Nurs Forum	Oncological Nursing Forum
Osteo Int	Osteoporosis International

Abbreviation	Title
Path Res Pract	*Pathology, Research and Practice*
S Afr Med J	*South African Medical Journal*

Bibliography

Abdalla HI, et al. Endometrial thickness: a predictor of implantation in ovum recipients? *Hum Reprod.* 1994; 9: 363-365. (App. 5)

Adam SA, Sheaves JK, et al. A case-control study of the possible association between oral contraceptives and malignant melanoma. *Br J Cancer.* 1981; 41: 45-50. (Ch. 14)

Adami HO, Bergstrom R, Lund E, Meirik O. Absence of association between reproductive variables and the risk of breast cancer in young women in Sweden and Norway. *Br J Cancer.* 1990; 62: 122-126. (Ch. 1, 2, 7)

Ahlert T, et al. Tumor-cell number and viability as quality and efficacy parameters of autologous virus-modified cancer vaccines in patients with breast or ovarian cancer. *J Clin Oncol.* 1997; 15: 1354-1366. (Ch. 17)

Alderson Reporting Company. Transcripts of oral arguments before court on abortion case. *The New York Times.* April 27, 1989; B12. (Ch. 2, 8, App. 5)

Alexander FE, et al. Risk factors for breast cancer with applications to selection for the prevalence screen. *J Epidemiol Community Health.* 1987; 41: 101-106. (Ch. 9)

Allen S, et al. Human immunodeficiency virus infection in urban Rwanda. *JAMA.* 1991; 266: 1657-1663. (Ch. 12, 14)

Altman LA. Drug shown to shrink tumors in type of breast cancer. *The New York Times.* May 18, 1998. (Ch. 17)

Altman LK. Studies show 2nd drug can prevent breast cancer. *The New York Times;* April 21, 1998. (Ch. 17)

American Academy of Pediatrics. Contraception and adolescents. *Pediatrics.* 1990; 86: 134-138.

American Academy of Pediatrics. The adolescent's right to confidential care when considering abortion. *Pediatrics.* 1996; 97: 746-751. (Ch. 5, App. 2)

American Cancer Society. *Cancer Statistics.* Jan/Feb. 1997: 47.

American Fertility Society. Assisted reproductive technology in the U.S. and Canada: 1992 results generated from The American Fertility Society/Society for Assisted Reproductive Technology Registry. 1994; 62: 1121-1128.

An Emergency contraceptive kit. *The Medical Letter.* October 23, 1998; 40: 102-103.   (App. 5)

Anderson TJ, Battersby S, et al. Oral contraceptive use influences resting breast proliferation. *Hum Pathol.* 1989; 20: 1139-1144.   (Ch. 2, 8, 12, App. 4)

Andrieu N, Clavel F, et al. Variations in the risk of breast cancer associated with a family history of breast cancer according to age at onset and reproductive factors. *J Clin Epidemiol.* 1993; 46: 973-980.

Andrieu N, Duffy SW, Rohan TE, Lé MG, et al. Familial risk, abortion and their interactive effect on the risk of breast cancer – A combined analysis of six case-control studies. *Br J Cancer;* 1995; 72: 744-751.

Andrieu N, et al. Familial risk of breast cancer and abortion. *Cancer Detection and Prevention.* 1994; 18: 51-55.   (Ch. 7)

Annegers JF. Patterns of oral contraceptive use in the U.S. *Br J Rheumatol.* 1989; 28: 48-50.

Anonymous. Another look at the pill and breast cancer. *The Lancet.* November 2, 1985: 985-987.   (Ch. 5)

Anonymous. Indian women condemn contraceptive vaccine. *Pittsburgh Catholic.* December 3, 1993:3.   (Ch. 7)

Anonymous. Oral contraceptives in the 1980s. *Population Reports.* May-June, 1982; X: A189-A222.   (Ch. 5, 15)

Anonymous. Pro-choice intolerance. *The New York Post.* Fall, 1996.

Asano Yoshizo, et al. Clinical and serologic testing of a live Varicella Vaccine and two-year follow-up for immunity of the vaccinated children. *Pediatrics.* 1977; V: 60.   (App. 3)

Bachrach C, Mosher W. Use of Contraception in the U.S., 1982. Vital and Health Statistics of the National Center for Health Statistics [U.S. Dept. of Health and Human Services]. Dec. 4, 1984; Number 102: 1-8.   (Ch. 11)

Bailie R, et al. A case-control study of breast cancer risk and exposure to injectable progestin contraceptives. *S Afr Med J.* 1997; 87: 302-305.   (Ch. 11, 12, 15)

Bain C, Hennekens C, et al. Oral contraceptive use and malignant melanoma. *J Natl Cancer Inst.* 1982; 68: 537-539.

Benagiano G. Long-acting systemic contraceptives. In: Diczfalusy E, ed. *Regulation of Human Fertility.* Copenhagen: Scriptor; 1977: 323-360.   (Ch. 9)

Beral V, et al. Breast cancer and hormone replacement therapy: collaborative reanalysis of data from 51 epidemiological studies of 52, 705 women with breast cancer and 108,411 women without breast cancer. *The Lancet.* 1997; 350: 1047-1043.   (Ch. 1)

Beral V, et al. Mortality associated with oral contraceptive use: 25 year follow up of cohort of 46,000 women from Royal College of General Practitioners' oral contraception study. *Br Med J.* 1997: 318. 1/99: 96-99.   (Ch. 2)

Beral V, Colwell L. Randomized trial of high doses of stilboestrol and ethisterone in pregnancy: long-term follow-up of mothers. *Br Med J.* 1980; 281: 1098-1101.   (Ch. 10)

Beral V, Evans S, et al. Oral contraceptive use and malignant melanoma in Australia. *Br J Cancer.* 1984; 50: 681-685.   (Ch. 14)

Beral V, Hannaford P, et al. Oral contraceptive use and malignancies of the genital tract. *The Lancet.* Dec. 10, 1988: 1331-1334.   (Ch. 13)

Bergkist L, Adami HO, et al. The risk of breast cancer after estrogen replacement and estrogen-progestin replacement. *N Engl J Med.* 1989; 321: 293-297.

Berne R, Levy M. *Physiology.* 3rd ed. St. Louis: CV Mosby Co; 1983.

Bibbo M, Haenszel W, et al. A twenty-five-year follow-up study of women exposed to diethylstilbestrol during pregnancy. *N Engl J Med.* 1978; 298: 763-767.   (Ch. 10)

Bogger-Goren S. Antibody response to Varicella-Zoster Virus after natural or vaccine-induced infection. *J Infect Dis.* 1982; 146: 260.   (App. 3)

Boyle P, Chilvers C, et al. Depot-medroxyprogesterone acetate (DMPA) and cancer: Memorandum from a WHO meeting. *WHO Bulletin OMS.* 1993; 71: 669-676.   (Ch. 12)

Brahams D. What must women be told about the pill? *The Lancet.* July, 1989: 285.   (Ch. 16)

Brind J. ABC down under. *Abortion Breast Cancer Quarterly Update.* Summer, 1997.   (Ch. 5, 6, 7, 15)

Brind J. The untold story of breast cancer and abortion. *Life Advocate.* February, 1993: 24-27.

Brind J. U.S. Congress to NCI Chief. *Abortion-Breast Cancer Quarterly Update.* Winter, 1998-1999.   (Ch. 6)

Brind J. U.S. Reps call for ABC hearings. *Abortion-Breast Cancer Quarterly Update.* Spring, *1998.*   (Ch. 6)

Brind J, Chinchilli M, et al. Induced abortion as an independent risk factor for breast cancer: a comprehensive review and meta-analysis. *J Epidemiol Community Health.* 10/ 1996; 50: 481-496.   (Ch. 1, 2, 3, 5, 6, 7, App. 2)

Brind J, et al. Induced abortion and the risk of breast cancer. *N Engl J Med.* 1997; 336: 1834.   (Ch. 2, 6)

Brinton LA, et al. Long-term use of oral contraceptives and risk of invasive cervical cancer. *Int J Cancer.* 1986; 38: 339-344.   (Ch. 13)

Brinton LA, et al. Risk factors for cervical cancer by histology. *Gynecologic Oncology.* 1993; 51: 301-306.   (Ch. 13)

Brinton LA, Daling JR, et al. Oral contraceptives and breast cancer risk among younger women. *J Natl Cancer Inst.* 6/7/1995; 87: 827-835.   (Ch. 1, 3, 7, 8, 9, 11, 14, 15, App. 4)

Brinton LA, Hoover R, et al. Reproductive factors in the aetiology of breast cancer. *Br J Cancer.* 1983; 47: 757-762. (Ch. 1, 2, 6, 7)

Brinton LA, Reeves WC, et al. Oral contraceptive use and risk of invasive cervical cancer. *Int J Epidemiol.* 1990; 19: 4-11. (Ch. 13)

Brown HK, et al. Uterine Junctional Zone: Correlation between Histologic Findings and MR Imaging. *Radiology.* 1991; 1798: 409-413. (App. 5)

Brunet J. Effect of smoking on breast cancer in carriers of mutant BRCA1 and BRCA2 genes. *J Natl Cancer Inst.* 1998; 90: 761-766.

Buehring GC. Oral contraceptives and breast cancer: What has 20 years of research shown? *Biomed Pharmacotherapy.* 1988; 42: 525-530.

Bustan MN, Coker AL, et al. Oral contraceptive use and breast cancer in Indonesia. *Contraception.* 1993; 47: 241-249.

Byers T, Graham S, et al. Lactation and breast cancer. *Am J Epidemiol.* 1985; 121: 664-674. (Ch. 1)

Calle EE, Mervis CA, Wingo PA, et al. Spontaneous abortion and risk of fatal breast cancer in a prospective cohort of U.S. women. *Cancer Causes and Control.* 1995; 6: 460-468. (Ch. 7, 9)

Campbell NB, et al. Abortion in Adolescence. *Adolescence.* 1988; 23: 813-823. (Ch. 7, 11)

Cancer Fact & Figures for African Americans. American Cancer Society. 1996. (Ch. 11)

Cancer Facts & Figures-1996. American Cancer Society, 1996. (Ch. 13, 14, 16)

Canty L. Breast cancer risk: Protective effect of an early first full-term pregnancy versus increased risk of induced abortion. *Oncol Nurs Forum.* 1997; 24: 1025-1031. (Ch. 2)

Carr B, Parker CR, et al. Plasma levels of adrenocorticotropin and cortisol in women receiving oral contraceptive steroid treatment. *J Clin Endocrinol Metab.* 1979; 49: 346-349.

Carr BR, Griffin JE. *Williams Textbook of Endocrinology.* 8th ed. Wilson JD, Foster DW. Philadelphia: WB Saunders Company; 1992: 1011.

Casagrande JT, Pike MC, et al. "Incessant ovulation" and ovarian cancer. *The Lancet.* July 28, 1979: 170-172.

Cascante E., et al. Aspectos epidemilogicos de la neoplamsa intraepithlieal e invasore del cuello utermo. *Acta Med Costa Ricense.* 1979; 22: 347-360.

Castro-Vazquez. Macome JC, et al. On the mechanism of action of oral contraceptives. Effect of Lynestrenol on ovum implantation and oviductal morphology in the rat. *Fertility and Sterility.* 1971; 22: 741-744. (App. 5)

Catherino WH, Jeng MH, et al. Norgestrel and gestodene stimulate breast cancer growth through an oestrogen receptor mediated mechanism. *Br J Cancer.* 1992: 945-952. (Ch. 12)

Celentano DD. The role of contraceptive use in cervical cancer: the Maryland cervical cancer case-control study. *Am J Epidemiol.* 1987; 126; 592-604. (Ch. 13)

Chang MC, Hunt DM. Effects of various progestins and estrogen on the gamete transport and fertilization in the rabbit. *Fertility and Sterility*. 1970; 21: 683-686. (App. 5)

Check JH, et al. Influence of endometrial thickness and echo patterns on pregnancy rates during in vitro fertilization. *Fertility and Sterility*. 1991; 56: 1173-1175.

Check JH, et al. The effect of endometrial thickness and echo pattern on in vitro fertilization outcome in donor oocyte embryo transfer cycle. *Fertility and Sterility*. 1993; 59: 72-75.

Chie, et al. Oral contraceptive and breast cancer risk in Taiwan, a country of low incidence of breast cancer and low use of oral contraceptives. *Int J Cancer*. 1998; 77:219-223. (Ch. 9)

Chilvers C. Breast cancer and depot-medroxyprogesterone acetate: a review. *Contraception*. 1994; 49: 211-222.

Chilvers C, McPherson K, et al. Oral contraceptive use and breast cancer risk in young women (UK National Case-Control Study Group). *The Lancet*. May 6, 1989: 973-982. (Ch. 1, 2, 3, 5, 7, 8, 9, App. 2)

Choi NW, Howe GR, et al. An epidemiologic study of breast cancer. *Am J Epidemiol*. 1978; 107: 510-521.

Clarck RM, Chua T. Breast cancer and pregnancy: the ultimate challenge. *J Clin Oncol*. 1989; 1: 11-18. (Ch. 2, 7, 17)

Clarck RM. (personal letter regarding "Breast cancer and pregnancy: the ultimate challenge.") February 10, 1995. (Ch. 7)

Clavel F, Andrieu N, et al. Oral contraceptives and breast cancer: A French case-control study. *Int J Epidemiol*. 1991; 20: 32-38. (Ch. 9, App. 2)

Clavel F, Benhamou E, et al. Breast cancer and oral contraceptives: a review. *Contraception*. 1985; 32: 553-569. (Ch. 5)

Clubb EM, et al. *A pilot study on teaching NFP in general practice: current knowledge and new strategies for the 1990s*. Washington, D.C.: Georgetown University; 1990: 130-132. (Ch. 3, 9)

Coezy E, et al. Tamoxifen and metabolites in MCF7 cells: correlation between binding to estrogen receptor and inhibition of cell growth. *Cancer Research*. 1982; 42: 317-323.

Colditz G. Epidemiology of breast cancer. *Cancer*. 1993; 71: 1480-1489. (Ch. 1, 7, 17)

Colditz G, Hankinson S, et al. The use of estrogens and progestins and the risk of breast cancer in postmenopausal women. *N Engl J Med*. 1995; 332: 1589-1693. (Ch. 1)

Colditz G, Willett W, et al. Family history, age and risk of breast cancer (Prospective data from the nurses' health study). *JAMA*. 1993; 270: 338-343.

Collaborative Group on Hormonal Factors in Breast Cancer. Breast cancer and hormonal contraceptives: collaborative reanalysis of individual data on 53,297 women with breast cancer and 100,239 women without breast cancer from 54 epidemiological studies. *The Lancet*. 1996; 347: 1713-1727. (Ch. 3, 5, 8, 9, App. 4)

Collaborative Group on Hormonal Factors in Breast Cancer. Breast cancer and hormonal contraceptives: further results. *Contraception*. 1996; 34: S1-S106.   (Ch. 1, 3, 5, 8, 9, 12, 14, 15, 16, App. 1, 4)

Colton T, Greenberg ER, et al. Breast cancer in mothers prescribed diethylstilbestrol in pregnancy. *JAMA*. 1993; 269: 2096-3000.   (Ch. 1, 3, 5, 10, App. 4)

Commonwealth of PA. *1994 Abortion statistics*. 1994.

Cooper C, et al. Oral contraceptive pill use and fractures in women: a prospective study. *Bone*. 1993; 14: 41-45.   (Ch. 14)

Coste J, Job-Spira N, Fernandez H, Papiernik E, Spira A. Risk factors for ectopic pregnancy: a case-control study in France, with special focus on infectious factors. *Am J Epidemiol*. 1991; 133: 839-849. (App. 5)

Croxatto HB, Diaz S, et al. Plasma progesterone levels during long-term treatment with levonorgestrel silastic implants. *Acta Endocrinologica*. 1982; 101: 307-311.   (Ch. 7, App. 5)

Cunningham DS, Brodnik RM, et al. Suboptimal progesterone production in pathologic pregnancies. *J Reprod Med*. 1993; 38: 301-305.

Cunningham FG, et al. *Williams Obstetrics*, 20th ed. Stanford, CT: Appleton & Lange; p 580-581, 1339-1356.   (Ch. 7, App. 5)

Cunningham FG, et al. *William's Obstetrics*. Stamford, CT: Appleton & Lange; 1993: 1321-1340.   (Ch. 12)

Daling J, Brinton L, et al. Risk of breast cancer among white women following induced abortion. *Am J Epidemiol*. 1996; 144: 373-380.   (Ch. 1, 6, 7)

Daling J, Malone K, et al. Risk of breast cancer among young women: relationship to induced abortion. *J Natl Cancer Inst*. 1994; 86: 1584-1592.   (Ch. 1, 2, 5, 6, 7, 8, 11, 15, App. 2)

Daling JR, et al. The relationship of HPV-related cervical tumors to cigarette smoking, oral contraceptive use, and prior herpes virus type 2 infection. *Cancer Epidemiology, Biomarkers & Prevention*. 1996; 5: 541-548.   (Ch. 13)

Dallenbach-Hellweg. On the origin and histological structure of adenocarcinoma of the endocervix in women under 50 years of age. *Path Res Pract*. 1984; 179: 38-50.   (Ch. 13)

Damjanov I, Linder J. *Anderson's Pathology*. New York. Mosby. 1996.

Danforth. *Obstetrics and Gynecology*. 7th ed. Philadelphia, PA: JB Lippincott Company; 1994.

Davies M. RU-486 and Post Coital Contraception. Lecture at Hershey Medical Center, 11/13/97.   (Ch. 15)

De Leizaola MA. De premiere d'une etude prospecive d'efficacite du planning famillial naturel realisee en Belgique francophone. *J Gyncol Obstet Biol Rev*. 1994; 23: 359-364.   (Ch. 3, 9)

DeCherney AH. In vitro Fertilization and embryo transfer: a brief review. *The Yale Journal of Biology and Medicine*. 1986; 59: 409-414.

DeCook J, et al. *Hormonal Contraceptives, Controversies and Clarification.* February, 1999. Pro-Life Obstetrician. PO Box 81, Fennville, MI 49408. (App. 5)

DeCook JL, McIlhaney J, et al. *Hormonal Contraceptives: Are they Abortifacients.* Sparta, MI: Frontllines; 1998. For contact information call 1-616-887-6256. Email: order@frontlines.org (App. 5)

DeFriend DJ, et al. Effects of 4-hydroxytamoxifen and a novel pure antioestrogen (ICI 182780) on the clonogenic growth of human breast cancer cells in vitro. *Br J Cancer.* 1994; 70: 204-211.

Delgado-Rodriguez M, Sillero-Arenas, et al. Oral contraceptives and cancer of the cervix uteri. *Acta Obstet Gynecol Scand.* 1992; 71: 368-376. (Ch. 13)

Denton AS, et al. AIDS-related lymphoma: an emerging epidemic. *Br J Hosp Med.* 1996; 55: 282-288.

Dickey RP, et al. Relationship of endometrial thickness and pattern to fecundity in ovulation induction cycles: effect of clomiphene citrate alone and with human menopausal gonadotropin. *Fertility and Sterility.* 1993; 59: 756-760. (App. 5)

Diczfalusy E. The worldwide use of steroidal contraception. *Int J Fertility.* 1989; 34: 56-63.

Dorairaj K. The modification mucus method in India. *Am J Obstet Gynecol.* 1991; 165: 2066-2067. (Ch. 3, 9)

Durand JL, Bressler R. Clinical Pharmacology of the Steroidal oral contraceptives. In: *Steroidal Oral Contraceptives.* Year Book Medical Publishers, Inc. 1979: 97-125.

Earl DT, et al. Calcium channel blockers and dysmenorrhea. *Journal of Adolescent Medicine.* 1992; 13: 107-108. (Ch. 3, 9)

Ebeling K, et al. Use of oral contraceptives and risk of invasive cervical cancer in previously screened women. *Int J Cancer.* 1987; 39: 427-430. (Ch. 3, 13)

Eden JA, et al. The effect of Clomiphene citrate on follicular phase increase in endometrial thickness and uterine volume. *Obstet Gynecol.* 1989; 73: 187-190. (App. 5)

Ehmann R. Problems in Family Planning. International Congress of the World Federation of Doctors who Respect Life. 1990; 1-32.

Eley JW, Hill HA, et al. Racial differences in survival from breast cancer. *JAMA.* 1994; 272: 947-954. (Ch. 11)

Ellery C, MacLennan R, et al. A case-control study of breast cancer in relation to the use of steroid contraceptive agents. *The Medical Journal of Australia.* 1986; 144: 173-176. (Ch. 5, 15)

Elliot Institute. New study confirms link between abortion and substance abuse. *The Post-Abortion Review.* Fall, 1993; 1: 1,6. (Ch. 7)

Elliot Institute. The abortion/suicide connection. *The Post-Abortion Review.* Summer, 1993; 1: 1-2.

Elstein M, et al. Studies on low dose oral contraceptives: cervical and plasma hormone changes in relation to circulating d-norgestrel and 17alpha-ethyniyl estradiol concentrations. *Fertility and Sterility*. 27; 1976: 892-899.   (App. 5)

Enachescu D, Lemneanu S. Associated mammary neoplasm risk factors considered by means of retrospective epidemiologic investigations. *La Sante' Publique*. 1984; 27: 225-231.

Ewertz M. Oral contraceptives and breast cancer risk in Denmark. *Eur J Cancer*. 1992; 28A: 1176-1181.   (Ch. 1, 9, 15)

Ewertz M, Duffy SW. Risk of breast cancer in relation to reproductive factors in Denmark. *Br J Cancer*. 1988; 58: 99-104.   (Ch. 1, 2, 7)

Fauci AS, et al. *Harrison's: Principles of Internal Medicine*. 14th ed. New York, NY: McGraw Hill; 1998.   (Ch. 3, 14, 16)

Faust JM. Image change for condoms. ABC News Report. [Internet Website]. 6/8/97.   (Ch. 8, App. 5)

Fechner RE. Influence of oral contraceptives on breast diseases. *Cancer*. 1977; 39: 2764-2771.

Feldman G. Is genetic testing right for you? *Self*. October,1996; 187-190.   (Ch. 1)

Fessenden F, Slatalla M. Blacks and breast cancer. *New York Newsday*. Dec. 12, 1994.

Figa-Talamanca I, et al. Epidemiology of legal abortion in Italy. *Int J Epidemiol*. 1986; 15: 343-351.

Fitzpatrick AL, Daling JR, et al. Use of calcium channel blockers and breast carcinoma risk in postmenopausal women. *Cancer*. October 15th, 1997; 80: 1438-1447.

Fleischer AC, et al. Sonography of the endometrium during conception and nonception cycles of in vitro fertilization and embryo transfer. *Fertility and Sterility*. 1986; 46: 442-447.   (App. 5)

Fleischer AC, et al. Sonographic depiction of endometrial changes occurring with ovulation induction. *J Ultrasound Med*. 1984; 3: 341-346.   (App. 5)

Forrest D, Singh S. The sexual and reproductive behavior of American Women, 1982-1988. *Family Planning Perspectives*. 1990; 22: 206-214.

Frank-Hermann P, et al. Effectiveness and acceptability of the symptothermal method of NFP in Germany. *Am J Obstet Gynecol*. 1991; 165: 2052-2055.   (Ch. 3, 9)

Freedman AM. Why teenage girls love the shot; Why others aren't too sure. *The Wall Street Journal*. October 14, 1998.   (Ch. 11, 12)

Fujimoto I, et al. Epidemiological study of the preinvasive cervical cancer. *Japanese J of Cancer Research*. 1987; 33: 651-660.   (Ch. 7)

Gabutti G, et al. AIDS related neoplasms in Genoa, Italy. *Eur J Epidemiol*. 1995; 11: 609-614.   (Ch. 5)

Gallagher RP, Elwood JM, et al. Reproductive factors, oral contraceptives and risk of malignant melanoma: Western Canada melanoma study. *Br J Cancer*. 1985; 52: 901-907.   (Ch. 14)

Gans, et al. American Medical Association report: Induced termination of pregnancy before and after Roe versus Wade. *JAMA*. 1992; 268: 3231-3239.   (Ch. 7)

Garfinkel, et al. *Stress, Depression and Suicide: A Study of Adolescence in Minnesota*. Minneapolis: University of Minnesota Extension Service; 1986.   (Ch. 7)

Garrett L. Contraceptives linked to AIDS risk. *Pittsburgh Post-Gazette*. May 7, 1996.   (Ch. 12)

Gay JW, et al. Oral contraceptives and breast cancer. *Missouri Medicine*. 1990; 87: 763-766.   (Ch. 8)

Geil, et al. FDA studies of estrogen, progestogens, and estrogen/ progesterone combinations in the dog and monkey. *J Toxicol Environ Health*. 3: 1979.   (Ch. 1, 3, 8)

Gershon, AA. Live attenuated Varicella Vaccine: protection in healthy adults compared with leukemic children. *J Infect Dis*. 1990; 161: 661-666.   (App. 3)

Gerstman BB, Gross TP, et al. Trends in the content and use of oral contraceptives in the United States, 1964-1988. *Am J Public Health*. 1991; 81: 90-96.   (Ch. 8)

Ginsburg ES, Mello NK, et al. Effects of alcohol ingestion on estrogens in postmenopausal women. *JAMA*. Dec. 4, 1996; 276: 1747-1751.   (Ch. 7)

Giovanella BC, et al. Selective lethal effect of supranormal temperatures on human neoplastic cells. *Cancer Research*. 1976; 36: 3944-3950.   (Ch. 17)

Gissler M, et al. Suicides after pregnancy in Finland, 1987-1994: register linkage study. *Br Med J*. 1996; 313: 1431-1434.   (Ch. 7)

Gitsch G, Kainz C, et al. Oral contraceptives and human papillomavirus infection in cervical intraepithelial neoplasia. *Arch Gynecol Obstet*. 1992; 252: 25-30.   (Ch. 13)

Glissant A, et al. Ultrasound study of the endometrium during in vitro fertilization cycles. *Fertility and Sterility*. 1985; 44: 786-789.   (App. 5)

Goldzieher JW. Are low-dose oral contraceptives safer and better? *Am J Obstet Gynecol*. 1994; 171: 587-590.   (Ch. 14)

Gomes L, Guimaraes M, et al. A case-control study of risk factors for breast cancer in Brazil, 1978-1987. *Int J Epidemiol*. 1995; 24: 292-299.   (Ch. 1, 8, 9, 15)

Gonen Y, et al. Endometrial thickness and growth during ovarian stimulation: a possible predictor of implantation in in-vitro fertilization. *Fertility and Sterility*. 1989; 52: 446-450.   (App. 5)

Gorman C. Do abortions raise the risk of breast cancer? *Science*. Nov. 7, 1994: 61.

Gray RH, et al. Evaluation of NFP program in Liberia and Zambia. *J Biosoc Sci*. 1993; 25: 249-258.   (Ch. 9)

Greene MH. Genetics of Breast Cancer. *Mayo Clinic Proceedings*. Jan. 1997; 72: 54-64.   (Ch. 1)

Griffin PD. Immunization against HCG. *Hum Reprod.* 1994; 9: 88-95.

Grimes DA. Neoplastic effects of oral contraceptives. *Int J Fertility.* 1991; 36: 19-24.   (Ch. 9)

Grimes DA, et al. Ovulation and follicular development associated with three low dose oral contraceptives: A randomized controlled trial. *Obstet Gynecol.* 1994; 83: 29-34.   (App. 5)

Groenroos M. Etiology of premalignant cervical lesion in teenagers. *Acta Obstet Gynecol Scand.* 1980; 59: 79.   (Ch. 7)

Gwinn ML, et al. Pregnancy, breastfeeding and oral contraceptives and the risk of epithelial ovarian cancer. *J Clin Epidemiol.* 1990; 43: 559-568.   (Ch. 14)

Hadjimichael OC, et al. Abortion before first live birth and risk of breast cancer. *Br J Cancer.* 1986; 53: 281-284.   (Ch. 1, 2, 7)

Hall CB. Recommendations for the use of live attenuated varicella vaccine. *Pediatrics.* 1995; 95: 791.   (App. 3)

Hankinson SE, et al. A prospective study of oral contraceptive use and risk of breast cancer (Nurses Health Study, United States). *Cancer Causes and Control.* 1997; 8: 65-72.   (Ch. 3, 8)

Hankinson SE, et al. A quantitative assessment of oral contraceptive use and risk of ovarian cancer. *Obstet Gynecol.* 1992; 80; 708-714.   (Ch. 14)

Hannaford PC, et al. Oral contraceptives and malignant melanoma. *Br J Cancer.* 1991; 63: 430-433.   (Ch. 14)

Harlap S. Oral contraceptives and breast cancer. Cause and Effect? *J Reprod Med.* 1991; 374-395.   (Ch. 1)

Harris JR, Lippman ME, et al. Breast cancer. *N Engl J Med.* 1992; 327: 319-328.

Harris RW, et al. Characteristics of women with dysplasia or carcinoma in situ of the cervix uteri. *Br J Cancer.* 1980; 42: 359-369.   (Ch. 7)

Haskell CM. *Cancer Treatment.* 4th ed. Philadelphia, PA: WB Saunders Company; 1995.   (Ch. 1)

Hawley W, Nuovo J, et al. Do oral contraceptive agents affect the risk of breast cancer?: A meta-analysis of the case-control reports. *J Am Board Fam Pract.* 1993. 6: 123-135.   (Ch. 16)

Hayes CD. *Risking the Future.* Washington, D.C.: National Academy Press; 1987.   (Ch. 11)

Helmrich S, Rosenberg L, et al. Lack of elevated risk of malignant melanoma in relation to oral contraceptive use. *J Natl Cancer Inst.* 1984; 72: 617-620.   (Ch. 14)

Helmrich S, Shapiro S, et al. Risk factors for breast cancer. *Am J Epidemiol.* 1983; 117: 35-45.   (Ch. 1)

Henderson B, Bernstein L. The international variation in breast cancer rates: An epidemiological assessment. *Breast Cancer Research and Treatment.* 1991; 18: S11-17.   (Ch. 1)

Henderson BE, Ross R, et al. Do regular ovulatory cycles increase breast cancer risk? *Cancer*. 1985; 56: 1206-1208.

Henderson IC. Risk factors for breast cancer development. *Cancer* (Supplement). 1993; 71: 2127-2140.   (Ch. 1)

Henshaw SK. Induced abortion: a worldwide perspective. *Family Planning Perspectives*. 1986; 18: 250-254.   (Ch. 5, 15)

Henshaw SK. Abortion trends in 1987 and 1988: age and race. *Family Planning Perspectives*. 1992; 24: 85-86.

Henshaw SK. U.S. Teenage Pregnancy Statistics. The Alan Guttmacher Institute. May 30, 1996. [120 Wall Street, NY, NY 10005].

Henshaw S, Binkin N, et al. A portrait of American women who obtain abortions. *Family Planning Perspectives*. 1985; 17: 90-96.   (Ch. 7)

Henshaw S, Koonin L, et al. Characteristics of U.S. women having abortions, 1987. *Family Planning Perspectives*. 1991; 21: 75-81.   (Ch. 7)

Henshaw S, Kost K. Abortion patients in 1994-1995: Characteristics and contraceptive use. *Family Planning Perspectives*. 1996; 28: 140-158.

Henshaw SK, O'Reilly K. Characteristics of abortion patients in the United States, 1979 and 1980. *Family Planning Perspectives*. 1983; 15: 5-16.   (Ch. 6, 7, 15)

Herman R. New birth control pills increase clotting danger. *Pittsburgh Post-Gazette*. June 3, 1997. F4.   (Ch. 14)

Herrero, et al. Injectable contraceptives and risk of invasive cervical cancer: evidence of an association. *Int J Cancer*. 1990; 46: 5-7.   (Ch. 12, 13, 15)

Hiatt RA, et al. Exogenous estrogen and breast cancer after bilateral oophorectomy. *Cancer*. 1984; 54: 139-144.   (Ch. 9)

Hilliard GD, Norris HJ. Oral Contraceptives. *Pathologic Effects of Oral Contraceptives*. 1976: 50-71.

Hilliard GD, Norris HJ. *Pathologic Effects of Oral Contraceptives*, Recent Results in *Cancer Research*. 1979; 66; 49-71. (App. 5)

Hirohata T, et al. Occurrence of breast cancer in relation to diet and reproductive history: a case-control study in Fukuoka, Japan. *Natl Cancer Inst Monogr*. 1985; 69: 187-190.

Holly EA. Cutaneous melanoma and oral contraceptives: a review of case-control and cohort studies. *Recent Results in Cancer Research*. 1986; 102: 108-117.

Holly E, Cress R, Ahn DK. Cutaneous melanoma in women. *Am J Epidemiol*. 1995; 141: 943-950.   (Ch. 14)

Holly EA, Weiss NS, et al. Cutaneous melanoma in relation to exogenous hormones and reproductive factors. *J Natl Cancer Inst*. 1983; 70: 827-831. (Ch. 14)

Holmes, et al. Oral contraceptives: An assessment of their mode of action. *The Lancet*. June 2, 1962: 1174-1178.   (App. 5)

Horn-Ross PL. Multiple primary cancers involving the breast. *Epidemiological Reviews*. 1993; 15: 169-176.   (Ch. 1)

Hoskins J.M., Plotkin S.A. Behaviour of Rubella Virus in Human Diploid Strains. Wistar Institute of Anatomy and Biology, Philadelphia, PA. Jan 16, 1967. [The authors describe two cell lines, one developed from spontaneous abortions and one from induced abortions. Both were capable of sustaining growth of the rubella virus.] (App. 3)

Howe G, Rohan T, et al. The association between alcohol and breast cancer risk: evidence from the combined analysis of six dietary case-control studies. *Int J Cancer.* 1991; 47: 707-710.

Howe H, et al. Early abortion and breast cancer risk among women under age 40. *Int J Epidemiol.* 1989; 18: 300-304. (Ch. 5, 7, 15)

Hsieh C, et al. Twin membership and breast cancer risk. *Am J Epidemiol.* 1992; 136: 1321-1326. (Ch. 1)

Hulka BS. Risk factors for cervical cancer. *J Chron Dis.* 1982; 35: 3-11. (Ch. 7)

Hulka BS. Oral contraceptives, the good news. *JAMA.* 1983; 249: 1624-1625. (Ch. 5)

Hulka BS, Liu E, et al. Steroid hormones and risk of breast cancer. *Cancer Supplement.* 1994; 74: 1111-1124. (Ch. 8, 9)

Hulka BS, Stark A. Breast cancer: cause and prevention. *The Lancet.* Sept. 30, 1995; 346: 883-887. (Ch. 16)

Huse D, Childhood vaccination against chickenpox: An analysis of benefits and costs. *Pediatrics.* 1994; 124: 869-873. (Ch. 5, App. 3)

Imoedemhe DA, et al. Ultrasound measurement of endometrial thickness on different ovarian simulation regimens during in vitro fertilization. *Hum Reprod.* 1987; 2: 545-547. (App. 5)

Irwin KL, Rosero-Bixby L, et al. Oral contraceptives and cervical cancer risk in Costa Rica. *JAMA.* 1988; 259: 59-64. (Ch. 13)

Isaacs JH. Cancer of the breast in pregnancy. *Surgical Clinics of North America.* 1995; 75 (1): 47-51. (Ch. 7)

Jacobs Patrick, Jones C.M., Baille J.P. Characteristics of human diploid cell designated MRC-5. *Nature.* 1970; 227: 168-170. (App. 3)

Jeng MH, Parker CJ, et al. Estrogenic potential of progestins in oral contraceptives to stimulate human breast cancer cell proliferation. *Cancer Research.* 1992; Dec. 1: 6539-6546. (Ch. 8, 12)

Jick SS, et al. Oral contraceptives and endometrial cancer. *Obstet Gynecol.* 1993; 82: 931-935. (Ch. 14)

Jick SS, Walker AM, et al. Oral contraceptives and breast cancer. *Br J Cancer.* 1989; 59: 618-621. (Ch. 1, 5)

Job Spira N, Fernandez H, Coste J, Papiernik E, Spira A. Risk of Chlamydia PID and oral contraceptives. *JAMA.* 1990; 264: 2072-2074. (App. 5)

John EM, et al. Characteristics relating to ovarian cancer risk: Collaborative analysis of seven U.S. case-control studies. Epithelial Ovarian Cancer in Black Women. *J Natl Cancer Inst.* 1993; 85: 142-147. (Ch. 14)

Jordan A. Toxicology of depot medroxyprogesterone. *Contraception.* 1994; 49: 189-201.

Jordan C, Jeng MH, et al. The estrogenic activity of synthetic progestins used in oral contraceptives. *Cancer Supplement.* 1993; 71: 1501-1505.   (Ch. 8, 12)

Kahn RH, et al. Effect of long-term treatment with Norethynodrel on A/ J and C3H/HeJ mice. *Endocrinology.* 1969; 84: 661.   (Ch. 3, 8, 13)

Kaunitz A. Long-acting injectable contraception with depot medroxyprogesterone acetate. *Am J Obstet Gynecol.* 1994; 170: 1543-1549.   (Ch. 12, 15)

Kay CR. Oral contraceptives and cancer. *The Lancet.* October 29, 1983: 1018-1020.

Kay CR, Hannaford PC. Breast cancer and the pill-A further report from the Royal College of General Practitioners' oral contraception study. *Br J Cancer.* 1988; 58: 675-680.   (Ch. 5, 9)

Kelsey J. A review of the epidemiology of human breast cancer. *Epidemiologic Reviews.* 1979; 1: 74-109.   (Ch. 1, 9)

Kelsey J, Horn-Ross P. Breast cancer: Magnitude of the problem and descriptive epidemiology. *Epidemiologic Reviews.* 1993; 15: 7-16.   (Intro, Ch. 11)

Kenya PR. Oral contraceptive use and liver tumours: a review. *East African Medical Journal.* 1990; 67:146-153.   (Ch. 3, 14, 15)

Key TJA, Pike MC. The Role of oestrogens and progestagens in the epidemiology and prevention of breast cancer. *Eur J Clin Onc.* 1988; 24: 29-43.

Killick S, et al. Ovarian follicular development in oral contraceptive cycles. *Fertility and Sterility.* 1987; 48: 409-413.

King RM, Welch JS, et al. Carcinoma of the breast associated with pregnancy. *Surgery, Gynecology and Obstetrics.* 1985; 160: 228-232.   (Ch. 2, 7)

Kirschstein RL, et al. Infiltrating duct carcinoma of the mammary gland of a Rhesus monkey after administration of an oral contraceptive: a preliminary report. *J Natl Cancer Inst.* 1972; 48: 551-553.   (Ch. 1, 3, 8)

Kjaer SK. Risk factors for cervical neoplasia in Denmark. *Acta Pathol Microbio, Immunol Scand, Supplement* 80. 1998; 80: 5-42.   (Ch. 13)

Kjaer SK, Engholm G, et al. Case-control study of risk factors for cervical squamos-cell neoplasia in Denmark. Role of oral contraceptive use. *Cancer Causes and Control.* 1993; 4: 513-519.

Klassen A, Wilsnack S. Sexual experience and drinking among women in a U.S. national survey. *Archives of Sexual Behavior.* 1986; 15: 363-391.   (Ch. 7)

Kleerekoper M, et al. Oral contraceptive use may protect against low bone mass. *Arch Intern Med.* 1991; 151: 1971-1976.   (Ch. 14)

Koetsawang S. Once-a-month injectable contraceptives: efficacy and reasons for discontinuation. *Contraception.* 1994; 49: 387-398.   (Ch. 12)

Kohler U, et al. Results of a case control study on predisposing factors for cervical carcinoma (in German). *Zentralblatt fur Gynakologie.* 1994; 116: 405-409.

Krieger N. Social class and the black/white crossover in the age-specific incidence of breast cancer: A study linking census-derived data to population-based registry. *Am J Epidemiol.* 1990; 131: 804-814.

Kroman N, et al. Should women be advised against pregnancy after breast-cancer treatment? *The Lancet.* 1997; 350: 319-322.   (Ch. 7)

Kunz J, Keller PJ. HCG, hpl, oestoradiol, progesterone and AFP in serum in patients with threatened abortion. *Br J Obstet Gynaecol.* 1976; 83: 640-644.

Kupesic S. The first three weeks assessed by transvaginal color doppler. *J Perinat Med.* 1996; 24: 301-317.   (App. 5)

Kvale G, et al. A prospective study of reproductive factors and breast cancer. *Am J Epidemiol.* 1987; 126 (5): 831-41.

La Vecchia C. Depot-medroxyprogesterone acetate, other injectable contraceptives, and cervical neoplasia. *Contraception.* 1994; 49: 223-230.

La Vecchia C, et al. Breast cancer and combined oral contraceptives: an Italian case-control study. *Eur J Cancer.* 1989; 25 11-G; 1613-1618.   (App. 1)

La Vecchia C, et al. General epidemiology of breast cancer in northern Italy. *Int J Epidemiol.* 1987; 16: 347-355.   (Ch. 1, 7)

La Vecchia C, Decarli A, et al. Oral contraceptives and cancers of the breast and of the female genital tract. Interim results from a case-control study. *Br J Cancer.* 1986; 54: 311-317.   (Ch. 5, 15)

La Vecchia C, Negri E, et al. Long-term impact of reproductive factors on cancer risk. *Int J Cancer.* 1993; 53: 215-219.

La Vecchia C, Negri E, et al. Oral contraceptives and breast cancer: A cooperative Italian study. *Int J Cancer.* 1995; 60: 163-167.   (Ch. 9, 15)

Laarsson, KS, et al. Predictability of the Safety of Hormonal Contraceptives from Canine Toxicology Studies. In: Michal, F. ed. *Safety Requirements for Contraceptive Steroids.* Cambridge: Cambridge University Press; 1989: 203-269.   (Ch. 1, 5, 12)

Lagnado L. Study on abortion and cancer spurs fight. *The Wall Street Journal.* Oct. 11, 1996.   (Ch. 2, 6)

Lagnado L. Abortion study fuels debate on cancer link. The *Wall Street Journal.* Jan. 9, 1997: B1, B5.   (Ch. 6, App. 1)

Laing AE, Bonney GE, et al. Reproductive and lifestyle factors for breast cancer in African-American women. *Genet Epidemiol.* 1994; A300.   (Ch. 11)

Laing AE, Demenais FM, et al. Breast cancer risk factors in African-American women: The Howard University tumor registry experience. *Journal of the National Medical Association.* 1993; 85 (12): 931-939.   (Ch. 11)

Lambe M, Hsieh C, et al. Transient increase in the risk of breast cancer after giving birth. *N Engl J Med.* 1994; 331 (1): 5-9.

Lanari C, Molinolo AA, et al. Induction of mammary adenocarcinomas by medroxyprogesterone acetate in balb/c female mice. *Cancer Letters.* 1986; 33: 215-223. (Ch. 1, 8, 12)

Landis SH, Murray T, Bolden S, Wingo PA. Cancer statistics, 1999. *CA Cancer J Clin.* 1999; 49: 8-31. (Intro)

Lantz PM, Remington P, et al. Mammography screening and increased incidence of breast cancer in Wisconsin. *J Natl Cancer Inst.* 1991; 83: 1540-1546.

Lé MG, Bachelot A, et al. Oral contraceptive use and breast or cervical cancer: preliminary results from a French case-control study. In Wolff JP, Scott JS. eds. *Hormones and Sexual Factors in Human Cancer Aetiology. Excerpta Medica.* New York: Elsevier Science Publishers; 1984: 139-147. (Ch. 7)

Lé MG, Cabanes PA, et al. Oral contraceptive use and risk of cutaneous malignant melanoma in a case-control study of French women. *Cancer Causes and Control.* 1992; 3: 199-205. (Ch. 7, 14)

Leary WE. Sickle cell trial called success, halted early. *The New York Times.* January 13, 1995: B5.

Lee HP, Gourley L, et al. Risk factors for breast cancer by age and menopausal status: a case-control study in Singapore. *Cancer Causes and Control.* 1992; 3: 313-322. (Ch. 9, 15)

Lee NC, Rosero-Bixby L, et al. A case-control study of breast cancer and hormonal contraception in Costa Rica. *J Natl Cancer Inst.* 1987; 6: 1247-1254. (Ch. 5, 9, 12, 15, App. 1, 2)

Lehrer S, Levine E, et al. Diminished ration of estrogen receptors to progesterone receptors in breast carcinomas of women who have had multiple miscarriages. *Mount Sinai Journal of Medicine.* 1992; 59 (1): 28-31. (Ch. 7)

Leishman K. On the abortion front line. *Health and Medicine for Physicians.* March 1997: 22-26. (Ch. 5)

Levi F, et al. Oral contraceptives and the risk of endometrial cancer. *Cancer Causes and Control.* 1991; 2: 99-103. (Ch. 14)

Lewis NA. Ban on method of late abortion passes house despite veto threat. *The New York Times.* October 9, 1997: 1,29.

Lin TM, Chen KP, MacMahon B. Epidemiologic characteristics of cancer of the breast in Taiwan. *Cancer.* 1971; 27: 1497-1504. (Ch. 1, App. 2)

Lindefors-Harris BM, Edlund G, et al. Risk of cancer of the breast after legal abortion during the first trimester: a Swedish register study. *Br Med J.* 1989; 299: 1430-1432. (Ch. 4, 5, 6, 9)

Lindefors-Harris BM, Eklund G, et al. Response bias in a case-control study: analysis utilizing comparative data concerning legal abortions from two independent Swedish studies. *Am J Epidemiol.* 1991; 134: 1003-1008. (Ch. 2, 5, App. 2)

Lipworth L, Katsouyanni K, et al. Abortion and the risk of breast cancer: a case-control study in Greece. *Int J Cancer.* 1995; 61: 181-184. (Ch. 6, 7)

Longman SM, et al. Oral contraceptives and breast cancer. *Cancer.* 1987; 59: 281-286.   (Ch. 8)

Longnecker MP. Alcoholic beverage consumption in relation to risk of breast cancer: meta-analysis and review. *Cancer Causes and Control.* 1994; 5: 73-82.   (Ch. 1)

Longnecker MP, Newcomb PA, et al. Risk of breast cancer in relation to lifetime alcohol consumption. *J Natl Cancer Inst.* 1995; 87: 923-929. (Ch. 1)

Lowe CR, MacMahon B. Breast cancer and reproductive history of women in South Wales. *The Lancet.* Jan. 24, 1970: 153-157.   (Ch. 1)

Lund E, et al. Oral contraceptive use and premenopausal breast cancer in Sweden and Norway: Possible effects of different pattern of use. *Int J Epidemiol.* 1989; 18: 527-532.   (Ch. 9)

Malone K. Diethylstilbestrol (DES) and breast cancer. *Epidemiologic Reviews.* 1993; 15: 108-109.   (Ch. 1)

Malone K, Daling J, et al. Oral contraceptives in relation to breast cancer. *Epidemiologic Reviews.* 1993; 15: 80-94.   (Ch. 5)

Mantel N, Haenszel. Statistical Aspects of the analysis of data from retrospective studies of disease. *J Natl Cancer Inst.* 1959; 22: 719-748.   (Ch. 4)

Marquardt H. Cell cycle dependence of chemically induced malignant transformation in vitro. *Cancer Research.* 1974; 34: 1612-1615.

Marubini E, Decarli A, et al. The relationship of dietary intake and serum levels of retinol and beta-carotene with breast cancer. *Cancer.* 1988; 61: 173-180.

Marx PA, et al. Progesterone implants enhance SIV vaginal transmission and early virus load. *Nature Medicine.* 1996; 2: 1084-1089.   (Ch. 12, 14)

Mati, et al. Contraceptive use and the risk of HIV in Nairobi, Kenya. *Int J Gynecol Obstet.* 1995; 48: 61-67.   (Ch. 14)

Maybery RM. Age-specific patterns of association between breast cancer and risk factors in black women, ages 20 to 39 and 40 to 54. *Ann Epidemiol.* 1994; 4: 205-213.   (Ch. 1, 9, 11)

Mayberry RM, Stoddard-Wright C. Breast cancer risk factors among black women and white women: similarities and differences. *Am J Epidemiol.* 1992; 136: 1445-1456.   (Ch. 1, 11)

McCredie MER, et al. Breast cancer in Australian women under age of 40. *Cancer Causes and Control.* 1998; 9: 189-198.   (Ch. 9)

McGinnis J. The politics of cancer research. *The Wall Street Journal.* Feb. 28, 1997.   (Ch. 6)

McGregor DH, et al. Breast cancer incidence among atomic bomb survivors, Hiroshima and Nagasaki 1950-1969. *J Natl Cancer Inst.* 1977; 59: 799-811.   (Ch. 1, 4)

McPherson K. The pill and breast cancer: why the uncertainty? *Br Med J.* Sept. 20, 1986; 293: 709-710.   (Ch. 5, App. 1)

McPherson K, Vessey MP, et al. Early oral contraceptive use and breast cancer: Results of another case-control study. *Br J Cancer.* 1987; 56: 653-660.   (Ch. 5, 9, App. 1)

McTiernan A, Thomas DB. Evidence for a protective effect of lactation on risk of breast cancer in young women. *Am J Epidemiol*. 1986; 124: 353-358.   (Ch. 1)

Meirik, et al. Relationship between induced abortion and breast cancer. *J Epidemiol Community Health*. 1998; 52 (3).   (App. 2)

Meirik O, Lund E, Adami HO, et al. Oral contraceptive use and breast cancer in young women. *The Lancet*. Sept. 20, 1986: 650-653.   (Ch. 9, 15)

Melbye M, Wohlfahrt J, et al. Induced abortion and the risk of breast cancer. *N Engl J Med*. 1997; 336: 81-85.   (Ch. 2, 4, 5, 6, 7, 9, App. 1)

Mendelson, J. Lukas S, et al. Acute alcohol effects on plasma estradiol levels in women. *Psychopharmocology*. 1988; 94: 464-467.   (Ch. 7)

Merck: Drug insert of VARIVAX, 1995.   (App. 3)

Michels K, Hsieh C, et al. Abortion and breast cancer risk in seven countries. *Cancer Causes and Control*. 1995; 6: 75-82.

Miller BA, et al. Cancer Statistics Review: 1973-1989. Bethesda MD: National Cancer Institute, 1992. [NIH Publication Number 92-2289]   (Ch. 11)

Miller DR, Rosenberg L, et al. Breast cancer before age 45 and oral contraceptive use: new findings. *Am J Epidemiol*. 1989; 129: 269-279.   (Ch. 3, 5, 9, 16, App. 1, 4)

Miller DR, Rosenberg L, et al. Breast cancer risk in relation to early contraceptive use. *Obstet Gynecol*. 1986; 68: 863-868.

Mills PK, et al. Prospective study of exogenous hormone use and breast cancer in seventh day Adventists. *Cancer*. 1989; 64: 591-597.   (Ch. 9)

Mirra AP, Cole P, et al. Breast cancer in an area of high parity: Sao Paulo, Brazil. *Cancer Research*. 1971; 31: 77-83.   (Ch. 1)

Mol BWJ, Ankum WM, Bossuyt PMM, Van der Veen F. Contraception and the risk of ectopic pregnancy: a meta analysis. *Contraception* 1995; 52: 337-341.   (App. 5)

Molina R, et al. Oral contraceptives and cervical carcinoma in Chile. *Cancer Research*. 1988; 48: 1011-1015.   (Ch. 7)

Morabia A, et al. Consistent lack of association between cancer and oral contraceptives using either hospital or neighborhood controls. *Preventive Medicine*. 1993; 22: 178-186.

Morabia A, Cole P, et al. Epidemiology and Natural History of Breast Cancer. *Surgical Clinics of North America*. 1993; 70 (4): 739-752.

Moseson M, Koeneg K, et al. The influence of medical conditions associated with hormones on the risk of breast cancer. *Int J Epidemiol*. 1993; 22: 1000-1009.

Mosgaard BJ, et al. The impact of parity, infertility and treatment with fertility drugs on the risk of ovarian cancer. *Acta Obstet Gynecol Scand*. 1997; 76: 89-95.

Moshur WD. Contraceptive practices in the United States, 1982-88. *Family Planning Perspectives*. 1990; 22: 198-205.

Mostad SB, et al. Hormonal contraception, vitamin A deficiency and other risk factors for shedding HIV-1 infected cells from the cervix and vagina. *The Lancet.* 1997; 350: 922-927.   (Ch. 12, 14)

Nagasawa H. Causes of age-dependency of mammary tumour induction by carcinogens in rats. *Biomedicine.* 1981; 34: 9-11.

National Cancer Institute. *SEER Cancer Statistics Review.* 1973-1992: Tables and Graphs. Bethesda, MD. Incidence rates of breast cancer in black and white women age 20-44.   (Ch. 11, App. 1)

Newcomb PA, et al. Lactation and a reduced risk of premenopausal breast cancer. *N Engl J Med.* 1994; 330: 81-87.   (Ch. 1)

Newcomb PA, Lantz PM. Recent trends in breast cancer incidence, mortality, and mammography. *Breast Cancer Research and Treatment.* 1993; 28: 97-106.   (Ch. 7)

Newcomb PA, Longnecker MP, et al. Recent oral contraceptive use and risk of breast cancer (United States). *Cancer Causes and Control.* 1996; 7: 525-532.   (Ch. 5, 9, App. 1)

Newcomb PA, Storer BE, et al. Pregnancy termination in relation to risk of breast cancer. *JAMA.* 1996; 275: 283-322.   (Ch. 5, 7)

Nischan P, et al. Comparison of recalled and validated oral contraceptive histories. *Am J Epidemiol.* 1993; 138: 697-703

Nixon A, Neuberg D, et al. Relationship of patient age to pathologic features of the tumor and prognosis for patients with stage I or II breast cancer. *J Clin Oncol.* 1994; 12: 888-894. (Ch. 7)

Norman RJ, et al. Inhibin and relaxin concentration in early singleton, multiple, and failing pregnancy: relationship to gonadotropin and steroid profiles. *Fertility and Sterility.* 1993; 59: 130-137.   (Ch. 3, App. 5)

Nullis C. WHO OKs birth control injections. *Pittsburgh Post-Gazette.* June 5, 1995.   (Ch. 15)

Ober WB. The effects of oral and intrauterine administration of contraceptives on the uterus. *Hum Pathol.* 1977; 8: 513-527.   (App. 5)

Olsson H. Hypothesis: Risk for malignant tumors after oral contraceptive use: is it related to organ size while taking the pill? *Med Oncol Tumor Phamacother.* 1990; 7: 61-64.

Olsson H, Borg A, et al. Early oral contraceptive use and premenopausal breast cancer-A review of studies performed in southern Sweden. *Cancer Detection and Prevention.* 1991; 15: 265-271.   (Ch. 5, 9, 11, App. 4)

Olsson H, et al. Her-2/neu and INT2 prot-oncogene amplification in malignant breast tumors in relation to reproductive factors and exposure to exogenous hormones. *J Natl Cancer Inst.* 1991; 83: 1483-1487.   (Ch. 5, 9)

Olsson H, Moller TR, Ranstam J. Early contraceptive use and breast cancer among premenopausal women: Final report from a study in southern Sweden. *J Natl Cancer Inst.* 1989; 81: 1000-1004.   (Ch. 5, 9, 15, App. 1)

Olsson H, Ranstam J, et al. Letter on CASH. *The Lancet*. November 23, 1985; 1181.   (Ch. 5, App. 1)

Olsson H, Ranstam J, et al. Proliferation and DNA ploidy in malignant breast tumors in relation to early contraceptive use and early abortions. *Cancer*. 1991; 67: 1285-1290.   (Ch. 2, 5, 7, 9, App. 4)

Orthocept: Drug Insert. Ortho Pharmaceuticals. 1996.   (Ch. 14)

Ory HW, et al. Combination oral contraceptive use and the risk of endometrial cancer. *JAMA*. 1987; 257: 796-800.   (Ch. 14)

Ory HW, et al. Long-term oral contraceptive use and the risk of breast cancer (CASH Study). *JAMA*. 1983; 249: 1591-1595.   (Ch. 5, 8)

Ory HW, et al. Oral contraceptive use and the risk of ovarian cancer. *JAMA*. 1983; 249: 1596-1599.

Ory HW, et al. Oral-contraceptive use and the risk of breast cancer (CASH Study). *N Engl J Med*. 1986; 315: 405-411.   (Ch. 8)

Ory HW, et al. The reduction in risk of ovarian cancer associated with oral-contraceptive use. *N Engl J Med*. 1987; 316: 650-655.

Osterlind A. Hormonal and reproductive factors in melanoma risk. *Clinics in Dermatology*. 1992; 10: 75-78.   (Ch. 14)

Osterland A, et al. The Danish case-control study of cutaneous malignant melanoma *Int J Cancer*. 1988; 42: 821-824.   (Ch. 14)

Ownby HE, et al. Interrupted pregnancy as an indicator of poor prognosis in T1,2, N0, M0 primary breast cancer. *Breast Cancer Research and Treatment*. 1983; 3: 339-344.   (Ch. 7)

Paffenbarger R, Kambert J, et al. Characteristics that predict risk of breast cancer before and after the menopause. *Am J Epidemiol*. 1980; 112: 258-268.

Palmer JR. Oral contraceptive use and gestational choriocarcinoma. *Cancer Detection and Prevention*. 1991; 15: 45-48.   (Ch. 14)

Palmer JR, Rosenberg L, et al. Oral contraceptive use and breast cancer risk among African-American women. *Cancer Causes and Control*. 1995; 6: 321-331.   (Ch. 3, 9, 11, App. 4)

Palmer JR, et al. Oral contraceptive use and risk of cutaneous malignant melanoma. *Cancer Causes and Control*. 1992; 3: 547-554.   (Ch. 14)

Parker Sheryl L, et al. *Cancer Statistics*, 1997. American Cancer Society. 1997; 47: 19.

Parker S, Tong T, et al. *Cancer Statistics*, 1996. *American Cancer Society*. 1996; 46: 1-23.   (Ch. 1)

Parkin DM, Pisani P., Ferlay J. Global cancer statistics. *CA Cancer J Clin*. 1999; 49: 33-64.

Parkin, et al. Estimates of the worldwide frequency of sixteen major cancers in1980. *Int J Cancer*. 1988; 41: 184-197.   (Ch. 3, 13, 14, 15)

Parkins T. Does abortion increase breast cancer risk? *J Natl Cancer Inst*. 1993; 85: 1987-1988.   (Ch. 6)

Parrazini F, et al. Determinants of risk of invasive cervical cancer in young women. *Br J Cancer*. 1998; 77: 838-841.   (Ch. 13)

Parrazini F, et al. Oral contraceptive use and invasive cervical cancer. *Int J Epidemiol.* 1990; 19: 259-263.   (Ch. 13)

Parrazini F, La Vecchia, et al. Menstrual and reproductive factors and breast cancer in women with family history of the disease. *Int J Cancer.* 1992; 51: 677-681.   (Ch. 7)

Parrazini F, La Vecchia, et al. Spontaneous and induced abortions and risk of breast cancer. *Int J Cancer.* 1991; 48: 816-820.

Parrazini F, et al. Risk factors for adenocarcinoma of the cervix; A case-control study. *Br J Cancer.* 1988; 57: 200-204.   (Ch. 7)

Pater A, Bayatpour M, et al. Oncogenic transformation by human papillomavirus type 16 deoxyribonucleic acid in the presence of progesterone or progestins from oral contraceptives. *Am J Obstet Gynecol.* April, 1990; 162: 1099-1103.   (Ch. 13)

Paul C, Skegg DC, et al. Oral contraceptive use and risk of breast cancer in older women (New Zealand). *Cancer Causes and Control.* 1995; 6: 485-491.   (Ch. 9)

Paul C, Skegg DC, et al. Oral contraceptives and breast cancer: a national study. *Br Med J.* 1986; 293: 723-726.   (Ch. 1, 15)

Paul C, Skegg DC, et al. Oral contraceptives and risk of breast cancer. *Int J Cancer.* 1990; 46: 366-373.   (Ch. 5, 9, App. 1, 2)

Paul C, Skegg DC, Spears GFS. Depot medroxyprogesterone (Depo Provera) and risk of breast cancer. *Br Med J.* 1989; 299: 759-762.   (Ch. 12)

Peters K, et al. Risk factors for Invasive cervical cancer among Latinas and non-Latinas in Los Angelos County. *J Natl Cancer Inst.* 1986; 77: 1063-1077.   (Ch. 13)

Peterson L. Contraceptive use in the United States: 1982-1990. Advance Data (U.S. Dept. of Health and Human Services). 1995; 260: 1-16.

Peto J. Oral contraceptives and breast cancer: Is the CASH study really negative? *The Lancet.* March 11, 1989: 552.   (Ch. 8)

Physicians' Desk Reference (1995). Description Ortho-Cyclin & Ortho Tri-Cyclen. 49th ed.   Montvale, NJ: Medical Economics: 1782.

Physicians' Desk Reference (1997). Description of Clomid (R). (Ch. 10)

Physicians' Desk Reference (1997). (The noted information can be found when looking up any oral contraceptive. Failure rate for "typical use" is noted to be 3 percent.) (App. 5)

Pike MC, Bernstein L. Oral contraceptives and breast cancer. *The Lancet.* July 15, 1989: 158.   (Ch. 5, 8, App. 1)

Pike MC, Bernstein L. Oral contraceptives and breast cancer. *The Lancet.* March 18, 1989: 615-616.   (Ch. 5, App. 1)

Pike MC, Henderson BE, et al. Breast cancer in young women and use of oral contraceptives: possible modifying effect of formulation and age at use. *The Lancet.* October 22, 1983: 926-929.   (Ch. 9, 12)

Pike MC, Henderson BE, et al. Oral contraceptive use and early abortion as risk factors for breast cancer in young women. *Br J Cancer.* 1981; 43: 72-76.   (Ch. 1, 2, 3, 5, 6, 7, 8, 9)

Plourde, et al. Human immunodeficiency virus type 1 infection in women attending a sexually transmitted disease clinic in Kenya. *J Infect Dis.* 1992; 166: 86-92.   (Ch. 12)

Population Council. Entwisle B, Kozyreva P. Induced abortion in Russia. *Studies in Family Planning.* March 1997; 28: 14-23.

Potter LA. How effective are contraceptives? The determination and measurement of pregnancy rates. *Obstet Gynecol.* 1996; 88: 13S-23S.   (Ch. 9, 10, App. 5)

Preblud S. Varicella: complications and costs. *Pediatrics.* Supplement 1986; 78: 728.   (App. 3)

Prentice RL. Epidemiologic data on exogenous hormones and hepatocellular carcinoma and selected other causes. *Preventive Medicine.* 1991; 20: 38-46.   (Ch. 14)

Primic-Zakelj, et al. Breast-Cancer risk and oral contraceptive use in Slovenian Women aged 25-54. *Int J Cancer.* 1995; 62: 414-420.   (Ch. 9)

Rabe T, et al. Liver tumors in women on oral contraceptives. *The Lancet.* 1994; 344: 1568-1569   (Ch. 14)

Rabinowitz R, et al. The value of ultrasonographic endometrial measurement in the prediction of pregnancy following in vitro fertilization. *Fertility and Sterility.* 1986; 45: 824-826.   (App. 5)

Ranstam J, et al. Oral contraceptives and breast cancer. *Dissertation Abstracts International.* 1992; 53: 705C.   (App. 4)

Ranstam J, Olsson H, et al. Survival in breast cancer and age at start of oral contraceptive usage. *AntiCancer Research.* 1991; 11: 2043-2046.   (Ch. 9, App. 4)

Rao DN, Ganesh B, et al. Role of reproductive factors in breast cancer in a low-risk area: a case-control study. *Br J Cancer.* 1994; 70: 129-132.   (Ch. 1)

Ravnihar B, et al. A case-control study of breast cancer in relation to oral contraceptive use in Slovenia. *Neoplasma.* 1988; 35: 109-121.   (Ch. 9)

Reardon. *A survey of psychological reactions.* Elliot Institute. 1987.   (Ch. 7)

Recer P. Women's response casts doubt on abortion-breast cancer link. *Pittsburgh Post-Gazette.* December 4, 1996.

Register TC, et al. Oral contraceptive treatment inhibits the normal acquisition of bone mineral in skeletally immature young adult female monkeys. *Osteo Int.* 1997; 7: 348-353.   (Ch. 14)

Remennick L. Induced abortion as cancer risk factor: a review of epidemiological evidence. *J Epidemiol Community Health.* 1990; 44: 259-264.

Remennick L. Reproductive patterns and cancer incidence in women: a population-based correlation study in the USSR. *Int J Epidemiol.* 1989; 18: 498-510.   (Intro, Ch. 7, 15)

Reuter KL, et al. Sonographic appearance of the endometrium and ovaries during cycles stimulated with human menopausal gonadotropin. *J Reprod Med*. 1996; 41: 509-514.

Risch HA, Weiss NS, et al. Events of reproductive life and the incidence of epithelial ovarian cancer. *Am J Epidemiol*. 1983; 117: 128-139.

Ritchie WGM. Ultrasound in the evaluation of normal and induced ovulation. *Fertility and Sterility*. 1985; 43: 167-181.   (App. 5)

Robbins S, Coltran R, Kumar V, et al. *Pathologic Basis of Disease*. 5th ed. Philadelphia, PA: WB Saunders Company; 1994.

Rohan, et al. *Am J Epidemiol*. 1988; 128: 478-489.   (Ch. 5, 6)

Rohan T, McMichael A. Oral contraceptive agents and breast cancer: a population-based case-control study. *The Medical Journal of Australia*. 1988; 149: 520-526.   (Ch. 9, 15)

Roland M, et al. Sequential endometrial alterations during one cycle of treatment with synthetic progestagen-estrogen compounds. *Fertility and Sterility*. 1966; 17: 339.   (App. 5)

Rombauts L, et al. Cumulative pregnancy and live birth rates after gamete intra-Fallopian transfer. *Hum Reprod*. 1997; 12: 1338-1342.

Romieu I, Berlin J, et al. Oral contraceptives and breast cancer. Review and meta-Analysis. *Cancer*. 1990; 66: 2253-2263.   (Ch. 1, 3, 5, 8, 9, 11, 15)

Romieu I, Willett W, et al. Prospective study of oral contraceptive use and risk of breast cancer in women. *J Natl Cancer Inst*. 1989; 81: 1313-1321.   (Ch. 9)

Rookus MA, Leeuwen FE. Oral contraceptives and risk of breast cancer in women ages 20-54 years. *The Lancet*. 1994; 344: 844-851.   (Ch. 1, 2, 3, 5, 6, 9, 15, App. 2)

Rookus MA, Leeuwen FE. Induced abortion and risk for breast cancer: reporting (recall) bias in a Dutch case-control study. *J Natl Cancer Inst*. 1996; 88: 1759-1764.   (Ch. 1, 2, 6, 7, 8, App. 2)

Rosenberg L. Induced abortion and breast cancer: more scientific data are needed. *J Natl Cancer Inst*. 1994; 86: 1569-1570.   (Ch. 6)

Rosenberg L, et al. A case-control study of oral contraceptive use and invasive epithelial ovarian carcinoma. *Am J Epidemiol*. 1994; 139: 654-661.   (Ch. 14)

Rosenberg L, Miller D, et al. Breast cancer and oral contraceptive use. *Am J Epidemiol*. 1984; 119: 167-176.

Rosenberg L, Palmer JR, et al. Breast cancer in relation to the occurrence and time of induced and spontaneous abortion. *Am J Epidemiol*. 1988; 127: 981-989.   (Ch. 1, 2, 5, 6, 7, App. 1)

Rosenberg L, Palmer JR, et al. A case-control study of the risk of breast cancer in relation to oral contraceptive use. *Am J Epidemiol*. 1992; 136: 1437-1944.   (Ch. 3, 5, 9)

Rosenberg L, Palmer JR, et al. Case-control study of oral contraceptive use and risk of breast cancer. *Am J Epidemiol*. 1996; 143: 25-37.   (Ch. 5, 8, 9, App. 4)

Rothman K, et al. Teratogenicity of high vitamin A intake. *N Engl J Med.* 1995; 333: 1369-1373. (Ch. 1)

Rubin R. Debating abortion and breast cancer. *US News and World Report.* Oct. 26, 1996: 96.

Rushton L, et al. Oral contraceptive use and breast cancer risk: a meta-analysis of variations with age at diagnosis, parity and total duration of oral contraceptive use. *Br J Obstet Gynaecol.* 1992; 99: 239-246. (Ch. 16)

Russell-Briefe R, et al. Prevalence and trends in oral contraceptive use in premenopausal females ages 12-54 years, United States, 1971-1980. *Am J Public Health.* 1985; 75: 1173-1176.

Russo J, Russo IH. Susceptibility of the mammary gland to carcinogenesis. *Am J Pathol.* 1980; 100: 497-512. (Ch. 1, 2, 6)

Russo J, Russo IH. Development pattern of human breast and susceptibility to carcinogenesis. *European Journal of Cancer Prevention.* 1993; 2 supplement: 85-100.

Russo J, Russo IH. Toward a physiological approach to breast cancer prevention. *Cancer Epidemiology, Biomarkers and Prevention.* 1994; 3: 353-364. (Ch. 1, 2, 6, 7)

Russo J, Tay TK, et al. Differentiation of the mammary gland and susceptibility to carcinogenesis. *Breast Cancer Research and Treatment.* 1982; 2: 5-73. (Ch. 1, 6)

Rutteman GR. Contraceptive steroids and the mammary gland: is there a hazard? *Breast Cancer Research and Treatment.* 1992; 23: 29-41. (Ch. 12)

Ryder RE. Natural Family Planning: effective birth control supported by the Catholic Church. *Br Med J.* 1993; 307: 723-726. (Ch. 3, 9)

Ryder RE, Campbell H. Natural family planning in the 1990s. *The Lancet.* 1995; 346; 233-234.

Schenker MB, et al. Self-reported stress and reproductive health of female lawyers. *Journal of Occupational and Environmental Medicine.* 1997; 39: 556-568. (Ch. 7)

Schildkraut J, Hulka B, et al. Oral contraceptives and breast cancer: A case-control study with hospital and community controls. *Obstet Gynecol.* 1990; 76: 395-402.

Schlesselman J. Cancer of the breast and reproductive tract in relation to use of oral contraceptives. *Contraception.* 1989; 40: 1-39.

Schlesselman J, Stadel B, et al. Breast cancer detection in relation to oral contraception. *J Clin Epidemiol.* 1992; 45: 449-459. (Ch. 9)

Schlesselman J, Stadel B, et al. Consistency and plausibility in epidemiologic analysis: application to breast cancer in relation to use of oral contraceptives. *J Chron Dis.* 1987; 40: 1033-1039.

Schonborn I, Nischan P, et al. Oral contraceptive use and the prognosis of breast cancer. *Breast Cancer Research and Treatment.* 1994; 30: 283-292. (Ch. 9)

Schoonen W, et al. Effects of two classes of progestagens, pregnane and 19-nortestosterone derivatives, on cell growth of human breast tumor cells: II. T47D cell lines. *J Steroid Biochem Mol Biol.* 1995; 55: 439-444. (Ch. 12)

Schuurman A, et al. Exogenous hormone use and the risk of postmenopausal breast cancer: results from the Netherlands Cohort Study. *Cancer Causes and Control.* 1995; 6: 416-424. (Ch. 9)

Schwartz LB, et al. The embryo versus endometrium controversy revisited as it relates to predicting pregnancy outcome in in-vitro fertilization-embryo transfer cycles. *Hum Reprod.* 1997; 12: 45-50. (App. 5)

Segal S, Faundes A, et al. Norplant implants: the mechanism of contraceptive action. *Fertility and Sterility.* 1991; 55: 273-277.

Segala C, Gerber M, et al. The pattern of risk factors for breast cancer in a southern France population. Interest for a stratified analysis by age at diagnosis. *Br J Cancer.* 1991; 64: 919-925.

Segi M, et al. An epidemiological study on cancer in Japan. *GANN.* 1957; 48: 1-63. (Ch. 2, 6)

Severyn, K. Children to be used as guinea pigs for drug company profits. Ohio Parents for Vaccine Safety: May 10, 1995. [251 West Ridgeway Drive, Dayton, Ohio 45459]. (App. 3)

Shoham Z et al. Is it possible to run a succesful ovulation induction program based solely on ultrasound monitoring: The importance of endometrial measurements. *Fertility and Sterility.* 1991; 56: 836-841. (App. 5)

Shoupe D, Haseltine FP. *Contraception.* New York: Springer-Verlag, 1993.

Shubik P. Oral contraceptives and breast cancer: laboratory evidence. In: Interpretation of Negative Epidemiological Evidence for Carcinogenicity. *IARC Sci Pub.* 1985; 65: 33. (Ch. 1, 3, 8)

Shy KK, et al. Oral contraceptive use and the occurrence of pituitary prolactinoma. *JAMA.* 1983; 249: 2204-2207. (Ch. 9)

Simonsen et al. HIV infection among lower socioeconomic strata prostitutes in Nairobi. *AIDS.* 1990; 139-144. (Ch. 14)

Siskind V, Schofield F, et al. Breast cancer and breastfeeding: results from an Australian case-control study. *Am J Epidemiol.* 1989; 130: 229-236.

Skegg DCG, et al. Progestogen-only contraceptives and risk of breast cancer in New Zealand. *Cancer Causes and Control.* 1996; 7: 513-519. (Ch. 9, 12)

Skegg DCG, Noonan EA, et al. Depot medroxyprogesterone acetate and breast cancer [A pooled analysis of the World Health Organization and New Zealand studies]. *JAMA.* 1995: 799-804. (Ch. 1, 3, 11, 12, 15, App. 4, 5)

Smith, J. *Contraception, Why Not?* ©One More Soul. Dayton, OH (513-279-5433) 1995. (App. 5)

Snell, R. *Clinical and Functional Histology for the Medical Student.* Boston, MA: Little, Brown & Co.; 1984: 586-591. (App. 5)

Soini I. Risk factors of breast cancer in Finland. *Int J Epidemiol.* 1977; 6: 365-373. (Ch. 1)

Somerville S. Before you choose: The link between abortion and breast cancer. Purcellville, VA. *Ann Intern Med.* 1993. (Ch. 5)

Somkuti SG, et al. The effect of oral contraceptive pills on markers of endometrial receptivity. *Fertility and Sterility.* 1996; 65: 484-488. (App. 5)

Speckhard A. *Psycho-Social Stress Following Abortion,* Ph D Thesis, University of Minnesota, 1985. (Ch. 7)

Speroff L, Glass RH, et al. *Clinical Gynecologic Endocrinology and Infertility.* 5th ed. Philadelphia, PA: Williams & Wilkins; 1994.

Spice B. Drug used to battle breast cancer may help heart. *Pittsburgh Post-Gazette.* June 4, 1997. (Ch. 17)

Spiritas R, et al. Fertility drugs and ovarian cancer: Red alert or red herring: *Fertility and Sterility.* 1993; 59: 291. (Ch. 10, 14)

Stadel B, Lai S, et al. Oral contraceptives and premenopausal breast cancer in nulliparous women. *Contraception.* 1988; 38: 287-299. (Ch. 5, 8, 9, App. 1)

Stadel B, Rubin G, et al. Oral contraceptives and breast cancer in young women. *The Lancet.* November 2, 1985: 970-973.

Stadel B, Rubin G, et al. Oral contraceptives and breast cancer in young women. *The Lancet.* February 22, 1986: 436.

Staffa JA, Newschaffer CJ, et al. Progestins and breast cancer: an epidemiologic review. *Fertility and Sterility.* 1992; 57: 473-491. (Ch. 12, 16)

Stanford J. Larimore WL. Postfertilization effects of oral contraceptives and their relationship to informed consent. *Arch Fam Med.* 9; 2000: 126-133.

Stanford JL. Combined oral contraceptives and liver cancer. *Int J Cancer.* 1989; 43: 254-259. (Ch. 14)

Stanford JL, et al. Oral contraceptives and endometrial cancer: Do other risk factors modify the association? *Int J Cancer.* 1993; 54: 243-248. (Ch. 14)

Stanford JL, et al. Oral contraceptives and breast cancer: results from an expanded case-control study. *Br J Cancer.* 1989; 60: 375-381.

Stanford JL, Weiss N, et al. Combined estrogen and progestin hormone replacement therapy in relation to risk of breast cancer in middle-aged women. *JAMA.* 1995; 274: 137-142.

Stavraky K, et al. Breast cancer in premenopausal and postmenopausal women. *J Natl Cancer Inst.* 1974; 53: 647-654.

Stehlin JS, Giovanella BC, et al. Results of hyperthermic perfusion for melanoma of the extremities. *Surgery, Gynecology and Obstetrics.* 1975; 140: 339-348. (Ch. 17)

Stewart DR, Overstreet JW, et al. Enhanced ovarian steroid secretion before implantation in early human pregnancy. *J Clin Endocrinol Metab.* 1993; 76: 1470-1476. (Ch. 3, 8)

Stewart H, Dunham LJ, et al. Epidemiology of cancers of uterine, cervix, and corpus, breast, and ovary in Israel and New York City. *J Natl Cancer Inst.* 1966; 37: 1-95.

Sun M. Panel says Depo-Provera not proved safe. *Science.* 1984; 226: 950-951.   (Ch. 12)

Talamini R, La Vecchia C, et al. Reproductive and hormonal factors and breast cancer in a northern Italian population. *Int J Epidemiol.* 1985; 14: 70-74.

Talan J. Alcohol linked to estrogen increase. *Pittsburgh Post-Gazette.* December 4, 1996: A21.

Talwar, et al. Phase I clinical trials with three formulations of anti-human Chorionic Gonadotropin vaccine. *Contraception.* 1990; 41: 301-316.   (Ch. 7, 15)

Tavani A, Negri E, et al. Oral contraceptives and breast cancer in northern Italy. Final report from a case-control study. *Br J Cancer.* 1993; 68: 568-571.

Tavani A, et al. Female hormone utilisation and risk of hepatocellular carcinoma. *Br J Cancer.* 1993; 67: 635-637.   (Ch. 14)

The WHO Task Force on intrauterine devices for fertility regulation. A multinational case-control study of ectopic pregnancy. *Clin Reprod Fertil.* 1985; 3: 131-143.   (App. 5)

Thomas DB. Oral contraceptives and breast cancer: review of the epidemiologic literature. *Contraception.* 1991; 43: 597-643.   (Ch. 1, 3, 8)

Thomas DB. Oral contraceptives and breast cancer. *J Natl Cancer Inst.* 1993; 85: 359-364.   (Ch. 5, 8, App. 1, 4)

Thomas DB, et al. Breast cancer and depot-medroxyprogesterone acetate: a multinational study. *The Lancet.* 1991; 338: 833-838.   (Ch. 12)

Thomas DB, et al. Invasive squamos-cell cervical carcinoma and combined oral contraceptives: Results from a multinational study. *Int J Cancer.* 1993; 53: 228-236.   (Ch. 3, 13)

Thomas DB, et al. Oral contraceptives and invasive adenocarcinomas and adenosquamos carcinomas of the uterine cervix. *Am J Epidemiol.* 1996; 144: 281-289.   (Ch. 3, 7, 13)

Thomas DB, Noonan EA. Breast cancer and combined oral contraceptives: results from a multinational study [The WHO collaborative study of Neoplasia and steroid contraceptives]. *Br J Cancer.* 1990; 61: 110-119.   (Ch. 1, 3, 5, 9, App. 2)

Thomas DB, Noonan EA, et al. Breast cancer and specific types of combined oral contraceptives. *Br J Cancer.* 1992; 65: 108-113.   (Ch. 9)

Thorburn J, Berntsson C, Philipson M, Lindbolm B. Background factors of ectopic pregnancy. I. Frequency distribution in a case-control study. *Eur J Obstet Gynecol.* 1986; 23: 321-331.   (App. 5)

Tietze C. *Induced Abortion: A World Review.* 5th ed. Population Council; 1983.   (Ch. 5, 15)

Tomasson H, et al. Oral contraceptives and risk of breast cancer: [A historical prospective case-control study]. *Acta Obstet Gynecol Scand.* 1996; 75: 157-161.   (Ch. 15)

Tretli S, et al. The effects of premorbid height and weight on survival of breast cancer patients. *Br J Cancer.* 1990; 62: 299-303. (Ch. 1)

Tryggvadottir L, et al. Oral contraceptive use at a young age and the risk of breast cancer: an Icelandic, population-based cohort study of the effect of birth year. *Br J Cancer.* 1997; 75: 139-143. (Ch. 15)

Ueno J, et al. Ultrasonographic appearance of the endometrium in natural and stimulated in-vitro fertilization cycles and its correlation with outcome. *Hum Reprod.* 1991; 6: 901-904. (App. 5)

Ungchusak, et al. Determinants of HIV infection among female commercial sex workers in northeastern Thailand: Results from a longitudinal study. *J Ac Immune Defic Syn Hum Retro.* 1996; 12: 500-507. (Ch. 12, 14)

Ursin G, Aragaki C, et al. Oral contraceptives and premenopausal bilateral breast cancer: a case-control study. *Epidemiology.* 1992; 3: 414-419. (Ch. 9)

Ursin G, et al. Does oral contraceptive use increase the risk of breast cancer in women with BRCA1/BRCA2 mutations more than in other women? *Cancer Research.* 1997; 57: 3678-3681. (Ch. 9, 15)

Ursin G, Peters RK, et al. Oral contraceptive use and adenocarcinoma of cervix. *The Lancet.* November 19, 1994; 344: 1390-1393. (Ch. 13)

Ursin RK, et al. Use of oral contraceptives and risk of breast cancer in young women. *Breast Cancer Research and Treatment.* 1998; 50: 175-184. (Ch. 9)

U.S. Government statistics regarding OCP use in black and white women. Source cannot be specifically cited until government publication is made public (work currently in progress). (Ch. 11)

Van der Kooy K, Rookus MA, et al. P53 protein overexpression in relation to risk factors for breast cancer. *Am J Epidemiol.* 1996; 144: 924-933. (Ch. 1, 9)

Van der Vange N. Ovarian activity during low dose oral contraceptives. In: Chamberlain G. ed. *Contemporary Obstetrics and Gynecology.* London: Butterworths; 1988: 315-326. (App. 5)

Ventura S, Taffel S, et al. Trends in pregnancies and pregnancy rates, United States, 1980-1988. *Monthly Vital Statistics Report.* 1992; 41: 1-12.

Ventura S, Taffel S, et al. Trends in pregnancies and pregnancy rates, United States, 1980-1992. *Monthly Vital Statistics Report.* 1995; 43: 1-24. (Ch. 11)

Vessey M, Baron J, et al. Oral contraceptives and breast cancer: Final report of an epidemiological study. *Br J Cancer.* 1983; 47: 455-462.

Vessey MP, et al. Patterns of oral contraceptive use in the United Kingdom. *Br J Rheumatol.* 9; 28 (Suppl): 46-47.

Vessey MP, McPherson K, et al. Breast cancer and oral contraceptives: findings in Oxford-Family planning Association contraceptive study. *Br Med J.* 1981; 282: 2093-2094.

Vessey MP, McPherson K, et al. Oral contraceptive use and abortion before first term pregnancy in relation to breast cancer risk. *Br J Cancer.* 1982; 45: 327-331. (Ch. 9, 16)

Wang Q, Ross R, et al. A case-control study of breast cancer in Tianjin, China. *Cancer Epidemiology.* 1992; 1: 435-439.   (Ch. 3, 9, 15)

Weed D, Kramer B. Induced abortion, bias, and breast cancer: why epidemiology hasn't reached its limit. *J Natl Cancer Inst.* 1996; 88: 1698-1699.   (App. 2)

Weed D, Kramer B. Breast cancer studies aren't "political." *The Wall Street Journal.* March 26, 1997.   (Ch. 6)

Weinstein A, Mahoney M, et al. Breast cancer risk and oral contraceptive use: results from a large case-control study. *Epidemiology.* 1991; 2: 353-358.   (Ch. 3, 9)

Weisburger JH, et al. Reduction in carcinogen induced breast cancer in rats by an anti-fertility drug. *Life Sci.* 1968; 7: 259.   (Ch. 3)

Weisse AB. Barry Marshall and the resurrection of Johannes Fibiger. *Hospital Practice.* September 15, 1996: 105-112.

Welsch CW, et al. 17B-Oestradiol and enovid mammary tumorigenesis in C3H/HeJ female mice. *Br J Cancer.* 1977; 35: 322.   (Ch. 3, 8)

Westerdahl J, et al. Risk of malignant melanoma in relation to drug intake, alcohol, smoking and hormonal factors. *Br J Cancer.* 1996; 73: 1126-1131.   (Ch. 14)

White E, Daling J, et al. Rising incidence of breast cancer among young women in Washington State. *J Natl Cancer Inst.* 1987; 79: 239-243.   (Ch. 1, 7, 11)

White E, Lee C, et al. Evaluation of the increase in breast cancer incidence in relation to mammography use. *J Natl Cancer Inst.* 1990; 82: 1546-1552.   (Ch. 7)

White E, Malone K, Weiss N, Daling J. Breast cancer among young U.S. women in relation to oral contraceptive use. *J Natl Cancer Inst.* 1994; 86: 505-514.   (Ch. 1, 3, 5, 7, 8, 9, 12, App. 1)

Whittemore AS. Personal characteristics relating to risk of invasive epithelial ovarian cancer in older women in the United States. *Cancer Supplement.* 1993; 71: 558-564.   (Ch. 14)

Whittemore AS, et al. Characteristics relating to ovarian cancer risk: collaborative analysis of 12 U.S. case-control studies. II. Invasive epithelial ovarian cancers in white women. Collaborative Ovarian Cancer Group. *Am J Epidemiol.* 1992; 136: 1184-1203.   (Ch. 10, 14)

Willett WC, Bain C, et al. Oral contraceptives and risk of ovarian cancer. *Cancer.* 1981; 48: 1684-1687.

Willett WC, Hunter DJ. Vitamin A and cancers of the breast, large bowel, and prostate: Epidemiologic Evidence. *Nutrition Reviews.* 1994; 52: S53-S59.

Williams G, Anderson E, et al. Oral contraceptive (OCP) use increases proliferation and decreases oestrogen receptor content of epithelial cells in the normal human breast. *Int J Cancer.* 1991; 48: 206-210.   (Ch. 8)

Wingo PA, et al. The risk of breast cancer following spontaneous or induced abortion. *Cancer Causes and Control.* 1997; 8: 93-108.

Wingo PA, Lee NC, et al. Age-specific differences in the relationship between oral contraceptives use and breast cancer. *Cancer* (supplement). 1993; 71: 1506-1517. (Ch. 3, 7, 8, 9)

Witt B, Wolf G, et al. Relaxin, CA-125, progesterone, estradiol, Schwangerschaft protein, and human Chorionic Gonadotropin as predictors of outcome in threatened and nonthreatened pregnancies. *Fertility and Sterility.* 1990; 53: 1029-1036. (Ch. 6, App. 5)

Wolf DP, et al. Human cervical mucus v. oral contraceptives and mucus rheologic properties. *Fertility and Sterility.* 1979; 32: 166-169. (App. 5)

Wolfe JN. Risk for breast cancer development determined by mammographic parenchymal pattern. *Cancer.* 1976; 37: 2486-2492. (Ch. 1)

Yagel S, et al. The effect of ethinyl estradiol on endometrial thickness and uterine volume during ovulation induction by clomiphene citrate. *Fertility and Sterility.* 1992; 57: 33-36. (App. 5)

Yang CP, Daling JR, et al. Noncontraceptive hormone use and risk of breast cancer. *Cancer Causes and Control.* 1992; 3: 475-479. (Ch. 1)

Yuan J, Yu M, et al. Risk factors for breast cancer in Chinese women in Shanghai. *Cancer Research.* 1988; 48: 1949-1953. (Ch. 9, 15)

Yuasa S, MacMahon B. Lactation and reproductive histories of breast cancer patients in Tokyo, Japan. *Bull World Health Org.* 1970; 42: 195-204. (Ch. 1)

Zanmetti P, et al. Characteristics of women under 20 with cervical intraepithelial neoplasia. *Int J Epidemiol.* 1986; 15: 477-482. (Ch. 7)

Zelnik M, Kantner J. Sexual activity, contraceptive use and pregnancy among metropolitan-area teenagers: 1971-1979. *Family Planning Perspectives.* 1980; 12: 230-237. (Ch. 11)

Zhang DW, et al. The effectiveness of the ovulation method used by 688 couples in Shanghai. Reprod. *Contraception.* 1993; 13: 194-200. (Ch. 9)

Zondervan KT, Carpenter LM, et al. Oral contraceptives and cervical cancer-further findings from the Oxford family planning association contraceptive study. *Br J Cancer.* 1996; 73: 1291-1297. (Ch. 7)

Index